CLINICAL CHILD PSYCHOLOGY

CURRENT PRACTICES AND FUTURE PERSPECTIVES

CLINICAL CHILD PSYCHOLOGY

CURRENT PRACTICES AND FUTURE PERSPECTIVES

Edited by
Gertrude J. Williams, Ph. D.
Sol Gordon, Ph. D.
for the Section on Clinical Child Psychology
American Psychological Association

Behavioral Publications
New York

All royalties derived from the sale of this book will
go to further the work of the Section on Clinical
Child Psychology.

Library of Congress Catalog Number 73-13511
ISBN, 0-87705-125-9
Copyright© 1974 by Behavioral Publications

BEHAVIORAL PUBLICATIONS 72 Fifth Avenue, New York 10011

Printed in the United States of America
This printing 4567 987654321

Library of Congress Cataloging in Publication Data
Williams, Gertrude Joanne, comp.
Clinical child psychology.

1. Clinical psychology—Addresses, essays, lectures.
2. Child psychiatry—Addresses, essays, lectures.
I. Gordon, Sol, 1923-   joint comp. II. American Psychological Association,
Division of Clinical Psychology. Section on Clinical Child Psychology.   III. Title.
(DNLM: 1. Child psychology. WS105 C641 1974)
RJ503.5.W54 1974   155.4   73-13511

TO ALL CHILDREN

To Gilbert B. Williams and Gilbert E. Williams
and
To Judith P. Gordon

There is in every child at every stage a new miracle of vigorous unfolding, which constitutes a new hope and a new responsibility for all.

Erik Erikson
Childhood and Society

CONTENTS

Foreword ix

The Authors xi

PART ONE. THE EMERGING FUTURE

1. Human Treatment and Public Policy
   Burton Blatt 3
2. The 1970 White House Conference on
   Children and Youth
   *White House Conference Committee,
   Erwin Friedman, Chairman* 19
3. Children's Needs in the Seventies:
   A Federal Perspective
   Edward Zigler 24
4. I. Forecasting the Future (1968)
   II. Four Years After the Forecast
   Alan O. Ross 35
5. The Psychologist as Child Advocate:
   Reflections of a Devil's Advocate
   Gertrude J. Williams 45

PART TWO. THE CONCEPTUAL REVOLUTION

6. The Sickness Model of Mental Disorder
   Means a Double Standard of Care
   George W. Albee 53
7. A Clinical Child Psychologist "Examines"
   Retarded Children
   Alan O. Ross 67
8. Parents, Peers, and Child Patients
   Make the Best Therapists
   Paul W. Clements 81
9. The Journey Beyond Trips: Alternatives to Drugs
   Allan Y. Cohen 98
10. Psychologist and Pediatrician: A Mental
    Health Team in the Prevention and
    Early Diagnosis of Mental Disorders
    Lee Salk 110

PART THREE.   FROM RESEARCH IN CHILD
DEVELOPMENT TO DEVELOPMENTAL CHILD CARE

11. Psychological Assessment, Developmental
    Plasticity, and Heredity, with
    Implications for Early Education
        J. McV. Hunt   119
12. Infant Development Projects:
    Problems in Intervention
        Alice S. Honig   142
13. Programs of Child Care: The United States
    Need and What Should Be Done
        Dorothy S. Huntington   168
14. Preschool Enrichment and Learning
        Jerome Kagan   179
15. Psychological Services in Project Head Start
        Paul Wohlford   197

PART FOUR.   ADVANCES IN EDUCATION

16. Family Style Education: A New Concept for
    Pre-School Classrooms Combining Multi-Age Grouping
    with Freedom of Movement Among Classrooms
        J. Ronald Lally and Lucille Smith   213
17. The Three-Pipe Problem: Promotion of Competent
    Human Beings Through a Pre-School Kindergarten
    Program and Sundry Other Elementary Matters
        Eli M. Bower   224
18. Emotional Education in the Classroom:
    The Living School
        Albert Ellis   242
19. Developing Understanding of Self and Others
    Is Central to the Educatı nal Process
        Don Dinkmeyer   252
20. Learning Problems
        Howard S. Adelman   258
21. Health and the Education of
    Socially Disadvantaged Children
        Herbert G. Birch   266
22. Compensating, Remediating, Innovating, and
    Integrating: Illusions of Educating the Poor
        Sol Gordon   292

PART FIVE. THE CONCEPT OF "INTELLIGENCE"

23. Intelligence Testing of Minority Group
Children: A Symposium
Danger: Testing and Dehumanizing Black Children
    Robert L. Williams   309
Danger: Chauvinism, Scapegoatism, and Euphemism
    Norman A. Milgram   312
Danger: Attacks on Testing Unfair
    Richard L. Wikoff   315
Testing Minority Group Children
    T. Ernest Newland   318
From Dehumanization to Black Intellectual
Genocide: A Rejoinder
    Robert L. Williams   320
Clinicians Must Listen!
    Florence C. Halpern   324
24. Social Responsibilities and Failure in Psychology:
The Case of the Mexican-American
    Manuel Ramirez III   326
25. Exit IQ: Enter the Child
    Constance T. Fischer   333

PART SIX. YOUTH IN PERSPECTIVE

26. Why Use Comic Books to Teach about Sex?
    Sol Gordon and Roger Conant   351
27. Alternatives to the Family
    Thomas Linney   363
28. Higher Learning in the Ignorant Society
    Michael Marien   371
29. Youth and Jobs: Educational, Vocational,
and Mental Health Aspects
    Milton Shore   381
30. Identity Group Psychotherapy with Adolescents
    Arnold W. Rachman   391

PART SEVEN. SEX, SEXISM, AND SEXUAL
STEREOTYPES

31. Gadflying the Sex Thing
    Gertrude J. Williams   419
32. Liberated Women = Liberated Children
    Margaret M. Horton   425

33. Children and Fathers
    Robert S. Pickett   437
34. Family Planning in the 1970s — A Dynamic
    Force Affecting the Status of Children
    Naomi T. Gray   443
35. Second Thoughts About Sex Education
    in the Schools
    Sol Gordon   453

PART EIGHT. PROFESSIONAL TRAINING

36. The Training of Clinical Child Psychologists
    Loretta K. Cass   463

PART NINE. CLINICAL CHILD PSYCHOLOGY
REASSESSED

37. Is Traditional Clinical Child Psychology Obsolete?
    S. Thomas Cummings   485
38. Is Clinical Child Psychology Obsolete?
    Some Observations on the Current Scene
    Ira Iscoe   507
39. The Death and Rebirth of Clinical
    Psychology — Tragicomical Reflections
    Gertrude J. Williams   515

Index   523

FOREWORD

Clinical child psychology is a young profession as witnessed by the paucity of universities offering specific training in this field. The needs of children, however, have not waited for academia. Moreover, traditionally trained clinical and child psychologists have taken the initiative in contributing to the ever changing, ever expanding needs of children and youth. Clinical child psychologists now have significant roles in family planning centers, pediatric wards, Head Start, hotlines, free schools, community-controlled services, street clinics and, indeed, the entire child care movement. Clinical child psychologists are becoming increasingly involved in changing traditional social structures that obstruct the fullest development of children and youth, professional isolationism is giving way to child advocacy.

In this book, we have deliberately strayed from the beaten track. In the main, we have omitted materials which are readily available elsewhere or which present conventionally accepted commentary on children and youth. We have selected articles that represent a broad spectrum of practices and viewpoints in clinical child psychology. In fact, we hope that this departure from traditional practices and ideas will help to define for the future the inchoate profession of clinical child psychology in terms of the active promotion of every child's well-being.

G. J. W.
S. G.

THE AUTHORS

George W. Albee, Ph.D., past President of the American Psychological Association is Professor of Psychology at the University of Vermont. He was formerly George Trumbull Ladd Distinguished Professor of Psychology at Case Western Reserve University.

Herbert G. Birch, M.D., Ph.D.,* was Research Professor at the Albert Einstein College of Medicine at Yeshiva University. An important contributor to the field of biosocial factors in the development and learning of disadvantaged children, he also served as member of the Task Force of the Joint Commission on Mental Health of Children.

Burton Blatt, Ph.D., is Centennial Professor and Director of the Division of Special Education and Rehabilitation at Syracuse University. He is the author of *Exodus From Pandemonium—Human Abuse and a Reformation of Public Policy.*

Eli M. Bower, Ed.D., is Professor of Educational Psychology at the University of California at Berkeley. A long-time activist in behalf of children, he has also served as President of the American Orthopsychiatric Association.

Loretta K. Cass, Ph.D., a Diplomate in Clinical Psychology, is Chief Psychologist of the Child Guidance Clinic of the Washington University School of Medicine and Associate Professor in the Graduate Program in Clinical Psychology, Washington University.

Paul W. Clement, Ph.D., is Associate Professor of Psychology and Director of Clinical Training at the Fuller Graduate School of Psychology in Pasadena, California.

Allan Y. Cohen, Ph.D., is Associate Professor of Psychology and Director of the Institute for Drug Abuse Education and Research, John F. Kennedy University, Martinez, California.

Roger Conant is a freelance journalist and cartoonist.

S. Thomas Cummings, Ph.D., a Diplomate in Clinical Psychology, is Director of Psychology, Children's Division, The Menninger Foundation. He is largely occupied with practicing traditional clinical methods and in teaching them to postdoctoral fellows in psychology and psychiatry.

Don C. Dinkmeyer, Ph.D., is Professor of Educational Psychology and Counseling at DePaul University and is a Consultant at the Illi-

*Deceased.

nois Psychiatric Institute and at the Illinois State Department of Education and Department of Guidance Services.

Albert Ellis, Ph.D., a Diplomate in Clinical Psychology, is Executive Director of the Institute of Advanced Study in Rational Psychotherapy and is the creator of the technique of Rational-Emotive Therapy.

Constance T. Fischer, Ph.D., is Associate Professor in the Department of Psychology at Duquesne University. She has written extensively on humanistic approaches to children and youth.

Sol Gordon, Ph.D., is Professor of Child and Family Studies and Director of the Marriage and Family Counseling Program at the College for Human Development, Syracuse University.

Naomi T. Gray, M.S.W., ACSW, is President of Naomi Gray Associates, San Francisco, a national family planning consultant firm. She was formerly Vice-President of Planned Parenthood-World Population, New York.

Alice S. Honig, Ph.D., is Assistant Professor in the Department of Child and Family Studies in the College for Human Development at Syracuse University where she also serves as Program Director for its Children's Center, a research program which provides developmental day care for low income infants.

Margaret M. Horton, Ph.D., is a Staff Psychologist at the Malcolm Bliss Mental Health Center and an adjunct Professor at Lindenwood College in St. Louis. She is a member of the Policy Council of the Association for Women in Psychology and is active in the Women's Movement.

J. McV. Hunt, Ph.D., is a former president of the American Psychological Association. He is a Professor of Psychology and Education at the University of Illinois and is a Diplomate in Clinical Psychology.

Dorothy S. Huntington, Ph.D., is Program and Research Director of the Family Developmental Center, a research and demonstration project sponsored by the Office of Child Development. She was representative of the American Psychological Association to the American Academy of Pediatrics Committee on Standards for Day Care of Children Under Three Years Old.

Ira Iscoe, Ph.D., a Diplomate in Clinical Psychology, is Professor of Psychology and Education, Director of Graduate Training in Community Mental Health, and Director of Counseling and Psychological Services at the University of Texas. He is a former President of the Division of Community Psychology of the American Psychological Association.

Florence C. Halpern, Ph.D., a Diplomate in Clinical Psychology, is an activist child psychologist who is Professor of Psychology at New York University. She was formerly on the staff of the Tufts-Delta Health Center in Mound Bayou, Mississippi and was the recipient of the Hughes Memorial Award for Distinguished Service in Education and School Psychology.

Jerome Kagan, Ph.D., is Professor of Psychology at Harvard University. He is an important contributor to the field of child development.

J. Ronald Lally, Ph.D., is Director of the Children's Center and Associate Professor of Child Development and Education at Syracuse University. He is Consultant to various agencies and programs dealing with daycare and preschool education and was Appalachian Regional Commission Consultant at the 1970 White House Conference on Children.

Thomas Linney is an independent writer and consultant to various groups concerned with education and mental health since 1968. His current interest is alternate life styles.

Michael Marien, Ph.D., was Research Fellow at the Educational Policy Research Center at Syracuse University. He is the author of *Alternative Futures for Learning: An Annotated Bibliography*. Currently he is on the staff of the World Institute.

Norman A. Milgran, Ph.D., is Professor and Chairman of the Department of Psychology at Tel Aviv University in Israel. He is a Diplomate in Clinical Psychology and was formerly the Editor of *The Clinical Psychologist*.

T. Ernest Newland, Ph.D., is a Diplomate in School Psychology and Professor of Educational Psychology at the University of Illinois.

Robert S. Pickett received a Ph.D. in history and is a specialist on the history of the family. He is Associate Professor and Chairman of the Department of Child and Family Studies in the College for Human Development at Syracuse University.

Arnold W. Rachman, Ph.D., is a Faculty Member at the Postgraduate Center for Mental Health Group Psychotherapy Clinic and a Clinical Associate at Columbia University Teachers College. He is a Consultant in Group Psychotherapy at the Beth Israel Hospital and at Encounter, Inc., in New York City.

Manuel Ramierez III, Ph.D., is Associate Professor of Mexican-American Studies and Psychology at the University of California at Riverside and Director of the Bicultural/Bilingual Educational Program, a follow-through project for Mexican-American elementary

school children which is subsidized by the U.S. Office of Education.
Alan O. Ross, Ph.D., is Professor of Psychology and Director of
the Doctoral Program in Clinical Psychology at the State University
of New York at Stony Brook and Vice-President of the American
Board of Professional Psychology. He is a member of the Board of
Directors of the National Academy of Professional Psychology.

Lee Salk, Ph.D., is Director of the Division of Pediatric Psychology
and Clinical Professor at the New York Hospital-Cornell Medical
Center and is in private practice in New York City.

Milton Shore, Ph.D., a Diplomate in Clinical Psychology, is a
Clinical Psychologist at the Mental Health Study Center, National
Institute of Mental Health and is on the faculties of the University
of Maryland and Catholic University of America.

White House Conference Committee: *Erwin Friedman*, Ph.D., is
Director of the National Children's Center and is on the faculty of
the George Washington University Medical School Department of
Pediatrics and Psychiatry.

Lucille Smith is Principal of the Children's Center at Syracuse University and is responsible for on-going training.

Richard L. Wikoff, Ph.D., is Associate Professor of Psychology at
the University of Nebraska. He is a consultant for public schools
with interests in Psychological testing.

Gertrude J. Williams, Ph.D., a Diplomate in Clinical Psychology, is
in independent practice of clinical and consulting psychology in St.
Louis and is the Editor of the *Journal of Clinical Child Psychology*.

Robert L. Williams, Ph.D., is Director of the Deparment of Black
Studies and Professor of Psychology at Washington University. He
was formerly National Chairman of the Association of Black Psychologists.

Paul Wohlford, Ph.D., who is now with the National Institute of
Mental Health Division of Manpower and Training, was formerly
Director of Psychological Services of National Head Start, Office
of Child Development.

Edward F. Zigler, Ph.D., is Professor of Psychology at Yale University. Until 1972, he was Director of the Office of Child Development and Head of the Children's Bureau in the Department of
Health, Education and Welfare.

Part One

THE EMERGING FUTURE

Ways to help children in the future have already been documented in the past. Every ten years, the White House Conference presents its recommendations for the benefit of children. National commissions report their findings on issues vital to children and youth such as: population growth, pornography, civil disorders, discrimination, drugs, juvenile crime . . . They begin with a bang; they end with a whimper. Recommendations are neglected and/or rejected. Have these commissions merely served as channels for the ventilation of anger, frustration, and despair? Or will their recommendations be implemented for the benefit of children?

Child advocates, don't give up!

1. Human Treatment and Public Policy[1]

Burton Blatt

It has been said that artists distort reality to present reality. Most of us must distort reality to preserve it. Things are not what they are but rather how they appear. Each person views his world in his own way, and each perception is a special perception. If, in this paper, you believe my lens has become distorted, please attempt to adjust your focus, not my vision. In this special way, permit me to behave as though things are how I see them.

My thesis is that society will not eradicate institutional back wards, will not guarantee human rights, and will not eliminate hunger by tearing down back wards or "guaranteeing" human rights or feeding hungry people. Mankind must change if we are to reduce inhumanity, if humanity is to survive.

You and I have experienced too much. We observe and record the devastation and consequences of mankind's mad excesses and, in bewilderment, we grope to comprehend this sickness infecting normal people. In despair, we must conclude that, while humanity is imperiled, life continues to flourish heedlessly. In anger, we realize that while man perseveres, his soul dies. In frustration, we observe that, during our evolution, we have camouflaged the body but accomplished little on behalf of the spirit. We have smoothed the skin but not the conscience, brought dignity to the carriage but hardly any to the carrier.

In humility, and with knowledge that I am no better qualified as accuser than those to whom I speak, I seek redress for certain acts committed by and against mankind.

I am a collector of injustices. Is there a profession as vilified, held more in contempt? I appear as a modern-day Pharisee, and enjoy my role less than those upon whom I intrude. I cringe with embarrassment, presuming to tell you what you must become. Yet I abandon caution, not to save my brothers, but to preserve myself. And,

---

[1]This article is based on an address in celebration of the 100th Anniversary of Syracuse University in April 1970.

to preserve myself, I ask you to please hear this review of a small segment of human history.

Have you been to Dachau? Can you add all of the Dachaus to all of the Siberias? Is there anyone willing to catalogue our own Southern history, life in demented mental hospitals, Vietnam, and the world of man-made subhumans some call state institutions? In his own manner, each man thinks about evil. And, in his curious mind, there are times and situations where he is comforted by its presence. But, is there one who will tolerate a flood that is endless and fathomless and senseless?

In his own manner, each man dreams about clean, happy, laughing people. And, watching a lively girl stroll the avenue on a clear morning, a day that is perfect for mankind, is there a soul who can think about beaten and made-ugly humanity? Yet I am driven to remind you that the moon does have its dark side; the human spirit does entice the inhuman act; man does not always please. Without credentials for these responsibilities, I seek to preserve the precarious thread between each of us and the humanness that we are fast losing. Without credentials, I make demands—yet prefer to follow. I am forced to enjoin my betters, for you have rejected the wisdom of your betters. While the time is long past when mankind ceased his climb upward, there is yet a chance to revive that destined goal and divert ourselves from this faithless journey to nowhere. And, today at least, I believe our one chance lies not in extolling the glories and virtues of that dreamed-of ascendancy, but in describing, dissecting, and comprehending our debasements and agonies. We may save ourselves, not with promises of a new good life to goad us, but with plain accounts of the real/unreal world we have fashioned for ourselves. For now, we must either change it or eternally wallow in its slime.

What must we change? Where shall we do battle? Who are the people responsible for Dachau and Song My, for Hitler and Stalin, for some now nameless forgotten German officer and for our own, for the Cancer Ward and the State School, for bloated starving Biafran children and too many of our children, for wars and killings and hunger and slavery and avarice and dehumanization and inhumanity? Who are the people responsible? You are the only person and I am the only person responsible and accountable. If you do not change, all is lost, and if I do not change, nothing will change. If I blame an evil world, a stupid system, blind leaders, or man's obvious imperfections, I may be right. But if it means I do not have to change, I contribute to the evil.

You and I are all that is needed to change the world. Our necessary confrontation is not social. It is personal. The battle is not against society but with oneself. It is not political but psychological, not within the group but in the mind, not to safeguard one's civilization but oneself, not legal but moral. The final confrontation will not be among groups such as those seated at the United Nations but within the depths and images and mazes that comprise and consume the substance of each man. The race to eternity will be between a civilization moving toward its infamy and each person weighing his belief in its glory or his worship of its obscenity. In whatever way the race concludes—win or lose, the survival of humanhood or the triumph of savagery—the individual will determine the outcome.

My thesis is, and must be, expressed with repeated use of such terms as "I" and "my." This cannot be an objective discourse concerning ambiguous Man. It must be the subjective revelation of someone who is forced to flee the safety and comfort of dispassionate exchange. Both this report and whatever you and I do in reaction to it must be personal—in the profound sense—not social.

During my travels through Germany, I had often wondered,
 "Was *he* guilty? Was *she* involved?"
Having never encountered one who was guilty or involved,
I realized that I had been asking
 the wrong questions.
Can a man be guilty just because he is not involved?

Where were those 50 million uninvolved Germans?
Where are the 150 million (175 million?) unbigoted Americans?
Were the good Germans innocent?
Is liberal America racist?

They were guilty.
We are racists,
 not because we abuse and destroy, but because
 our voices are silent.
The silent Americans are guilty!

The racist tells the coon joke and the kike joke and
The racist listens without rancor.
The racist does not rent to blacks and
The racist does not protest.

Every German who lived unharmed was guilty.
Every American—white and black—who is comfortable in this society
 is racist.

All who have experienced or know of Purgatory, asylums, and
totalization—
and are untroubled—
Dehumanize their brothers.

To observe sorrow untouched is to cause it to continue.

I ask you to change humanity by changing yourself, to solve the
riddle "I" before you attempt to solve the human puzzle, to commit
yourself before you commit mankind. I ask you to think of yourself,
not society, and how you must evolve, not what civilization must
endure. And for the one who concludes that I ask the chicken to
change the egg when I say that the individual must change himself
first and then society, does he still doubt that man one day will
change his genes?

It is clear that, ultimately, each man must account for his personal
behavior and the behavior of those he influences. And, it is clear
that each point has its counterpoint. For each deed there is another
deed or a misdeed. And, all these fulfill a grand design for man to alter
and improve. As man comprehends his mission and destiny, the
design for each of us will reveal as much as he wishes. Man is able to
judge and determine his future, and the condition in which he will
achieve it. Man is capable of understanding *how* the human world
is the sum and the substance of infinite points and counterpoints.

As each point has its counterpoint, each paradox can unfold
understanding. To study human behavior is to study apparent
paradoxes—just as it is to seek truth. If to know all is to accept all,
to know people is to bring one closer to understanding and accepting
them and their weaknesses as well as what makes them unique and
marvelous. In the profound sense, there is no paradox to:

the thief who is honest,
the harlot who is virtuous,
the noble man who is ignoble,
the wait for Godot that is the wait for God.

And, knowing that to be comfortable in a mad universe one must
operate in a state of discomfort.

In the profound sense, it may not be paradoxical that, as we grope
toward an understanding of dehumanization, we may be led to
accept the puzzle of humanity. In the process, we may learn that,
while living is a pardox, life is a simple and self-revealing truth.

Since time immemorial, man has heard—and done little—about

starving and tortured children. However, even the cleverest among us is unable to conceal or justify mankind's historical denial of fundamental human rights to some among his brothers. There is a difference between truth and fantasy, and whoever does not appreciate this difference can be dangerous. Such a person finds his truth as it conveniences him and as it fits his behavior. To that individual, truth is operational belief, a kind of functionalism; if I do it or believe it, by my definition of the infinite it is the correct thing to do or to believe. Even such a person is unable to conceal or justify our sorrowful heritage.

Despite my belief that we, in America, no more—or less—than other nations sanction human indignities, what I have to report draws its reference from the historical antecedants and the contemporary character of life in America. For, we must admit that the *Zeitgeist* of our obese society is menacing:

> Fat, indolent, oppressive
> America, America
> God shed thee of your waste
> Plunder and spoil
> You destroy
> And that which you destroy
> Destroys
> And much that you conserve
> Destroys

> Busy, ingenious, submissive
> America, America
> Your crown has thorns
> With paradoxes that have paradoxes
> Our days are better
> As they grow worse
> We become more affluent
> As we sink
> Lower

> Our obese and hungry together average where we should be
> Not where we were or what we are
> All of our wars have been righteous and we fight mental illness
> As we continue to kill and be killed
> In foreign lands and at home
> We are confused and inept with the Blacks
> The Reds, The Yellow, (not Yellows?)
> No not Yellow, never Yellows
> Always the Yellow Menace, the Yellow Horde

And, in our crises with the Blacks
And the Yellow Horde
We lose what we know of ourselves
And what man can make of himself
While bright young Ph.Ds and other Ds engage themselves
And prove to us
That ants are elephants
That the world is a marvel
That society brings me happiness

That I cannot change the world
That I am not responsible

Our pioneering forefathers carved out a great and mighty civilization from an indomitable wilderness that required billions of years to form and but a mere hundred or so to conquer. And the price of that wondrous achievement was destroyed Indian civilizations, exploited and brutalized Oriental field workers, victimized Italian railroad laborers, hollow-eyed children working in Manhattan sweatshops and, probably, the longest and most continuous and most systematic dehumanization program known to mankind—American slavery. Through some quirk, we are as careful to record for posterity our sicknesses as well as our spiritual victories. There has never been a scarcity of injustice collectors and, in view of our behavior through the years, they should have been kept quite busy. It would benefit each of us to review recorded descriptions of the auction block. Read about men, fighting and crying, begging not to be separated from wives and children; a girl, no more than fifteen, her dress torn away to show that she has no whiplash scars, to demonstrate she isn't a "mean nigger." Slaves branded on the thigh, head, or breasts, or back—chained together and marched from one state to another—and those too old or too tired or not caring to live anymore, left by the wayside to die. Generations of blacks, engulfed and mired in a culture so inhumane that—only now—can some appreciate the myth of their inferiority and natural subservience. And, although there will always be the rebel leader and heroic freedom fighter, America's humanscape will long bear the scars of a system that taught human beings to believe they were not human while they were taught to pray to, and believe in, a merciful God. From the beginning, our history is not unspoiled.

In New York, recently, the papers reported the arrest of a man and his wife for murdering the woman's daughter. The child was starved and beaten and, eventually, thrown into a river, anchored to forty-five pounds of rocks. However, it is not about child-beaters, insane killers, pathological rapists, and humanity gone berserk that I address myself. Horrifying and painful as those situations are, for thousands and thousands of years civilization has upheld the illegality of such behavior and, thus, society has recognized and accepted its responsbility to exact an "eye for an eye" or to impose whatever punishment or retribution it finds necessary to protect itself. Rather, I ask you here to consider our legally or quasilegally sanctioned policies and practices that lead to and encourage the denial of human rights to human beings. I ask you to consider the public's will, not the criminal's code; society's ethics, not its prohibitions.

I ask you to reflect upon the consequences of our unique American slave system, injustice in our schools, and the evil perpetrated within our mental hospitals and state schools for the mentally retarded. I ask you to view contemporary American life and your personal activities and convictions with the same diligence and remorselessness we in America judged Hitler's policies in the Warsaw Ghetto, Stalin's at Lubyanka, and Mao's, Castro's and Mussolini's. To our misfortune, the American list is not unlike most other nations'. Here I will focus particularly on children and their treatment in institutions.

As I exhort you to change and as I remind myself that reform will not come unless I change, I am compelled again to seek a form more personal than prose to communicate beliefs concerning man and his interrelatedness.

> For mankind must believe that:
> Each man's life means everything,
> Or it means nothing,
> He is the only man,
> Or no man exists.
> Each life and each death
> Is a profound event,
> Or no life—not a single life ever—
> Was of any consequence.
> Everything matters or nothing has mattered.

But to account for oneself as one accounts for his brother, to speak of personal anguish so as to deal better with the anguish of others, is a severe test. To do this and to be optimistic in the face of reality—in spite of reality—is *the* test of poets.

> For, who can describe beauty in institutions
> Who can pay honest tributes to their buccolic scenes

of lush fields and clear streams
Who can so reduce the terror inside
  to permit its physical appreciation outside
Who can view the scatalogical in relation to its
  tautological—not its villainy

Who will attempt to discuss the humanitarian ethos
  in terms of:
  asylums
  custody
  totalization
Who is so capable that he may bring dignity to such
  words as:
  inmate
  patient
  material
Who is so sensitive, and insensitive, as to drive from
  his mind:
  the back ward
  the day room
  the nonschool school

Is there a poet—has there ever been one—so brave or
  wise that he dared:
  to squeeze out the truth until it appeared as a lie
  to be so objective as to be beyond reality
  to stare down evil and find goodness

Are there men—is there a human being—who can
  detach themselves from passion and prejudice
Who can write a true account of life in the institution;
    who can write about:
  the good as well as the evil
  the beauty with the horror
  the profound asylum and the vivid confinement

Is there one person not of the establishment—
  and not of the reformists—whose axes are ground and whose
  battles are won:
  who can take distance and yet have compassion
  who is neither frightened of evil nor awed by goodness
  who can forgive everything and nothing

Is there a poet with words so true, with a mind so clear
  and soul so deep that:
  he comprehends the incomprehensibility of asylums

his language permits new understandings
we accept his words as deeds

If there is such a poet
he would appear

Some day, a man will be known
Who will teach us of life, of beauty, and evil
Who will help us unfold the meanings of things
And will cause us to learn that there is a design

He will teach us that:
 in spite of the back wards
 in spite of the inmates
 in spite of the evil
The design for each us holds nothing but good

In Paris, on December 10, 1948, the United Nations General Assembly adopted a Universal Declaration of Human Rights. Its preamble spoke of dignity and equality and freedom, once-revered concepts that in recent years have fallen upon evil days. I am compelled today, more than two decades after adoption of the Universal Declaration, to review some of the Articles, thereby assessing the state of humanity as I have experienced it and as I judge it to be.

If *"All human beings are born free and equal in dignity and rights,"* then why have I seen, in dormitories for the severely mentally retarded, solitary confinement cells that are continuously filled and with waiting lists for their use?

If *"Everyone has the right to life, liberty and security of person,"* then why have I seen a female resident at the state school for the mentally retarded who has been in a solitary cell for five years, never leaving—not for food or toileting or sleep?

If *"No one shall be held in slavery or servitude,"* then why have I seen men who have been held in state school custody for twenty or thirty years, neither having been granted a review of their cases nor genuine consideration of the possibility that they may be capable of discharge and community placement?

If *"No one shall be subjected to torture or to cruel, inhuman or degrading treatment or punishment,"* then why have I seen two young women in one solitary cell at the state school, lying nude in a corner, their feces smeared on the walls, ceiling, and floor—two bodies huddled in the darkness, without understanding the wrongs they have committed or those committed against them?

If *"Everyone has the right to recognition everywhere as a person before the law,"* then why have I seen another young woman, in solitary confinement, day after day and year after year, nude and assaultive, incontinent and nonverbal—except for one day each month when her parents call for her, and when she is washed and dressed and, then, taken home or for a ride in the country—except for one day each month when her clothes remain on her, when she communicates, when she is a human being?

If *"No one shall be subjected to arbitrary arrest, detention or exile,"* then why have I seen men and women—residents of state schools for half a century—never knowing why they were placed originally, no longer caring to experience the outside world, and with no possibility that anyone outside is either interested in them or knows that they exist as human beings?

If *"Everyone is entitled in full equality to a fair and public hearing by an independent and impartial tribunal, in the determination of his rights and obligations and of any criminal charge against him,"* then why have I seen a boy at a state school in continuous seclusion twenty-four hours a day, described by the dormitory physician as a "monster"?

If *"No one shall be subjected to arbitrary interference with his privacy, family, home or correspondence, nor to attacks upon his honor and reputation,"* then why have I seen incoming mail to state school residents, and their outgoing mail, read and censored by institutional supervisors?

If *"Everyone has the right to freedom of movement and residence within the borders of each state. (If) Everyone has the right to leave any country, including his own, and to return to his country,"* then why have I seen human beings who have never—in ten or twenty or thirty or seventy years—left the one hundred or two hundred or a thousand acres of the state school—they who were delivered there at birth and only whose souls will leave?

If *"Men and women of full age, without any limitation due to race, nationality or religion, have the right to marry and to found a family,"* then why have I seen the mentally retarded , the epileptic, and others denied such rights by state statutes; why have I seen young women sterilized as a condition for their release from the state school?

If *"Everyone has the right to own property alone as well as in association with others. (If) No one shall be arbitrarily deprived of this property,"* then why have I seen residents of the state school deprived of their personal possessions and their entitlements under public assistance?

If *"Everyone has the right to freedom of thought, conscience and religion,"* then why have I seen some residents at the state school required to attend church services and other residents prohibited from such attendance?

If *"Everyone has the right to freedom of opinion and expression,"* then why have I seen a child berated by his state school teacher because of the opinions he expressed and why did I hear her tell him how ungrateful, how wicked he was, in light of the bountiful state, that had given this unwanted child everything and expected only loyalty and gratitude in return?

If *"Everyone, as a member of society, has the right to social security,"* then why have I seen more securing than security, more solitary than social, more indignity than dignity, more enchainment than freedom?

If *"Everyone has the right to work, to free choice of employment, to just and favorable conditons of work and to protection against unemployment,"* then why have I seen residents of state schools in custody long beyond that time when they merited community placement, in custody because they were performing essential and unpaid work at the institution?

If *"Everyone has the right to education,"* then why have I seen children at state schools for the mentally retarded permanently denied any semblance of education, treatment, or training?

If *"Nothing in this Declaration may be interpreted as implying for any state, group or person any right to engage in any activity or to perform any act aimed at the destruction of any of the rights and freedoms set forth herein,"* then why have I seen human beings who have been given nothing, who have nothing and who, tomorrow, will have less?

Why have I seen a state school superintendent who did not call for a postmortem, an inquiry, or even a staff conference to determine the possibility of negligence or other unusual circumstances surrounding the death of a severely retarded child who choked when an attendant fed her a whole hard-boiled egg?

Why have I seen a state school director of nursing leave suddenly for a three-day vacation, without assigning additional staff or someone to succeed him in his absence, during the midst of a hepatitis epidemic where, in one building alone, twenty-seven of seventy-one patients were diagnosed as having this dreaded disease?

Why have I seen a severely retarded ambulatory resident, stabbed in the testicles by an unknown assailant while he slept, who almost died because the night attendant bandaged him as best she could, with no one doing anything else for the wound until ten hours later?

Why have I seen children at the state school go to bed each night wearing dungarees instead of pajamas, on mattresses without sheets, without pillows, and not one child "owning" even a single article of clothing?

Why have I seen children nude and bruised, sitting, sleeping, and eating with moist or dried feces covering them and their surroundings?

Why have I seen children lying on filthy beds, uncovered, flies crawling all over them?

Why have I seen children playing in and eating garbage?

Why have I been forced to view my brothers, and the world in which they live, as if I were standing in garbage, as if it were to consume me?

Form in your mind's eye this scene, this continuation, this last vulgar ounce of value squeezed from those least valued. Visualize this short true story. [2]

Fine grains of snow fall gently on the roughly hewn gray stone fort. Inside, amid the harsh lives and broken thoughts, a procession silently and fleetingly mourns. Those who comprehend learn that one has passed and they mourn, not for him, but for themselves and for each other.

They mourn for lives lived without hope, that end without meaning.

They mourn for a soul used in his lifetime as material, whose bones and meat continue to serve science.

They mourn for those deadly years and, now, this restless death, swirling in gleaming vats in Boston and Syracuse, waiting for bright lively boys in white to perform one final necessary obscenity.

They mourn for their wasted lives that shall end as this one ends, not cleanly, neither in sympathy for the living survivors nor with respect for the immortal spirit.

But, they mourn more for the creations of God and obstetricians than the final indignities imposed by chairmen of medical school cadaver committees.

For, the law requires that their bloated, mutilated, and sewn flesh

---

[2] Based on infrequent involvements with medical school cadaver committees, experiences the reader may wish to forego. I have observed that certain deceased state school residents are selected for medical study as they were selected for institutionalization, and are treated in death as they were treated in life. On the average, each selected corpse involuntarily contributes one year of his eternal life to society before he is permitted his rest; he, of all people, who owes so little to society, from whom society has exacted so much, and from whom society has made his entire life— and now his death—a sacrifice.

must be scooped together someday and returned to the earth they long for, the earth that will treat them more gently than the world that spawned them.

For is there a law, is there an authority that can do for one—in life —what all beings achieve in death?

Is there a mundane justice that, however infinitesimally, compares with the equality and brotherhood of the ground?

Dare we believe that there is a faithful conclusion, even for one whose life is as faithless as his mortal mission is senseless, whose life is a violation of his right to be faithful?

Dare we hope that dead people bear no grudges, even as the living remorsefully pursue the unforgiven unblessed departed?

I have brought up the past and now the deceased. What of the living, and how may we predict the future? For the living confound us as we are drawn to them. Can there be a better world for the mentally retarded? Asking the question implies that, indeed, there can be a better world, that, in retrospect, this is a better world. Asking the question denies the inevitable answer.

Some among you may conclude than an insuperable chasm lies between this discourse and evidence. Some may claim that I bring the softest data to support these words. In truth, I need no data, for everything reported here is well known to those who know about such matters; and anyone who requires data is unlikely to put such evidence to useful purposes. We need no data to conclude that there never was, there is not now, and there will not be a better world for the mentally retarded.

There cannot be a better world for the mentally retarded, or a poorer world, or any world. Worlds and futures are for the living, not for labels and nomenclatures and retards or defectives. Worlds are for lives, not for things or prejudices or administrative configurations. The mentally retarded are no more people than is the photograph a person. To understand this permits one to appreciate the beauty of Helen Keller and to realize that—while she was not mentally retarded—before she was not mentally retarded and before Anne Sullivan, she *was* mentally retarded.

We are trapped. Now that man has created the "mentally retarded" (and the "mentally ill") he must label and categorize him, not only as he seeks to help him—irony of ironies—even as he struggles to wipe away the effects of his evil taxonomy, even as he strives to erase forever the taxonomy itself. As I entreat you to destroy the concept "mental retardation," I find myself using the term as you use it, adding to the layers of inhumanity heaped upon those souls so foully designated. As I tell you there is no future for the mentally retarded—there will not be any until they are returned to their brothers as men and women—as I tell you these things, I meander about human beings as "mentally retarded." We are trapped by civilization's penchant for creating insane problems. And, our brothers and sisters and we will not be rescued by psychologists or sociologists or special educators—and, although they will better describe and teach us about the benchmarks of civilization, not even by poets or historians. We have a modest chance to permit the now-retarded, the now-disturbed, the now-abused to enter our world—albeit an imperfect world—and, I believe, that chance depends upon a decision society must make, but only insofar as each individual must make his personal decision.

People can no longer hide their faith and their souls in the United Nations or with any other group. What we have done to each other no nation and no group can rectify. What I have done to you, only I can repay and correct. Before each man seeks to change the world, he must change. Before these words become more than just words, I must become more than I am now. As I lament on the plight of mankind, I must account for my own plight:

> For, who can tell a man, "We will make up to you for the lost years?"
> Who can return to a man the sweet pleasures of a summer day,
> His wife and carefree children at his side—
> To a man destroyed before his marriage,
> With children never to be conceived?
> Who can describe the fragrant sensation of a pine-covered hill in May,
> Backdropping a neat farmhouse overlooking
>   fields and streams,
> And living things—
> To one who had hardly lived and had barely been given time
>   to stop
> And gather in these wonders?
> Is there a man who can claim, "I have seen these times restored,
> I have been given back the years that were taken,
> The flesh that was ravaged,
> The being that once ceased to be?"
> Who will unfold the years that are gone,
> The times that are past,
> The moments that are wasted,
> This instant that will never again be?
> When a man thinks about these questions, he cries.
> He doesn't cry for mankind, nor for you.
> He cries for himself and for the wasted times in a
> desolate and plundered
> Cosmos.

Man is a wise fool and a sentimental sadist. Is this his natural manner? The fundamental question is whether man is able—and, if as I believe he is able, is he willing—to change? Both fearfully and hopefully, I conclude that, if he doesn't change, nothing will matter. And, if he doesn't, all of our past could not have mattered. If he doesn't, he will have become an example of the Rabbis' ancient saying that God gives wisdom only to those who have wisdom.

Further, I believe that what each individual does—and how his every act causes and effects—is more than a reflection of his selfhood. It is a re-creation of it. But, what has he fashioned?

Man differentiates himself from other beings.
He has speech.
He can protect himself from the elements.
He can leave the old and adapt to a new environment.

Man's speech, his clothing, and the ingenious ways he travels and
    migrates.
Allows him to be freer than:
 The Eagle
 The Jungle Beast and
 Even
 The Wind.

Man is capable of controlling the forces of nature more than they
    are capable of controlling him.
But man has not demonstrated his capability to control himself.
And that which permits him to fly, to build, to shape his destiny.
Causes him to impede and destroy other men.
That which gives some men their freedom gives enslavement to
    others.
That which makes man uniquely free,
Makes him uniquely harrassed.

Our gifts are our demons.
Never having spoken, the lion rules with a roar.
Hardly moving, the snail endures.
In his pond, the fish is free.

But man, prideful and eloquent man!
He disdains the mute and struggles against a relationship with them.
He binds the crippled and increases their spasticity.
He restrains the weak and incompetent and guarantees their infirmity.
He envelopes the old and feeble and insures their loneliness.
He segregates the ill and recreates their mental and spiritual
    disabilities.

Man enforces his retribution on those who do not speak by incar-
cerating them.
On those who do not think by enchaining them.
On those who do not conform by denuding them.
On those who will not be broken by breaking them.

The animals have fewer gifts than man but
  fewer imperatives
  fewer options but
  fewer requirements
  fewer accomplishments but
  fewer needs.

Animals are less civilized than man, but have more civilization.
Animals have less freedom.
But the animal world has more freedom.

Mankind has enslaved his brothers and himself.

Some may wonder why I wrote this paper. There is a compelling
Israeli dialogue, where a visitor asks, "Why did you come here?"
The Israeli replies, "I came to Israel to forget." "To forget what?"
"I forgot."

I wrote this paper to remind those who have forgotten and to help
instruct those who claim not to know. For there are other compelling words, born and nurtured and, forevermore, carved in the soil
of Dachau:
          "Remember us. Do not forget."

Our Jerusalem will be the back ward. We must not forget its existence—and all of mankind's ideological back wards—until civilization makes it unnecessary for us to remember.
    Most of all, I wrote this paper to remind myself. I must not forget.

2. The 1970 White House Conference on Children and Youth

Position Paper of the Section on Clinical Child Psychology, American Psychological Association

by the White House Conference Committee

Erwin Friedman, Chairman
Charlotte H. Altman, Paul W. Clement, Milton F. Shore,
Addison W. Somerville, Zanwil Sperber

Clinical child psychologists have accumulated a body of knowledge about children with both social and individual problems from both the areas of service and research which is relevant to individual development and might be of value in planning the agenda for the White House Conference. There are three general areas in which clinical child psychologists have special expertise: (a) the understanding of the normal as well as deviant processes of development in children and youth (b) empirical experience in clinical and developmental services to children and in research with children and youth, and (c) sensitivity to and understanding of the intra-psychic and socio-cultural forces affecting the psychological and social development and growth of children and youth.

It is out of this three-fold approach to children and youth,—developmental, empirical, and psychosocial—that the following suggestions for the White House Conference are being made.

Youth in the United States have become more and more alienated from their social institutions and the community. In order to reverse this trend, the Committee of clinical child psychologists felt that the White House Conference should serve as a *model* of how adults and youth can work together in developing recommendations for national policy. Unfortunately, there are few models where such constructive interaction between adults and youth has occurred on a wide scale. Therefore, it becomes necessary to develop mechanisms so that the White House Conference can become a cooperative endeavor in which youth participate on various levels; both the adults and the youth have their special contribution to make. The initiation of this dialogue can indeed be the greatest contribution the Conference can make.

The participants in the 1970 White House Conference on Children and Youth should be representative of the society at large. Special attention must be given to assure that each minority group is fairly represented. This means especially minority groups such as Negroes, American Indians, Japanese, Chinese, Filipinos, Puerto Ricans, and Mexican Americans. These groups can have representatives in proportion to their number in the American population or one delegate if their number in the overall population is not significant. However, it is also important that the representatives of these groups be those who are effective and influential so that they not only reflect the concerns of these groups, but are able to implement any recommendations that might come out of the conference.

The Committee also felt that it was very important that the militant representatives of minority groups be included as well as those who are conservative in their orientation. The most recent U.S. census plus contemporary sampling techniques developed by social scientists could be applied in selection of representatives to the Conference.

All major social systems—the family, government, community, church, schools—should be reviewed by the Conference. The family is only one of the institutions and it is important that the Conference not limit itself to one such institution, but encompass the whole range of institutions that affect youth and children in their development and growth.

The Committee felt that a most crucial principle is that youth begin to be involved in some ways in the planning and programming process of all institutions that are concerned with their lives. The nature of their involvement will depend on the decisions that have to be made, the ages of the youth, and the social context. New role possibilities need to be developed and new ways of involving youth encouraged. Some suggestions might be: (1) a national magazine, published for youth, focusing on political and social issues; (2) a youth ombudsman; (3) youth be involved in apprenticeship activities in a variety of social institutions, playing a role in school administrations, police stations, courts and other areas.

As with adults, it is essential that in viewing children and youth certain general principles and psychological needs be taken into account. The techniques for meeting these needs must be geared to the developmental process, as well as (a) the need for control over one's destiny, (b) the need for involvement and commitment to a social purpose and feelings of belonging to a social order, (c) the need for adult models for identification, and (d) the need for self-esteem and self-worth. All techniques that are developed should be evaluated for involving youth in terms of how they meet these needs and if so, in what way.

Emphasis should be placed on community participation and local control of programs where possible. One of the purposes behind such a move would be the development of a feeling of involvement and a sense of community. The Conference should focus on the necessity for developing new neighborhood structures. The need for small intimate individual contacts within a community context are great, and it becomes necessary that certain community activities be developed around which feelings of meaningfulness can arise. (It is out of lack of such a community feeling that such activities as vandalism have been traced.) It is our belief that the school is more appropriate than the medical clinic, especially after the early years, as a center for community activity since the schools in principle foster growth and focus on the development of skills and competence rather than on remediation services and casualties. Thus, models for developing a community focus suggest that schools become more flexible in their activities and be brought more into line with needs of communities by such mechanisms as being open during evenings, weekends, and summers, and establishing many school-based community activities that were frequently previously associated with settlement houses.

Certain needs are not being met by the family at the present time and there appears to be little chance that the family can meet these needs in the foreseeable future. It therefore becomes necessary to recognize the limits of the family as the sole context of early childhood experiences and to develop new institutional structures. Examples of such structures are day-care centers to meet the needs of young children. But these centers should be set up with high standards. They should be staffed by a sufficient number of workers selected for interest in children and personal capacity to respond meaningfully and effectively to children's needs. Professional leadership should be available to help the workers develop programs and practices relevant to the needs of children at different ages, as established through empirical research and clinical experience. Along with this, emphasis should be placed on pre-school education with greater concern for instruction in effective child care in all medical settings. The importance of such pre-school care and stimulation for later development has been highlighted by much recent research.

It seemed for a short period during this present decade that we were going to bridge the service gap which was the legacy of a century of neglect in the area of retardation and handicapping conditions in children and youth. The interest in this particular area is waning and the Committee suggests a refocusing on these problems until the services for this group of children become acceptable and effective. The lack of adequate funding for these services is a most expensive luxury in which our society indulges itself.

The Joint Commission on the Mental Health of Children will be making a final report in 1969. Previous White House Conferences have not had such a fertile source of expert data and opinion in mental health with documents and recommendations originating from many disciplines. Therefore, the Committee strongly recommends that the White House Conference pay special attention to the report of the Joint Commission on the Mental Health of Children and perhaps use its material and recommendations as a major resource for discussion of national policy on children and youth.

Our society needs more people, both professional and non-professional, who are especially capable in working with children and youth. This includes not only assisting those young people who are ill but also encouraging positive growth experiences. We need more resources to train such individuals. We need greater rewards to those who are willing to participate in work with children (as is done in some other countries). The Conference must realize that if we are to meet the great needs, highly trained professionals will need to function more as consultants than as providers of direct service. These professionals need to be encouraged to involve people from all sources interested in children and youth. Lay personnel as well as sub-doctoral individuals have to be trained to carry the share of developing and participating in all youth programs—recreational, educational, social—and also therapeutic.

There is a great deal of empirical evidence that the mass-media, especially television and movies, may contribute to some of the recent problems in the development of adequate controls over aggressive behavior in youth. The Conference should address itself to studying the roles that mass-media are playing in stimulating violence within our society. The Conference should address itself also to the positive effects the mass-media can have on children and youth, encouraging research on how the media might be put to use in aiding the healthy development of children and youth.

There is a strong tendency in the United States toward a well-disguised punitiveness toward children. This takes many forms. For example, many laws relating to children have contained a strong punitive element rather than being designed to help the child develop his personal resources (e.g., laws concerning so-called "illegitimate" children). Children should not be punished for the legal or moral violations of their parents. In addition to removing the punitive clauses in our laws relating to children, laws relating to sexual behavior should also be re-evaluated in order to make them more compatible with contemporary knowledge in social sciences. Children should be taught their legal rights in schools. We strongly feel that a verbalized interest should not be used to disguise some basically punitive attitudes which have often taken over institutional settings, particularly settings such as the juvenile courts, reformatories and state institutions for the retarded.

Our society needs to educate children and parents so that decisions are based on psychological knowledge and information, not on ignorance and superstitution. All programs for children and youth should be designed with the psychological needs of the child taken into account. One cannot separate the legal and psychological, the educational and psychological, the medical and psychological, the recreational and psychological, etc.

One important aspect of the Conference, we feel, should be the focus on a dynamic, constantly evolving view toward children and the institutions that relate to children. There is a need for constant re-evaluation and self-correction. For example, mechanisms should be established for re-evaluating the role of the schools in regard to non-college bound youth, union practices with regard to youth, and the role of vocational ties alone of dubious motivating power. The trend toward shortened work weeks with its concomitant prolonged leisure periods and the above mentioned lack of motivation have important implications for the educational process. Education should strive to become preparation for *living* and should be geared to impart values rather than singular concentration on absorption of knowledge for the future job. The learned values should be applicable to leisure, community participation as well as work. A re-evaluation of the child-labor laws should be considered. These re-evaluations should be based on careful study and empirical foundations, not on the basis of fads or fancies. Constant empirical feedback is necessary with monitoring of programs and social accounting taking place so that there is a continuously growing picture of what is effective and what is not effective with regard to children and youth, and what changes are needed.

3. Children's Needs in the Seventies: A Federal Perspective*

Edward F. Zigler

I am delighted to have this opportunity to share with you some of my hopes and concerns regarding public policy towards children.

I must confess that I am far from content or sanguine about our nation's treatment of children. We are very fond of saying in this country that children are our most valuable natural resource. Unfortunately, it has been my experience that we treat this natural resource as badly as we have treated many of our other natural resources. In fact, I think that we tend to romanticize how much we do for children in the face of considerable evidence to the contrary. There is a myth abroad in this land that we are a child-oriented society, that nothing is too good for our children; however, the realities that we see all about us belie the myth. I don't think this country is going to make very much progress in its treatment of children until it sees with clarity, with open eyes, what the shortcomings of our country and society are in the treatment of our young.

Legalized Abuse and Dehumanization of Children

Let us consider our treatment of foster children. The statement has been made that concerns do not change; they just grow older. We have the same problem with foster children that we have always had. In fact, I was recently looking at the United Nations Charter on Children of 1959 in which it said that every child had a right to a home. I saw those same words in a Bill of Rights for Children that was produced by the White House Conference on Children of 1930. And yet, we still perpetuate a system in this country in which a child

*A version of this paper was presented at the convention of the American Psychological Association. September, 4, 1971, Washington, D.C., and published in the Journal of Clinical Child Psychology, I, 3, Fall 1972.

is permitted to be moved from home to home to home, when we all know that continuity, affection and solidity are what make for normal development. We are still satisfied with a system of foster care for children that permits a child to live one place for a few years and then be moved on to the next place for a few years. If one examines only the cost of this kind of care, the figure comes to 50 or 60 thousand dollars by the time the child reaches maturity. Yet our society is slow in spending the very few thousand dollars that would be involved in subsidized adoption.

But the problem goes beyond money. It goes to the very value system that we have with respect to children and their rights. Over and over, we see this nation so concerened with the rights of adults and biological parents that the rights of children do, indeed, come last. For instance, we have a situation in this country today where there are more families who would like to adopt children than there are children to be adopted. Yet, we still have foster children. That makes no sense. Why don't we have these children adopted? Well, it has been pointed out to me that the law in New York State says that you cannot adopt a child providing that the biological parent maintains some interest in the child. How great an interest? The rule in New York is that, if a parent will send that child one postcard a year, then that child cannot be adopted! We saw the clash between the rights of biological parents and children in a very dramatic way, again in New York State. A three-year old adopted child was taken from the arms of the only real mother, in my estimation, that child had ever had and handed back to the biological mother who, three years later, had changed her mind.

For any of you who must still be disabused about this nation's treatment of its children, I suggest you visit a few of the children's institutions in this country. This nation is the only one I know of that permits the legalized abuse and de-humanization of children in institutions. I hope you saw the television program "This Child Labelled X." Programs like that can make a difference, and I recommend it to you. I also recommend a book to you, essentially a book of pictures, entitled *Christmas in Purgatory,* by an old colleague and friend, Professor Burton Blatt, who is now at Syracuse University. On page after page you see children, young people, huddled in corners, filthy and neglected. What was the sin of these children? What did they do to deserve this kind of treatment by our society? In most cases, the only sin they perpetrated was that they happened to be mentally retarded.

Since I am a bureaucrat these days, you might interpret what I am saying as some kind of attack on the administration of which I am a part. That is not what I am doing here. I am not attacking this particular administration, or for that matter any administration that preceded it. What I am saying is, rather, an indictment of our nation.

Misplaced Attacks on Head Start

Another manifestation of this national indifference to children is the attack on Head Start. I discovered upon coming to Washington that probably the most innovative program our nation has ever mounted in behalf of needy children was being dismissed as a "failure." Head Start was yesterday's "thing;" now people could only say negative things about it, disparage it, say "well, the Westinghouse Report shows it's not very good, and it's not accomplishing very much, and what's the next thing we ought to be doing?" This is utter nonsense! The Jensen Report, Eysenck's book, the recent paper by Herrenstein, all lead to criticism of the compensatory education programs of this nation on the basis of the fact that some portion of intelligence is certainly inherited. That criticism is simply misplaced. I would say to you that if anyone looks at the evidence about the Head Start program, one would have no difficulty in asserting its success. What criteria should be used in evaluating such a program? First of all, one should look at the goals of the program itself. Head Start is a broad developmental program having many components and is certainly not directed exclusively at IQ raising. If one looks at what has been achieved with some of these components, Head Start is quite impressive.

Let's take health: figures indicate that of the children who show up at our Head Start centers, something on the order of 40 percent have an identifiable physical defect. If you now multiply that number by the some 400,000 children who have been in Head Start each of its five years, you are talking about hundreds of thousands of children. Of those children, over 75 percent have had their physical defects treated.

Or consider parent involvement. I had the honor of being the respondent to Senator Harris at the 1971 APA convention when he pointed out that our institutions are not responsive enough to people, and people must play an important role in shaping our institutions. I am proud to be one of the architects of Head Start, for which we enunciated the principle of parent participation, and parent participation remains a keystone of the Head Start program. Through such parent participation, one sees parents who get a new sense of dignity, a new sense of worth, a new sense of being able to control their destiny and that of their children. As a result we have children in homes that are much more conducive to the child's growth and development.

Let's look at the Kirschner Report on what happens when you have a Head Start program in a community. That report indicated that in 58 communities where Head Start was available, not only did it help the children in the Head Start program, but it changed the political and social ecology of the community. Something on the order of 1,500 changes have been made in the health and education delivery systems in those 58 communities.

How about parents' assessment of Head Start? They think it's great. They see what it is doing for their children; is this no longer a criterion for the worth of a program? Furthermore, although we have wrestled with the evaluation problem for a good number of years, one thing is very clear in the evaluations of Head Start; if you look at Head Start children versus an appropriate control group at the point of time at which they leave Head Start, those children are superior to the control children on any dimension—health, cognition, social development—anything you want to measure. What happens, of course, is that these gains seem to be lost as children proceed through the school system. There are many interpretations for this loss, but one hypothesis I would put to you is that these kinds of findings are much more an indictment of the American school system than they are of Head Start.

Why the negative view of Head Start? Well, I think we made some mistakes—I think the nation frequently does, and I think we experts often do. First of all, we were satisfied with too narrow an evaluation. We, ourselves, permitted Head Start to be painted into the IQ corner in which it was going to be assessed on the basis of whether we produced instant geniuses or not. But that was fallacious. That was never the goal of Head Start. Head Start had never been directed toward massive IQ changes. What it has been directed towards is improving the social competence of the child. Many of you have certainly heard me go on about this at some length, and those of you who have read my papers certainly know it is my conviction that the greatest good we can do in compensatory education—a fact totally overlooked by Jensen and by Herrenstein and by others—is to bring about changes in the motivational system of the child. The problems of many of our poor children are not problems of stupidity but rather, the problem of not using the intellect that they have. If we could just change their attitudes about themselves and create a sense of accomplishment and confidence in their ability to succeed, I think that you immediately see the kinds of gains that can occur through compensatory education programs.

The Environmental Mystique

In addition to this notion that what Head Start was all about was to produce a cadre of professors for Yale and Harvard, there was another mistaken view of Head Start that gained ascendency. Perhaps I should not use the word mistake because it is pejorative; rather, an argument concerning the relative importance of environment and heredity in intellectual development has been waging in the intellectual community for a good number of years, but in our thinking about Head Start one particular point of view prevailed. And that particular point of view, which I have referred to in the past as the environmental mystique, is characterized by the view that IQ is easy to change. Many believed it would be easy to hurry children along through the developmental sequence if we could just find the right gadget, the right mobile, the right something-or-other. Well, I do think that was a mistake. And those who have been writing for a good number of years about how easy it is to change the IQ and who report to us changes in IQs of 60 and 80 points, I think do a great disservice to social action programs because they are listened to by decision-makers.

Decision-makers listened to the "environmental mystiquers" at the inception of Head Start, and I saw this view manifested in the thinking of people who were indeed very powerful and really knew what power was all about. I remember standing in the Rose Garden next to President Johnson after the first summer of Head Start. We had gotten this program off the ground rather hurriedly, very slopily. We had given children something-or-other of varying quality for six or eight weeks and everyone liked it. It was the Sesame Street of 1965, and the President was there to announce that we would have a full year program. He said in effect, "We had six hundred thousand children in Head Start this summer, and as a result we will have six hundred thousand tax paying citizens whereas otherwise we would have had six hundred thousand more individuals on welfare." Well, what does this reflect? What it reflects is the kind of thinking that experts had instilled in decision-makers—that it is easy to develop the intellect—easy to develop social competence in children. And it reflects something else: it reflects a shortcoming that I think I have found in the national character, namely, a desire for simple solutions to complex problems. So we flit, and the nation flits, from "magic period" to "magic period". If you cannot do it with eight weeks, try a year. You didn't do it with a year, Head Start? Well, you got there too late. Now there is a new magic period, the first year of life, and we are in the "mobile" stage of child development. If we continue telling decision-makers this, we are probably the greatest enemies that our children have. I am convinced that we know better than that about child development, and the message we ought to be giving is: "Look, you are not going to get off on the cheap. The developing child is not that plastic a thing. There are no magic periods. Yes, the first year of life is critical. So is the second." I told President Johnson that I admired his position on the first five years of life. That is finally a step in the right direction. But I also informed him that if you do everything you can in the first five years of life and forget the next five, you're still not going to get the job done. You have to respect the continuity of human development. You have to make sure that the child has the environmental input at every stage to optimize his total development, and only by this kind of commitment will we ever be able to optimize the development of children.

I want to say one final thing about Head Start, something that is troubling me. Dr. Julius Richmond pointed it out most eloquently, and I would simply like to underline his remarks. We evaluators spend much time trying to demonstrate that if you do something for a child when he is four and maybe when he is seven, you can show that that child has got four more achievement points on a Metropolitan Reading Test which is correlated about .20 with something later in life. It is something *later* that we are shooting for. It is this kind of insidious thinking that I am here to attack; when we talk about the quality of the lives of citizens in this country, we always seem to be talking about the quality of the lives of adults, so that when we mount a program for children we always want to assess its future results. But if you go into a ghetto apartment in Harlem, or for that matter a shack in Mississippi, and see an over-burdened mother with no physical resources, under great stress; a child having little to do, not getting the proper nutrition, not getting health care, not getting the kind of experience that is in any way developmental; and then if you see the same child in a Head Start Center, opening up, smiling, sitting down to a balanced lunch, getting medical care—do you need much of an evaluation to tell you that programs such as this are worthwhile? If you let one of variables in your cost-benefit analysis be the happiness and the improvement in the quality of the lives of those children during their enrollment in your program, the program is indeed worth the cost.

Well, I do not think there has been an effort of mine that I take greater pride in than my role as a planner for Head Start. I am proud of that program, and I go on record again to tell you that I believe it is the most important social action effort ever mounted on behalf of needy children in this country. But after saying that, I will say to you that our country would be mistaken to stand pat. We cannot afford to stand pat on a program that only delivers these services to 10 to 15 percent of the nation's children who need them. We have to move on. Furthermore, the answer to the needs of many children is not just half-day programs. We have to move on into the day care area as well. I see us moving on from Head Start to types of centers that would provide a variety of services for children, with one very important new service being day care.

Heterogeneity: A Key to Future Child Centers

I also see the children's centers of the Seventies as different from the Head Start centers of the Sixties with respect to one very important phenomenon—namely, the mixing of children of different socio-economic groups. Looking back upon it now, I think that it was a mistake to set up a program just for poor children, to segregate these economically disadvantaged children at an early time in life. Again, we did not have enough money, so we chose to give the money to the most needy. Well, that really is not the solution. I think we know better now, and it is really interesting to me how the times have changed. I remember a year ago when I first started talking about the need for mixing socio-economic groups in children's centers, the New York Times took issue with me in an editorial in which they suggested very gently that I was probably some kind of a reverse Robin Hood—that what I had in mind was to take from the poor and give to the rich. That is not what I have in mind at all.

What I have in mind is centers most conductive to the growth of children, and there are at least three reasons why the children's centers of the future must be heterogeneous in terms of socio-economic classes. The first reason was pointed out by a far better politician than I am, and it is simply a pragmatic political reason—that as long as you have programs that are just directed at poor children, those programs are politically vulnerable. Senator Bayh, who is certainly no enemy of the poor, pointed out that you have got to have massive support to keep spending the literally billions of dollars that these programs are going to cost, and you will never get that support until the programs are providing services to more than just the poor.

The second reason is a little bit closer to my heart as a developmentalist: we know that children grow more optimally to the degree that they have a wide array of models after whom to model their behavior. I think that economically disadvantaged children can model after certain achievement traits, certain orientations, of the middle class child; and I think it would be equally valuable for the middle-class child to model after certain virtues of the child from poverty such as early independence, persistence, less fearfulness, and now there is evidence of even greater creativity—they are simply not as up tight as the middle class five year old, it appears.

The third reason is simply social-psychological. I am troubled by the quality of life in this country in many respects. I am troubled by the polarization; I am troubled by what we have witnessed over the last few years—whites against blacks; the old against the young; the academics aginst the hard-hats. The nation cannot long endure unless these groups find commonality. The social fabric can only stand so much pulling and hauling. If we want to produce the types of citizens, the types of adults who can indeed understand and respect one another, certainly the way to accomplish this is not to begin tracking children along socio-economic class lines at the age of 6 months. My social-pyschological training tells me that if you do so segregate groups, you will probably develop within these groups some in-group solidarity, and there is some value in that. But it is also accompanied by just too much out-group hostility. Given the values of our nation and what we would like our country to be, we must move to do all we can to bring children, at least, together. What I have in mind, then, are centers that have heterogeneous groups of children; that have a whole array of services, everything from day care to drop off service to overnight service to caring for a child for a few days while the family is in a period of stress. Obviously, we must protect what we have won for the poor to date in these centers, and the way to do this is pretty obvious. People who cannot afford these services will receive them as a right. People who can afford some of these services and want to avail themselves of them will pay a fee, with the fees being scaled to income.

Child Care Dilemmas for the Seventies

Now there is going to be another problem, and I think that it is going to be the battle of the Seventies; you are going to have to take sides on it and some of you will wind up on one side and some of you on another. But let me raise the problem: It would be very easy for me to sit in my office at Yale and devise the very best possible program for children that I could devise. I know what it would look like. But the cost is simply fantastic. We will have to find new ways of caring for children in this nation. The most important factor in the cost of care of a child in a Head Start center or the type of children's center that I envision is the amount of money that we pay the head teacher. The nation has tended to move in two directions on this cost issue. One direction you are all familiar with; I would refer to it as pristine professional purity—that is, if you want to have a very good center to help children, you should go to Bank Street and get one of their MA's. Well, there is little question in my mind that that is true, and I have a lot of friends who are MA's from Bank Street. But saying that Bank Street teachers will meet the child care needs of this nation is akin to saying that psychoanalysts will meet the needs posed by the mental health problems of this country. There are simply not enough of them. And there is another factor; when you start a children's center with an enrollment of thirty children, it is simply not economically viable to have such a person run it; it simply costs too much. So both from the view point of availability and from the view point of fiscal reality, we cannot staff our children's centers with the most highly trained professionals in child development.

There is another direction that the nation started to move in a few years ago, but it cannot be the solution. I am referring to the naive, romantic view that if you are just poor yourself, or have a good heart, or some combination of the two, you are ideally suited to train young children. This is not true. There is knowledge one should have about children. There are optimal ways to interact with children. There are many things that one should know. What we must do in this nation is develop an entirely new cadre of child care workers. This would be a group of certified people who have achieved their status through different pathways. The skills that we would want to require for certification would be circumscribed skills. I respect all of the things that go into a BA; I have spent much of my life training students for the BA. But really, much of what is taught in the university is not essential to caring for a child properly. What we need to do is develop more circumscribed training which will receive formal recognition. Is this a revolutionary concept? No! Other nations have done it. We are again behind. I would refer you to the children's nurse in Denmark, the up-bringer in Russia, the children's house worker in Israel—these are the kinds of models I have in mind; and the Office of Child Development will be moving over the course of the next year toward fleshing out this particular proposal.

I want to close by presenting one further trend I see for the Seventies. I am beginning to be a little troubled by the unidirectional stance that the nation is taking with respect to child care. We do a lot of talk about supplementing family life; we put a child into a day care center for 8, 10 or 12 hours a day so that the parents can earn the resources with which to provide an adequate home for the child; then we supplement family life a little bit more with an hour of good children's TV. Before long, at this rate, we will not be supplementing family life; we will be supplanting it. I think there is beginning to be a trend in this nation of parents handing children over to "experts," however they are trained, in the belief that they know what to do better than parents themselves. This budding trend will blossom in the Seventies as a full-blown problem. Dr. Urie Bronfenbrenner, per usual, is a little bit ahead of the thinkers in the field and is performing for us a great service, namely, analyzing what we now know about child development in centers. He comes out with the not terribly astounding, but nonetheless refreshing, conclusion that perhaps the best place to raise children is in the home. Be that as it may, there are new socil forms and society must provide choices. We are not going to stop the movement of women into the work force, and we must have good day care for the children of these women. But at the same time, we must not indicate to every parent, every mother, every father, every family, that optimal child development rests in handing the child over to some center.

Education for Parenthood

What I would recommend to this nation is that as we develop the kinds of centers I have been talking about, we develop alternate forms in which we do nothing but supplement family life by helping parents in the parenting function. I think we could do this in several ways. One way, which we should have begun a long time ago, is the training of young people in parenting. Parenting is tough. It is tough not just for the poor; it is tough for the rich. We all practice on our first child. We learn by some kind of trial and error, and it is becoming more and more difficult to care for our own children because we no longer have the extended family, a grandma or Aunt Susie to come help us. What we should do in this country is insist that, as part of high school life, every adolescent receive courses in parenting. These courses would involve adolescents in working with younger children—tutoring them, working in day care centers—to bring didactic materials on child development to life through particular young children. If our high schools can teach driver education and ancient history, we can certainly use that kind of learning center to help young people in assuming the most important role our society gives to an adult: namely, that of a parent.

We should do other things too, and we will. We should have not only center programs; we should begin—and we will begin in the Office of Child Development in the next few months—a program which I will label Homestart. In this program, we will have individuals go into homes upon the request of parents, not to give them great expertise but to ask a simple question: What kind of help do you want with your child? Then we will do our best to provide that kind of help. I have been intrigued by Homestart-like programs such as those of Ira Gordon, Susan Gray, and there are a number of them now. Let us begin utilizing this information to help mothers be mothers, because as Urie Bronfenbrenner puts it so well, it still appears that a mother will do for nothing what you cannot pay other people to do for a lot of money. In addition to courses in parenting and programs such as Home-start, I think we ought to have a "Sesame Street" for parents. Such programs are being developed now, and they will also contribute much to our efforts to help parents in the parenting function.

This has been a very brief view of where we have been the last few years, where I think we might be going over the next ten years, and what I believe the major problems to be. I have been a little severe, I think deservedly so in light of the track record of this nation. I would like to leave you on a somewhat more positive note, and that is that I think the nation is moving forward in respect to children. Workers have increasingly come out of the laboratories and have tried to see how we can use what we know in behalf of children, and I think that this will have great payoff to children. I think that the very establishment, for the first time in this nation, of an Office of Child Development is a very healthy step. I believe there is a real concern for children within the Administration and among leaders of both parties on the Hill. We now have knowledge, we now have expertise, we now have concern. There may be some obstacles ahead, but if we all keep up the momentum that I think we now have, I predict that we will indeed be able to say as we reach the Eighties that our nation has done the kind of job for children during the Seventies that children have a right to expect of us.

4. Part I: Forecasting the Future— 1968*

Alan O. Ross

Forecasting the future is at best an idle, at worst a dangerous occupation. Under present circumstances, it is also a depressing task, likely to bring out one's latent pessimism.

Many dedicated, well-informed, and well-meaning people have worked for the Joint Commission and those of us who have served on its Board of Directors have had the opportunity to see the prolific results of their labors. I have no doubt that great and exciting plans intended to deal with real and critical issues will be proposed in the Report of the Commission. What will be their impact? Two weeks from today, it will be three years since Mary Alice White and I attended the first organizational meeting of the Board of Directors of the Joint Commission on behalf of APA. I need hardly remind you that the past three years were not likely to inspire one's confidence in the soundness of our governmental process, the wisdom of our political leaders, or the flexibility of our social structure. Even those less inclined to cynicism than I have recently come to wonder whether things are likely to change without so radical an upheaval as to leave this society unrecognizably restructured.

Let me give you some samples of the source of my pessimism. I have been to a Joint Commission meeting where we discussed the desirability of setting up regional child development centers — and when I came back home, I learned that the community mental health center we were to have across the street would not be able to open because anticipated funds had not been made available.

I have been to a Joint Commission meeting where we discussed the urgent need for establishing Day Care and Parent-Child Centers — and when I came back home, I learned that the local Head Start

*Part I of this article was presented at the Symposium on *The Joint Commission on Mental Health of Children: Implications for Psychology as a Social Science*, American Psychological Association Convention, San Francisco, 1968. The entire article is reprinted from the Journal of Clinical Child Psychology, I, 3, Fall 1972.

Program had to curtail its services because operating funds had been cut.

I have been to a Joint Commission meeting where we discussed the importance of training child care specialists—and when I came back home, I learned that our training grant had been approved, but its budget reduced to the level of a symbolic gesture because needed funds were not available.

I could go on juxtaposing dream and reality, but I am sure that you get the idea. To those of you who look to the Report of the Joint Commission as bringing about major social changes, I feel impelled to say: "Don't get your hopes up!" I don't believe that this is an era of progress, and I feel that our Report will fall on deaf, hostile, or preoccupied ears. But maybe this jeremiad of mine simply reflects that my perception is distorted by my own choleric temperament. Is there a more objective basis on which to forecast the future?

The best way psychologists have for predicting future behavior is to extrapolate from past performance. Maybe the fate of the earlier Joint Commission on Mental Health and Illness will give us a basis for predicting the fate of our recommendation.

The Final Report of the old Joint Commission published in 1961, under the rousing title, "Action for Mental Health," carried the following as its first recommendations:

"1. A much larger proportion of total funds for mental health research should be invested in basic research as contrasted with applied research . . ."

If you are at all familiar with recent actions of Congress reported in such sources as *Science* and our own *Washington Report*, you will know how well that particular recommendation has fared.

Another key recommendation dealt with the fate of people in the mammoth custodial state mental hospitals hidden away in the countryside, many miles from the patients' homes. These institutions were to be decentralized and every effort made to provide treatment facilities as close as possible to the patients' homes. That was in 1961.

If I may be permitted to generalize from the couple of state institutions with which I am familiar, little has happened to change either their size or their dismal nature. Some have undergone a rechristening so as to put the words "community" or "mental health" into their name, but they maintain the same old cages in the same isolated remoteness. The salutary things that have happened in some mental hospitals are the result of research-based progress, unrelated to the recommendations of the Joint Commission. More of that later.

What may look to some like a major change in the nation's mental health picture—the development of Comprehensive Community Mental Health Centers—happens *not* to be the product of the Joint Commission's recommendations, although it is related to the concepts embodied in them. For that matter, I would hate to ask how many of you are acquainted with a well-functioning, fully-staffed, adequately-housed, competently-administered, truly *comprehensive* community mental health center that carries out all of its mandates and some of its optional functions in a responsible manner. I fear that a poll on this would reflect yet another sorry state of affairs, where a cynical travesty has been made of innovative and creative plans, simply in order to grasp newly available funds and to funnel them into the running of the same old psychiatric institutions, operating under the same management, serving the same privileged population, albeit with a new name over the door.

If I assess the history of the old Joint Commission even half-way correctly, an extrapolation from the past makes the future of the new Joint Commission look anything but promising. If you still can't share my pessimism about the chances for progress, I ask you to look at the present state of New Frontier or Great Society programs, started with such optimistic fanfare only a few short years ago. Where is the War on Poverty? Where is Head Start? Where is the Neighborhood Youth Corps? How healthy is Medicare? Or, for that matter, what happened to the recommendations contained in the President's own Commission on Civil Disorders?

On the basis of all these considerations, I am forced to make the prediction that the recommendations about to be made by the Joint Commission on Mental Health of Children will be ignored, distorted, or disparaged—or perhaps, enshrined in the National Archives next to other idealistic exhortations from the past. If any recommendations are implemented, I fear that they will be traduced or starved to death soon after birth, so that it can then be said, "We tried your ideas, but as we told you, they didn't work."

Whitney Young was recently forced to the conclusion that Americans do not respond to people who plead on moral grounds. Many of the Commission's recommendations will, of necessity, have to be based on moral grounds. Others will be based on logical grounds, but if the response to the data on smoking and health or the fate of gun control legislation is any guide, not much can be expected for these pleas either. As I see it, our country and its legislators spring into action for three reasons. These are fear, votes, and the profit motive. It is an unfortunate fact of life that children don't inspire such fear as does Communism, that they do not vote as do members of labor unions, and that they don't bring money into people's pockets as do river and harbor projects or road building programs. It is to the everlasting shame of this nation, that we find it easier to speed a man into outer space than to get food into the mouth of a child starving in our own country.

As if these socio-political obstacles to progress were not enough, there are some who believe that we may also be suffering from a dearth of new ideas. Dr. Sidney Werkman, a brilliant young child psychiatrist who is temperamentally more inclined to optimism than I, and who worked for a year as Deputy Director of the Joint Commission, said in the Spring of this year:

> "It may be that we are in a period of consolidation in the mental health enterprise, rather than one of a great surge forward . . . those who look for brilliant inventions, simple answers to overwhelming problems, will probably be disappointed. Our time is not in tune for such an approach. We seem to be in a period in which many opportunities for a systematic rearrangement of services exist. The community mental health centers, neighborhood service centers, and restructuring of cities are examples of such opportunities. We are not, however, blessed with ideological breakthrough or a new drug."

This from a man who was in the closest possible contact with the deliberations and workings of the Joint Commission and its task forces! Though I disagree with Dr. Werkman's conclusions, his words do not give me much comfort. If he is right, are we really condemned to the continued use of the same tired and ineffective approaches, simply adding some new slogan words like comprehensive, coordinated, and integrated? Are we to continue shifting our limited manpower around from one area and program to another much in the way we shift the urban poor from one slum to another under the auspices of "urban renewal"? Are we to continue rechristening the same incompetent institutions so that they can continue business as usual?

I surely hope that there are other answers than "consolidation." And here, I guess, I have used the word "hope" for the first time. Were I not able to use that word, you could rightfully ask me why on earth I spent three years serving on the Joint Commission. True, I have become disillusioned, but I can still see purpose in what the Joint Commission has done and to which I may have been able to contribute some infinitesimal part.

I do not believe that social progress comes because commissions write reports and make recommendations to Congress. Social progress comes when inspired, dedicated, or maybe simply opportunistic men who happen to be at the fulcrum of power, choose to lend impetus to given ideas. I think all our important social changes would have been impossible without such key figures as Lincoln, Franklin Roosevelt, George W. Norris, Jack Kennedy or Earl Warren. Two things are thus required for social progress: an influential man in the corridors of power, and an important idea. We can never tell who might be such a man or when he will come along. Since the important idea such a man might champion will not necessarily be his own, it seems to me that we had better have some ideas in readiness in case someone appears on the scene looking for something to sponsor. This, I believe, is how the Report of the Joint Commission might have a chance to make a difference. Dr. Werkman's assessment notwithstanding, you can be sure that the Report will contain a good many important ideas, and if we are lucky, some of these ideas will find their way to the right man at the right time. Then we might see progress. That's why I worked on the Joint Commission.

But social progress of the big-leap-forward variety is not the only way in which change can take place. In many smaller ways changes are occurring, usually as the result of an individual who dares to apply available knowledge. I referred earlier to the changes in the big custodial mental hospitals, changes that were unrelated to "Action for Mental Health." What I had in mind were the innovations resulting from the application of psychological research such as Fairweather's efforts with therapeutic communities, the token economy approaches of Krasner, and the operant work of Ayllon. In the child area we have seen similar movement as in project Re-Ed of Nick Hobbs, Susan Gray's work in pre-school education, Seymour Sarason's efforts with inner-city schools, or Ivar Lovaas' operant treatment programs. Change thus also comes about when relatively ordinary men and women apply ideas in their own small spheres of influence. While we wait for the great man who can move the country, we must look to the school down the street which can be improved by us. It is thus important that every one of us in his own way, and at his own place, do "his own thing." The discovery of knowlege and the sophisticated application of such knowledge, continue to be the first order of business for psychology and psychologists, regardless of what the Joint Commission might recommend or how its recommendations will fare in the market place of politics. Some of the supplementary material growing out of the work of the task forces and to be published under the auspices of the Joint Commission will contain valuable summaries of available knowleged that should greatly facilitate their application on local as well as national levels.

So far I have said three things: I have said that I am terribly pes-
simistic about anything meaningful resulting from the Report of the
Joint Commission on Mental Health of Children. I have said that we
must nonetheless promulgate the Report in hopes that it will give an
idea to some leader shopping for a worthwhile issue, and I have said
that we must increase and apply our available knowledge on whatever level we are individually able to influence. Before closing, permit me to ignore all I have said and to engage in some wishful thinking.

Assuming we can translate into reality some or all of the things the
Joint Commission is going to recommend, I want to list those I
would most like to see brought about.

First and foremost, I hope that the Commission Report will result
in sustained high-level support for every kind of good research in
human development. All but the most arrogantly artistic clinicians
admit how little we know and how much we are guessing when we
make broad recommendations designed to enhance the psychological development of children. Increasing available knowledge must
be given the highest priority.

Beyond this primary hope for more research support, I have
hopes for the establishment of certain programs, each of which
would have a tremendous impact on the lives of our children, and
each of which should include explicit plans for the evaluation of its
effectiveness.

Thus, I hope that the Joint Commission Report will lead to the
introduction of *meaningful* education for parenthood, starting in
childhood and continuing into the mature years. It is appalling that
we offer four-year college programs in animal husbandry but let
parents loose on their children without even the most rudimentary
training in the crucial skills of child rearing.

Next, I hope that we will see a total restructuring of our educational system with the emphasis placed on learning instead of
teaching, so that school failures will be viewed as failures of the
school and not as failures of the child. Such a restructuring should
result in maximizing the student's effectiveness by taking account of
individual differences in such areas as cognitive and learning styles.
Entailed in this is obviously a renewal of methods of teacher-train-
ing, teacher-recruitment, and teacher-employment so that the best
possible people can become and remain teachers.

I further hope that the Report will lead to a thorough and honest
re-examination of our values regarding the role and responsibility of
the family. We must ask ourselves where the responsibility of the
family ends and where the responsibility of society begins. Is the

worst family really better than the best institution? And what, for that matter, is to be called a "family"? Enmeshed in these questions is the issue of how to structure and deliver welfare services and how to assure adequate care for all children.

In relation to this, I hope that we will see an all-out effort to bring sophisticated physical and psychological care to the forgotten citizen, the child below age three. We need parent-child centers, readily accessible to all, which can provide well-child check-ups, day care services, and group foster homes. I would like to see the institutionalization of regular and routine health and mental health check-ups required for *all* children, just as we now by statute require small-pox vaccinations and school attendance. Between the legally required registration of the child's birth and the legally required registration for school, society has no knowledge as to the condition or whereabouts of a child. By the time he shows up in school with a handicap, disorder, or deficiency, it is often difficult to do anything about it, while with earlier access to the child, the condition might well have been prevented. It is meaningless to talk about prevention unless one is willing to assure universal access to all children.

I also hope that we can have the resources to train needed personnel at every level, from the baby sitter to the post-doctoral research scientist, for it is obvious that without this, all of my other hopes are not only dreams, but empty dreams.

My last hope is that we will come more and more to emphasize personal competence and social effectiveness instead of mental health and personality adjustment. To me, these concepts seem to have lost whatever utility they may once have had. Interestingly enough, we may be closer to this last hope than to any of the rest. Largely, I suppose, because it doesn't require legislation and it doesn't cost money to reconceptualize an approach. It is simply a matter of giving voice to the Zeitgeist. It is remarkable that a Commission with "mental health" in its name rarely mentions mental health in its reports and recommendations. In reading the various drafts, memoranda, and working papers, I was gratified to note that they generally reflected a recognition of the fact that environment controls behavior so that if we hope to improve what children do, we must improve and restructure the environment in which they live. The focus of the Joint Commission has clearly been on the interpersonal-environmental and not on the intra-psychic; it has been on the structure of society, not on the structure of the psyche. From my own point of view, I welcome this focus, for I think that it is a step in the right direction and, hence — at last — a basis for optimism.

Part II. Four Years after the Forecast

As I read over the comments I had prepared for the 1968 APA meeting in San Francisco, I realize that, in today's world, forecasting the future is a rather safe occupation; all one has to do is to paint the bleakest possible picture, events are bound to sustain the prophesy. I said in 1968, "Don't get your hopes up!" Now I can say, "I told you so!" Things turned out to be almost as bad as I had predicted. Wish it were otherwise.

The Joint Commission submitted its final report to Congress on June 30, 1969. I had naively expected that headlines all over the country would announce this epochal event, forgetting my own prediction that the Report would be ignored. There were no headlines; we had spent three years and a million dollars and the news media did not consider our conclusions worthy of note. The public version of the Report appeared later that year in the form of a 578-page hardcover edition, published by Harper and Row under the title, "Crisis in Child Mental Health, Challenge for the 1970's." Who recalls seeing this book advertised? How many have seen, let alone own, a copy of this ten-dollar volume? With my chronic tendency to attribute malevolence where only incompetence may be involved, I wonder why Harper & Row was so eager to get the publishing rights for this Report.

The key recommendation of the Commission calls for a Child Advocacy System which would range from the national to the local level where it would introduce Child Development Councils as "a new kind of institution." These Councils are to act as advocates on behalf of children with the responsibility to see to it that complete diagnostic, treatment, and preventive services are provided. They would have the responsibility for monitoring the effectiveness of existing agencies and for identifying mental health care needs in their jurisdiction. These Councils would, in other words, run interference with service agencies and make sure that a child in need of care was referred to and seen by an appropriate professional. What happened to these brave plans? I had predicted that they would be distorted and disparaged.

By November 1971 a Comprehensive Child Development Bill, modeled upon many of the Commission's recommendations, had passed the House and Senate in slightly different version. The Senate version contained a child advocacy provision that would have authorized the establishment of a series of pilot programs to test the concept in "no more than twenty different communities."

(The Joint Commission, compromising with what we thought was fiscal reality, had called for a pilot program in one hundred communities.) When the two versions of this Bill went to the House-Senate Conference Committee the entire child advocacy portion was deleted! What emerged as the Child Development Act of 1971 contained some sound provisions for Day Care Centers with quality safeguards and freedom of choice. This was the Bill that President Nixon chose to veto with the words: "Neither the immediate need nor the desirability of a national child development program of this character has been demonstrated." Had I predicted distortion and disparagement?

A separate attempt to implement the child advocacy recommendation was prepared by Senator Ribicoff who had sparked the Joint Commission. His Child Advocacy Bill (S. 1414) was still in the Senate Finance Committee when I checked with the Executive Director of the Commission in March of 1972. By the time these words are published the fate of this Bill should be known. I shall spare you another of my predictions.

Now for the Good News: The Office of Child Development, under the directorship of Ed Zigler,* had created a National Center for Child Advocacy to serve as a focal point from which to mobilize resources on behalf of children. This Office has also funded some studies in the area of child advocacy but the dollar amounts dedicated to these efforts are infinitesimal when measured against the enormity of the problem.

A little more has happened at the State level. North Carolina has enacted a Child Advocacy Bill which closely follows the recommendations of the Joint Commission. A similar law is now on the books of the State of Maine. Hawaii has established a Child Development Commission, and both Hawaii and Massachusetts have appointed a State Advocate for children. Several other States and some local communities are moving in similar directions. At this point, what remains of the Joint Commission cheers and tries to take credit each time the word "advocacy" appears in the news. These days, you have to find your good news wherever you can.

History, I suppose, will have to judge whether the effort of the Joint Commission was worthwhile. From my own jaundiced perspective, I consider this Commission, like White House Conferences and various Presidential Commissions, to have been a palliative for problems that have their solution in the political, not in the deliberative arena. Long ago, in another age and in another country,

---

*Editor's note: Dr. Zigler resigned from OCD in July, 1972.

I studied Greek as part of my "humanistic" education. There is one phrase I remember to this day; it translates, "When action is necessary, words are superfluous." The Joint Commission produced a lot of words.

5. The Psychologist as Child Advocate: Reflections of a Devil's Advocate*

Gertrude J. Williams

The time honored concept of advocacy is beginning to seep into clinical child psychology, and it will be interesting to see what happens to it. Will child advocacy become an active instrument for child power, or will it become just another one of the Brand X verbalisms that litter the field of psychology?

The paper of Alan Ross[1] and the position statement of the APA Ad Hoc Committee on Children and Youth refer frequently and favorably to the application of the advocacy concept to children which has been endorsed by the Joint Commission on Mental Health of Children. Briefly, as enunciated in these papers, child advocacy is an assertion of the rights of children to be wanted, to be born healthy, to live in a healthy environment, to receive basic need satisfaction and continuous loving care, to acquire optimal intellectual and emotional skills and appropriate treatment when required. Local Child Development Councils established throughout the nation would serve as agents of advocacy in order to guarantee these rights to every American child from conception through age 24.

Who but a villain could argue with such a proposal? In an age of population and garbage explosions in which war is perniciously equating the two, the unapologetic affirmation of human worth, while refreshing, is far from controversial. True, a statement of unequivocal support of human rights is especially welcome in psychology with its traditionally haughty view of involvement in public affairs as debasing the coinage, but it will hardly cause a stir. That APA, long guilty of child neglect, is becoming attentive to youth, clearly merits hosannas but certainly not debate. On the surface, child advocacy seems to fall within the limbo of those vacuously idealistic, hopelessly consensually validated concepts reflexly accepted by the zeitgeist. In actuality, however, advocacy refers to

*Reprinted from The Clinical Psychologist; Summer 1970, 7-8

a radical social process which requires tremendous courage to implement and incisive examination to implement wisely. Child advocacy in action would challenge and work to change existing institutions which are inharmonious with the fullest development of the child. Implicit in the concept is recognition of the serious damage produced in children by many obsolete but entrenched social and political structures and of the necessity to oppose these structures. Without active intervention, child advocacy becomes do-gooder lip service and the envisioned Child Development Councils little more than sites for grant hustlers. Whether psychology will risk the politics of intervention is uncertain.

The application of the concept in the field of social work will illuminate the hazards ahead. It is understandable that the concept of advocacy is already exerting a strong influence on the theory and practice of social work which, unlike psychology, has a tradition of professionalism and an ideology of activism. Nevertheless, an inspection of social work journals since 1965 when advocacy was first introduced into the social work literature[2] reveals the controversial nature of the concept even in this community-oriented field. The transition in social work from "enabling" to "advocating" the client has certain parallels in the recent history of clinical psychology. Briefly, enabling as opposed to advocacy refers to the ethically neutral facilitation of the client to work through his intrapsychic problems so that he can make effective decisions for himself. Enabling is reminiscent of the traditional medical model of psychotherapy. A client's continued lack of initiative or his inability to make constructive "choices" would tend to indicate that he is insufficiently motivated or that his problems require further working through. That the choices offered by society might be limited or unsatisfactory would not be a significant consideration. In short, the goal of enabling would be the internal adjustment of the client to an external world whose institutions are tacitly assumed to be fixed, proper and rarely subject to question. Misapplications of the concept of enabling to victims of destructive environmental forces are often incredible. For example, the absence from therapy of an ADC child who literally had no shoes to walk the mile to an agency with which I was formerly affiliated was interpreted as resistance by a well-meaning psychoanalyst. The therapist of a child who unquestionably verified that her psychotic mother was battering her was reluctant to cooperate with the court in parental severance proceedings. In addition to legalistic preoccupations about violating his patient's confidence, the therapist believed that a working through of the patient's hypothesized unconscious solicitation of brutal beatings would be more helpful than "merely changing the reality situation."

Environmental manipulation is still viewed by some social workers as a last resort for the "unmotivated" client, as an elementary procedure fit only for "untrained workers." Psychiatric social work with its intrapsychic emphasis is viewed as a means of creating *genuine* changes, and until recently, had more prestige than other social work specialties. Such elitism is even more prominent in clinical psychology. Manipulating the environment implies that genuine psychotherapy is not being undertaken and is disdainfully viewed as within the province of social work, some segments of which ironically also reject this process. In short, a focus on the environment and active intervention, however constructive, are viewed as tainted with an inferior brand of professionalism. Thus, a slum youth might be encouraged to explore the intrapsychic basis for repeated questioning by the police or even exhorted to behave himself. Until very recently, consideration by a therapist from any discipline of the possibility of police harassment and certainly the therapist's intervention in behalf of the youth would have seemed incredible, a hideous example of "overinvolvement in the case."

The inappropriateness of a neutral stance and an intra-individual focus in the context of increasingly obvious social injustice and brutality is currently being emphasized, and the appropriateness of the advocacy role for the social worker is being asserted:

> The dynamism of the times has resulted in dissatisfaction with such concepts as worker neutrality or adherence to enabling as a major tenet of method. Agencies that assist the poor to participate in community activities cannot, with equanimity, proclaim their neutrality when controversial issues are engaged. The contradiction of a community agency able and willing to help residents challenge community conditions, but unable or unwilling to put itself "on the line" as well, is not lost on its constituency.[3]

The intensified commitment of the National Association of Social Workers (NASW) to the championing of otherwise powerless victims of social neglect and injustice culminated in the establishment of an Ad Hoc Committee on Advocacy within this national professional organization. This Committee's Report[4] unequivocally affirms that social workers are bound by their Code of Ethics to assume the role of advocate:

> I regard as my primary obligation the welfare of the individual or group served, which includes action for improving social conditions.[5]

In addition to espousing action to change harmful social policies and institutions, this report recommends that NASW protect and assist the social worker-advocate against reprisals by agencies and communities.

In light of these crucial considerations, can psychology stretch its ideology to include the politics of intervention? Do psychologists have the courage and conviction to deal with the consequences of child advocacy? If the envisioned Child Development Councils materialize, the psychologists will be asked to participate as consultants, planners, advisors, resource persons, coordinators; whatever the title, they will be members of that sumptuous entourage which typically counsels the staff which actually works in the neighborhood to be served.

If, as Ross implies, advocacy refers to "eliminating the wrecking influences" on children's well-being, then the psychologist-advocate will have to oppose bureaucratic logrolling, police harassment, harmful policies of archaic social agencies, violations of health and safety codes, anachronistic school systems and entrenched school boards, illegal consumer practices, slum landlords who are powerful bulwarks of the community. These are the child-wreckers! And these representatives of institutionalized corruption are tough, and they brook no interference. Will the APA assist and protect the psychologist-advocate who receives retaliatory action for practicing what the profession preaches? Unless psychology uses its expertise to change the entrenched social structures which are destroying youth, child advocacy will be nothing more than "tinkling cymbals and sounding brass," merely a sentimental non-concept.

The poet, Housman, poignantly articulates the bewildering impact of a society out of touch with the individual:

> And how am I to face the odds
> Of Man's bedevilment and God's?
> I, a stranger and afraid
> In a world I never made.[6]

Child advocacy *in vivo* means changing the odds against the powerless child by actively challenging and remaking diabolical structures within our society. It will be interesting to see whether the tough-minded profession of psychology is tough enough to risk child advocacy in action.

References

1. Ross, A. O. An advocate for children. *The Clinical Psychologist,* Winter, 1970.
2. Grosser, C. Community development programs serving the urban poor. *Social Work,* Vol. 10, July, 1965.
3. Brager, G. A. Advocacy and political behavior. *Social Work,* Vol. 13, April, 1968, 5-15.
4. Ad Hoc Committee on Advocacy. The social worker as advocate: Champion of social victims. *Social Work,* Vol. 14. April, 1969, 16-21.
5. Code of Ethics of Social Workers.
6. Housman, A. E. *Last Poems,* XII.

Part Two

THE CONCEPTUAL REVOLUTION

Nothing's staying put these days. Antiquated ideas, worn out approaches, and obsolete professional practices are falling apart. Everything that's been nailed down is coming loose. There are too many decayed planks, too many rusty nails. In this section, the bracing winds of inquiry storm through the old ideological haunts, and disconcerting poltergeists smash some hoary professional stereotypes.

6. The Sickness Model of Mental Disorder Means a Double Standard of Care*

George W. Albee

Let me begin by arguing that the explanatory *model* used to account for disturbed and deviant human behavior determines the kind of *institutions* which society supports to provide intervention, and the nature of these institutions in turn determines the *kind of manpower* required for their staffing.

The explanatory model occupying the center of the stage today insists on the fiction that "mental illness is an illness like any other." It trims the stage with institutional trappings of sickness, beds, hospitals, and clinics. As a consequence, our manpower problems are defined as shortages of medical and paramedical professionals, which include the four major actors in the drama—the psychiatrist, clinical psychologist, psychiatric social worker, and psychiatric nurse. The bit players, or extras, we are seeking in large numbers include all the ancillary paramedical professionals needed to fill the depleted ranks in our "treatment institutions."

There is an everwidening gap between the growing manpower needs of our tax-supported treatment institutions and the shrinking supply of high-level professional workers. Partly this is due to an unwillingness to forego the benefits of status agency or private practice to take underpaid jobs in public agencies serving those most in need of help. As a result there is a great deal of talk today about training a new group of nonprofessionals, or semiprofessional people, to staff the places serving primarily the numerous emotionally-distressed poor. This third-rate idea, combined with a large dose of expert public relations, has almost convinced the public that there will soon be enough intervention to go around. Many people actu-

---

*From *Behavior Disorders: Perspectives and Trends*, by Ohmer Milton and Robert G. Wahler, published by J. B. Lippincott Company, Philadelphia.

ally believe that a large number of housewives actually are being trained to be counselors, that hundreds of storefront intervention centers already exist, and that highly successful intervention is being accomplished in the new comprehensive mental health centers. Actually, this whole show is going to fold in Boston, long before it reaches the Big Time!

What is required in this field is a whole reconceptualization of causation. Once the *sickness model* is replaced with a more valid *social-learning* explanation (which attributes most emotional disturbance to the dehumanized environment rather than to biological defect) there will follow a redefinition of intervention institutions as re-educational or rehabilitative centers which will call for a very different sort of manpower.

I want to develop the argument that this reconceptualization will lead to the establishment of centers staffed primarily by people educated at the bachelors level or less, with nursing, education, and social work as strong contenders for responsiblity and leadership.

A Gloomy Forecast

One of the several major myths which we must abandon before we can make any progress in closing the manpower gap suggests that somehow, someday, we will have enough traditional mental health professionals, and therefore, the need for nonprofessional, or middle-level, mental health workers is a temporary situation. This myth leads to all sorts of inconsistent behavior in approaching the training of these people. We hesitate to change our civil service requirements. We even fear that if we train *too* many they may organize, take over, and shut us out. The latter situation may come to pass, but we should welcome it.

Actually, there is *no* chance that psychiatry and psychology, as these disciplines are now defined, will ever provide the necessary amount of manpower for effective intervention[1]. Indeed, the number of people in these precious, highly-specialized disciplines will decrease rather than increase over the next couple of decades in proportion to population.

Let us take the field of psychiatry as an example. During the past two decades, as a result of an enormous financial investment in psychiatric training by the National Institute of Mental Health, together with the massive imporatation of foreign physicians, the membership of the American Psychiatric Asssociation has quadrupled. But during this same period, *the number of psychiatrists employed in tax-supported mental institutions has declined in absolute numbers!*

Today we have some 2,000 psychiatric clinics scattered throughout our land. However, more than two-thirds of these clinics do not have a single full-time psychiatrist on their staff! Obviously something at least equal to the miracle of the loaves and fishes will be required to staff the 2,000 comprehensive community mental health centers that are to be built by NIMH in the next decade.

Nor would a crash program to increase the number of psychiatrists trained have much effect. In the first place, the long-time policy of the American Medical Association to hold down medical school enrollments has resulted in a shortage of physicians which grows steadily greater. Each year we are at least 3,000 new M.D.'s behind the number that would be required simply to hold our own in ratio of physicians to population. And psychiatry must draw most of its recruits from the same limited pool where all the other medical specialities, equally hungry for residents, are seeking their neophytes.[2]

But suppose by some magic we could double the output of our medical schools and thereby double the number of young M.D.'s going into psychiatric residencies. It would still be a hopeless situation. When we look at the *distribution* of psychiatrists we find that more than 50 percent of our nation's total are to be found in the five favored (is that the right word?) states of Massachusetts, Pennsylvania, New York, Illinois, and California. Within these states, of course, the psychiatrists are concentrated in suburbia, where 80 percent of psychiatry is practiced in private offices (with a white, middle-class, largely female, non-Catholic clientele).[2]

I will not take time to recite comparable statistics for other mental health professions except to make it quite clear that I have no hidden agenda which intends somehow to advance *psychology* in the care-delivery field. Let me tell you quite bluntly that clinical psychology is going to disappear from the marketplace for the next 10-20 years, as the relative handful of people we are able to produce is recruited into academic teaching where serious shortages are developing, and where the psychologist is not a second-class citizen but breathes the air of academic freedom. It is also worth noting that there are 20 vacant positions for every graduate of social work, and that qualified psychiatric nurses are as close to extinction as the blue whale.

Training for New or Old?

Psychiatrist Moody Bettis[3] recently raised the crucial question when he asked whether solutions to "the manpower problem" involve training people for where we are trying to go, or for where we have been! Do we want to train people for new community programs or old institutional programs? Do we want to reconsider the adequacy of many of the institutions of the past or continue to regard them as somehow sacred and above change?

Generally we think of action programs aimed at reducing emotional disturbance in our society in terms that have traditionally been associated with institutional programs. We think of highly trained mental health porfessionals—medical and paramedical—intervening on a one-to-one basis in some specific physical place (clinic or hospital) in the community. It is very difficult for us to get over our belief that the things we have been doing for so long (and so ineffectively) in our clinics and public hospitals are wrong or worthless. Many programs achieve sanctification through use, a sacred cow status which requires that they continue to be used in the community.

Perhaps the most entrenched and pervasive attitude that influences our thinking about approaches to the preparation of new mental health workers has it that they are to be employed in existing agencies and institutions. Most of the accounts I have read of new training programs relieve senior people—"under careful supervision." The implication is quite clear that many of these workers are to fit into the conventional care-delivery structures as "assistants."

Behind this assumption, of course, lurks that old devil, the *sickness model*. Without beating further what is at least a sickening horse, if not a dead one, I think it is still important to point out that our professions' adherence to the sickness explanation of disturbed behavior ("mental illness is an illness like any other") puts us into a Procrustean model which binds us to hospitals (Procrustean beds?) and clinics as our primary intervention centers.

I would emphasize that a significant component of the enthusiasm for training middle-level workers originates among those seeking a solution for the glaringly inadequate staffing of our tax-supported public facilities. These new people are sought to staff, primarily, state hospitals, county-run child centers, retardation centers, etc. A cynical way of viewing this situation would be to suggest that there will always be just enough high-class, highly-trained mental health professionals to work in psychiatric wards in general hospitals, university hospitals and clinics, and in high prestige agencies, as well as private practice. We have known for years that the shortages become more and more acute in the facilities that serve the poor—the public agencies, public clinics, and public hospitals. Recently Mike Gorman[8] pointed out that in well over a third of the state hospitals in this country, little or no psychiatric time is available. My guess is that even this is a minimum estimate.

The Role of the CCMHC

The Comprehensive Community Mental Health Centers (CCMHC) movement, originally conceived as a shining hope for the poor and described as small intensive community-based centers in the heart of our cities, where the largest number of disturbed people is to be found, has now been captured and used to increase the resources of middle-class-serving general hospitals. The regulations for CCMHC's were written in such a way that a general hospital with a psychiatric unit could qualify for construction funds if it agreed to use even 10% of the beds for the indigent, beds newly built with tax dollars. This means that in a majority of the CCMHC's now being built in general hospitals, the poor will be largely excluded.

As a matter of fact this probably also means that middle-level mental health workers will be excluded too. General hospitals are not known for their eagerness to hire salaried people whose services are not billable. Indeed, most CCMHC's get by with a very minimum of psychological and social work help.[7] The whole emphasis in the funding of the CCMHC program has been on the granting of construction funds to add beds. General hospitals make their income from the use of beds, and the fortunate few psychiatrists who control bed privileges have a good thing. Does this sound cynical? Listen to the psychiatrist-director of the Los Angeles County Department of Mental Health (Harry R. Brickman, M.D.):

> Those responsible for mental health programs must soon decide whether they wish to build a vast new social machinery which will paradoxically "create" illness under the banner of health or whether they wish to grasp a real opportunity to help build a more humanistic community which is emotionally nutritive and which is increasingly tolerant and constructively helpful to social deviation in all forms.[6]

Dr. Brickman goes on to argue that the CCMHC's must not be considered an end in themselves. Rather they should be a means toward achieving a better and more humanistic society with intervention primarily carried out "by non-psychiatric agents." There is little evidence that this will happen.

Somehow, as our society becomes more dehumanized, more consumption-oriented, and more and more inbred with the philosophy: "I'll get mine, Jack," the more we seem to need "helping" professionals. For most of the world the mental health professions are unknown or unwanted. The Peace Corps does not receive requests for psychiatrists or clinical psychologists. In societies where families, neighborhood, religious institutions, and tradition provide comfort and support, relationship therapy is unneeded or unknown. It is only as we move toward a society of strangers, highly mobile, without roots, with little tradition, and few stable relationships that we develop a market for "the purchase of friendship" (William Schofield's apt name for psychotherapy). I would not argue against the fact that there are large numbers of lonely and lost people in our society who need help. It is simply that we can never solve our human problems by trying to put these people into hospitals or clinics, by calling them patients, and by giving them individual treatment by our traditional methods.

Effective Intervention

From one perspective the most effective interventions responsible for increasing and improving the mental health of millions of citizens need not be conventionally trained mental health workers at all. If we could reach newspaper publishers, TV advertisers, and disc jockeys—who have more input than most professional organizations—we might cause really effective intervention.

Let me suggest an example of what I have in mind.

Recently two black psychiatrists, Grier and Cobbs,[9] spelled out in searing and stark detail the tragic consequences of our racist white society's behavior for the mental health of black citizens.

Millions of black children grow up in a racist white society which thoughtlessly and chauvinistically equates attractiveness in children and adults with fair straight hair and regular features. The damaged self-concepts and damaged interpersonal relationships which result for black children might be eliminated very quickly if, for example, the federal government (Federal Communications Commission) were to order that at least 20% of all commercial advertisements use black models; that all actors in television dramas be employed without regard to skin color, and that our vast communication industry be rewarded with tax credits for effective techniques it develops to transmit the message that beauty and attractiveness can take many colors and forms.

As a matter of fact I find myself continually falling into the bad habit of thinking our mental health problems involve primarily schizophrenic and other serious conventional disorders. When I stop to consider, I do *not* believe that the most significant mental health problems of our society today are to be found in the population of our state hospitals, *nor* in the clientele of our outpatient psychiatric clinics, *nor* do I believe that our most serious mental health problems are to be found in the psychiatric wards of our general hospitals.

Our most significant mental health problems exist in middle-class people who rarely end up in a clinic or mental institution. I speak of the white racists identified in the Kerner Report, and their dehumanized fellows—perhaps most of us—who accept institutions that do not strengthen people but dehumanize them. It follows that a significant number of the mental health workers that I believe must be recruited and educated will hardly be identified as such, but rather as a cadre who may provide future leadership in combatting and reducing the amount of dehumanized aggression in our society and in our world, and increasing the amount of responsible human interaction of which humans are capable. These results are available in significant numbers in our undergraduate colleges. I believe the Kerner Report is right in reporting white racism to be the major cause of social unrest in our society. I believe also that we are moving (often with maddening delays and detours), toward an integrated society in which all human beings will be able to live and love more freely. The consequences of achieving such a society, in mental health terms, will far exceed any new treatment techniques, or new psychotropic drug discoveries, or any number of new mental health workers trained as interventionists.

The morally destructive forces in our society—forces that have polluted our environment, destroyed our lakes and streams, deforested our national parks, strip-mined our hills and fields, and turned our cities into a hideous blight—the same forces that have supported meaningless wars and have poured billions down the rat hole of accelerating militarism—they are also responsible for the dehumanization of our social environment. Our society is proselytized and propagandized into thinking that wasteful, meaningless consumption is the highest end of living. We are told that human sexuality is obscene but murder, violence, and aggression are entertaining. This obscene philosophy, which negates the importance of social relationships, produces dehumanized and irrational consumers unresponsive or refractory to violence and suffering whose fragmented emotional lives lead increasing numbers to go out of control.

Then the Establishment (the military-industrial complex that President Eisenhower warned us against) proceeds to explain away the increasing social pathology as being a result of individual defect (mental illness is an illness like any other) and escapes responsibility by well—publicized support of biochemical research aimed at discovering "causes and cures."

Most Needed Mental Health Workers

While a major contribution to the problems in our society originates in white racism, a significant amount of the actual resulting damage is done to the poor and the Black. While we are trying to change the pattern of racist behavior our society must also develop interventionists to ameliorate the damage already done. These interventionists should be drawn largely from the disadvantaged groups themselves. I think they should be essentially BA-level people, and we should make urgent efforts to recruit and train special interventionists from Black and from other disadvantaged groups. It is more and more difficult to separate mental health problems from welfare problems and from educational problems. The most needed middle-level mental health workers may turn out to be specially-selected teachers.

We also need bachelors-level social welfare workers in our public agencies serving the inner-city to do something about such problems as the high rate of "mental deficiency" revealed there by epidemiological studies. Most of these cases of retardation are not due to organic factors but are due to impoverished and demoralized conditions of life. Olshansky[10] studied 1,000 children in Boston whose families were receiving Aid for Dependent Children and discovered that nearly seven percent were functionally retarded. I believe that social welfare workers and pre-school teachers and visiting nurses (all primarily Black) must be the interventionists until we can reform our cities and eliminate slums and ghettoes.

I am not convinced that we need a new generic, all-purpose, middle-level mental health worker to work in institutions. We need a number of different kinds of mental health workers, trained primarily at the bachelors level, but many of them could develop out of existing professions.

A profession is distinguished from other occupations primarily by the fact that it has *theory* which the aspiring young professional must learn before he begins practice. There is also a sense of lifetime *career choice,* together with the learning of a special language, and ultimate responsibility for the indoctrination of the neophyte. With 40-50 percent of our college age youngsters enrolled in some kind of higher education, the new mental health workers are going to have to be professionals, or we are not going to recruit them.

One problem arises immediately. Bachelors-level professionals have high status when they run their own show. They have low status when they work as assistants to other higher status professions. Look, for example, at the profession of school teaching. It is a nice respectable BA profession because teachers control the schools and have clear-cut upwardly mobile paths available. On the other hand, bachelors-level people in hospitals are far down the pecking order and are recruited only with difficulty.

I would propose that some of our existing service professions should move quickly to take over or develop their own *care delivery institutions* which they would own and operate. The profession of nursing, for example, lacks just one thing to become a major force. It does not have a *care delivery setting* which it owns and controls. Many of the individuals in institutions for the insane and many of those in institutions for the mentally deficient could be cared for much better in institutions owned and operated by the nursing profession. (so could persons with any of the other chronic organic diseases.) As soon as nursing learns that it must have a setting of its own in which to train its own neophytes, and in which upward-bound career patterns are available, I anticipate that nursing will take over and do a much more effective job for the people now cared for in our antiquated state hospital program.

Psychiatric social work is another field that is on the verge of developing an effective independent service delivery system. Social group work is already intervening more frequently and more effectively with the emotionally disturbed poor than any other profession. As soon as psychiatric social workers free themselves from the psychiatric setting and establish their own crisis intervention centers that blend mental health and welfare programs, and that recruit staff from the inner-city people served—or better still as soon as they go to work with group workers in settlement houses located close to where the people are who need help—the sooner good care will be available. In truth, social work is doing most of the psychiatric care in the so-called mental hygiene clinics today. How long will it sit still and see the clinics directed by persons who give a few hours a week and take home high salaries for this limited service to the wrong target groups?

Clergy, Police and Students

In ranging over some of the current literature on mental health training for new groups of professional workers we frequently encounter mental health training for the clergy. Certainly it is true, as we discovered in William Ryan's survey of Boston's mental health services, that the clergy actually provide more counseling and psychotherapy within the American city than do the more traditional mental health professions. (Ryan[11] found that in Boston clergymen were doing more counseling than psychiatrists despite the fact that greater Boston is practically overrun with psychiatrists.) Mental health training for clergymen has usually come to mean training in psycho-dynamics and individual one-to-one intervention. But because most of the important, well-funded and heavily-supported churches and synagogues have moved to suburbia with the rest of the middle-class population, the one-to-one counseling of clergymen tends to be largely limited to middle-class parishioners. In talking with clergymen in my own neighborhood I discover that their counseling is most frequently with people with "drinking problems" and with families trying to cope with pregnant unmarried teenagers.

These clergymen could provide far more significant mental health intervention by leading their congregations toward a firm stand on fair housing and neighborhood integration, perhaps with an emphasis that prejudice and discrimination are grounds for excommunication from the church. This sort of "intervention" will require some significant break-throughs in religious dogma!

Let me cite another existing profession that, with a little change, might become more relevant.

This potential source of new and effective mental health professional workers is the police. I would suggest that we find ways to recruit to the uban police forces some of the same brave and socially motivated young people now attracted to the Peace Corps or the VISTA program. Most police forces are having trouble finding qualified recruits. Instead of such nonconstructive activities as many of our young people have engaged in viz-a-viz the police, why not find ways to help them volunteer to spend a few years on the police force trying to help teach the principles of democracy and respect for individual human dignity in this setting?

While on the subject of the police, why not use what we know about operants and reinforcement theory to single out those policemen who exhibit human relations skills? Policemen who complete training in human relations courses could be given a salary increment and a further increment or bonus each time they demonstrate that they practice behaviorally what they have learned.

Still another innovative source of people for intervention is the pool of high school students who could be spending time in the elementary school or even in kindergarten classes. In a few pilot projects around the country high school students are spending as much as one day a week working with one, two, or three children in a kindergarten or elementary school in their own district. High school boys, particularly, may be led to discover and experience the universal satisfaction to be derived from a consistent helping relationship with a young child. High school girls, too, may find new skills and satisfactions not available in conventional courses.

Under appropriate reinforcement conditions, high school boys and girls can not only help younger children to learn but can also serve (self-consciously) as role models. I find no convincing reason why a country that is able to spend $80 million a day in Southeast Asia cannot find a way to pay high school students to work with younger students.

Close State Mental Hospitals

We cannot limit our attention, either, to the pathology of our society and to preventive efforts without paying *some* attention to the unfortunate who have been damaged or destroyed by our system and who now sit out their empty lives in our "state institutions." What is to be done, and who is to do it? Obviously not the present Big Four mental health professions.

Two years ago[1] I suggested that our state hospitals and mental hygiene clinics should be closed and torn down—taken apart piece by piece and stone by stone and then, like the city of Carthage, plowed three feet under and sowed with salt. This proposal was widely reported by the press, and as a consequence I received many letters, some highly supportive and some highly critical. A number of writers were psychiatrists. Some of them were angry because my suggestion would eliminate their jobs in state hospitals, while others were angry (although they themselves were in private practice and knew relatively little about the state hospitals system) because it was inappropriate for a psychologist to butt into what was essentially a medical problem.

I continue to think the state hospitals should be abandoned, and I cite as supporting participants in this movement two recent presidents of the American Psychiatric Association, Harry C. Solomon[12] and Daniel Blain[5] both of whom suggested in their presidential addresses to their Association that the state hospitals are obsolete and should be eliminated.

The important point is that the state hospitals have come to be a dumping ground for the emotionally disturbed poor, for those who don't have Blue Cross Insurance or some kind of labor union coverage to pay for occupancy of a bed in a general hospital psychiatric ward.

Why bring up this whole matter of state hospitals and the double standard of care? Because much of the demand for the new mental health workers results from the need for such people to work in the state hospitals where medical and paramedical professionals refuse to work. State hospitals and clinics are tax-supported and that makes them socialized medicine and we all know how bad that is! So let's train a host of nonprofessionals to work in these places where we will dump the uninsured poor. Thus, we neatly separate our free-enterprise medical intervention with the affluent from our salaried subprofessional services for the poor. Training a corps of subprofessionals to staff the state hospitals would serve to prolong the existence of these antiquated institutions, and perpetuate the double standard of care. One way of blocking this neat but chauvinistic solution would be to close the state hospitals, thereby forcing the community, with good planning, into more effective nonmedical programs which might indeed be under the control of BA-level professional workers.

If the state hospitals are eliminated, what would happen to all of the present unfortunate inmates, and to those first admission cases who now wind up in the state hospital? It is instructive to look carefully at the poor people in these places now, and those entering them for the first time.

First of all, there is evidence that the unfortunate state hospital inmates are afflicted more by the desocialization that comes from the training these places give them in the role of inmate, than from any real disease process. What has happened for years to people in state hospitals is an almost perfect example of *the self-fulfilling prophecy.* When we admit them we predict that their condition is hopeless, and then we proceed to take away every vestige of humanity, self-respect, and pride, thus creating cases without hope. Then we congratulate ourselves that our original predictions were right.

We know now that at least half the first admissions really do not belong in a "mental hospital." Let me just cite the results of a recent study done by Moody C. Bettis and Robert E. Roberts of the Texas Research Institute of Mental Sciences.[4] Drs. Bettis and Roberts did a systematic study of more than 500 "proposed mentally ill patients" referred to an evaluation center for possible commitment. These people were studied for as much as a week at the center after which they were sent to a local state hospital or discharged back to the community. These scientists found that considerably more than half did *not* need mental hospital commitment, or would *not have* if community services had been available. It turns out that only about one-third of the pre-commitment group should have been put in a mental hospital if *their* need had been the major consideration. As it turns out, three-quarters of the group studied were actually committed to the state hospital, because no other solution was available. In a related study the same group of investigators found a significantly large number of persons trapped in the state hospital system who clearly did not belong there but for whom no appropriate intervention was available in the community.

If we were to close the state hospitals, what would happen to the people who presently are entering through their front door?

It is instructive to look at the nature of our first admission group in the state hospitals across the country. As indicated above, the majority of them should not ever be admitted to a state hospital. Half the first admissions are nonpsychotic but represent a mixed group of alcoholics, character disorders, neurotics, and lonely people who might be better dealt with in the community.

Of the remaining 50 percent who are admitted for the first time to state hospitals with the diagnosis of psychosis, half of them are diagnosed "chronic brain syndrome" which means that they are primarily elderly senile individuals who certainly do not deserve the horrible fate of being locked up in a state hospital. Again, better ways of dealing with elderly senile cases can be developed in the community, and in the case of those who require intensive care, general hospitals or nursing homes offer better solutions.

The remaining 25 percent of first admissions are functionally psychotic. But clearly a significant number of these could be dealt with in foster homes, half-way houses, day or night facilities, and with effective means of community support.

Ordinarily we tell legislators that we need our state hospitals for persons who are "dangerous to themselves or others." But when we look at our first admissions we find that the proportion that is dangerous is a very small number indeed.

We should develop small, tax-supported, comprehensive community mental health centers in the heart of the urban blight. But these centers cannot be medical or paramedical. They may take several forms—some owned and operated by nursing, some by social work, some by special education, and some by new child care professions. Most of the staff should be drawn from the same disadvantaged groups served. The rest of us should be working to bring about the social revolution we need to arrest our nation's pell-mell rush toward diaster.

References

1. Albee, G. W. 1968. Myths, models, and manpower. *Mental Hygiene*, 52, 2, April.
2. Albee, G. W. 1967. The relation of conceptual models to manpower needs. In: Cowen, E. L., Gardner, E. A., and Zax, M. (eds.): *Emergent Approaches to Mental Problems*. New York, Appleton-Century-Crofts, 63-73.
3. Bettis, Moody 1969. Personal Communication.
4. Bettis, Moody C. and Roberts, Robert E. 1969. Mental health manpower—the dilemma. *Mental Hygiene*. In Press.
5. Blain, Daniel 1965. Presidential Address. *American Journal of Psychiatry*.
6. Brickman, Harry R. 1967. Community mental health—means or end? *Psychiatric Digest*, 28, 43-50.
7. Glasscote, R., et al.: 1964. The community mental health center. An analysis of existing models. Washington, D.C., The Joint Information Service of the American Psychiatric Association and the National Association for Mental Health.
8. Gorman, Mike 1966. What are the facts about mental illness in the United States. National Committee Against Mental Illness. 66 pp. Pamphlet.
9. Grier, William H. and Cobbs, Price M. 1968. *Black Rage*. New York: Basic Books.
10. Olshansky, S. and Sternfield, L. A. 1963. A study of suspected cases of mental retardation in families receiving aid to dependent children. *American Journal of Public Health*, 53, 793.
11. Ryan, W.: 1969. *Distress in the City: A Summary Report of the Boston Mental Health Survey*. Cleveland: Case Western Reserve University Press.
12. Solomon, Harry 1958. Presidential Address to American Psychiatric Association. *American Journal of Psychiatry*.

7. A Clinical Child Psychologist "Examines" Retarded Children*

Alan O. Ross

My approach to retarded children is that of a *behaviorally* oriented *clinical child psychologist,* and each of these words has important implications for how I shall proceed. Let me elucidate each of these words—behavioral, clinical, child, and psychologist—so as to establish the boundaries of my discussion.

It is my contention that, for the psychologist, the proper study of mankind is man's *behavior.* I prefer to focus on phenomena I can observe, such as the responses a child makes, rather than worrying about inferred "mental" entities. With this orientation I am not even comfortable with the term "mental retardation" and would prefer Bijou's (1966) "developmental retardation" were it not for the semantic convention that makes the traditional phrase more readily communicative.

The adjective, *clinical,* is stressed in order to indicate that for purposes of this discussion, my interest is in the individual child and in how to help him. I am not interested in studying groups of children for the sake of finding some fictitious measure of central tendency, nor am I here concerned with establishing antecedents of maladaptive behavior in order to prevent its development in future children. I do not, for a moment, wish to disparage efforts at prevention but I maintain that the search for preventive measures requires a different approach from that appropriate to attempts at helping an individual casualty. Where these approaches are confounded, neither prevention nor treatment are optimally served.

The word *'child'* in clinical child psychology should tell you that I intend to discuss children as customarily defined. In addition, the word 'child' means to me that any study or discussion of phenomena related to children must have a developmental orientation. Hence I

---

*This paper was presented at a workshop on Research for the Educable Mentally Retarded, held at Harrisburg, Pennsylvania, May, 1970

look at mental retardation in developmental terms; not in some static sense that speaks of defect or inherent difference (Zigler, 1969).

Lastly, the implication of the term *psychologist* is that the questions I ask are questions relevant to psychology as the science of human behavior. There are many legitimate and important questions about mental retardation, only some of which fall into the purview of the psychologist's competence. For this reason many disciplines must cooperate in research and many professions must participate in treatment. When the psychologist asks questions the biochemist, the neurophysiologist, or the geneticist is best equipped to answer or, conversely, if the pediatrician, orthopedist, or psychiatrist tries to apply procedures which the psychologist is best trained to use, only confusion can result and the retarded child is the loser.

Diagnosis for What?

So much for my biases. Now I shall consider the kind of questions that I think a clinical child psychologist should ask when he is faced with a child whose adaptive behavior is impaired. Note that I do not say "a mentally retarded child" or "an autistic child." I say "a child whose adaptive behavior is impaired" because the questions to be asked are the same regardless of the chapter heading under which a given child's problems might be described in a textbook of abnormal psychology.

The questions to be asked are not "how shall I label this child?" nor are they "what caused his problem?" or "how did he get this way?" Instead, we must ask "where are we now?" "where do we go from here?" and "how do we get there?" In order to answer these questions, the psychologist must engage in a detailed and painstaking assessment of the child's *current* behavior and the conditions under which this behavior now occurs.

Such an assessment must look at three interrelated factors: the child's present response capabilities; the stimuli in his environment that are currently effective; and the reinforcers, both positive and negative, that are currently capable of maintaining his behavior. The assessment of the child's present response capabilities and behavioral repertoire should determine what responses he has learned up to this point and what responses he is capable of making. Tests of intelligence as traditionally used tend to focus on the available response repertoire in the circumscribed realm we deem relevant to "intelligence." The scores tell us a little about how much the child can do, but they do not tell us what the child might be able to do, and they totally hide the things he cannot do and what keeps him from doing them. As Bijou (1966) has so ably stated, responses "may be disadvantageously affected by impairments of the responding and coordinating systems of the individual. A physically impaired child cannot perform tasks involving response components which he cannot possibly execute . . . If he cannot physically perform a task, no amount of stimulation, exposure, or training will enable him to do so [p. 7]."

The assessment of currently effective stimuli not only ascertains the extent to which the child's sensory receptors are functioning, but also the extent to which his behavior has come under the control of available environmental stimuli. Not only must we find out whether the child can hear, but also whether he has learned to make the appropriate response to the verbal stimulus "please sit down."

The question about currently effective reinforcers must be answered before one can hope to modify the child's behavior by either teaching him new responses or by changing established patterns. Neither praise nor scolding, nor, for that matter, M & M candies are effective with all children all of the time. Hence we must find out for each individual child just which consequences do or can maintain his behavior.

The assessment, or functional analysis of behavior, so necessary for effective intervention, is unfortunately handicapped by an almost total lack of available tests that might permit a relatively quick cross-sectional survey. To date, the best approach is direct observation of actual behavior. Highly objective methods for such observations have been developed (e.g., Wahler, 1969) but since these require separate analysis for each behavior under study, they tend to be exceedingly time-consuming. At Stony Brook, we are currently developing survey techniques that should permit a clinician to arrive at an inventory of maladaptive behaviors and potent reinforcers in a relatively short time. What we need are instruments that will do for the behaviorally-oriented clinician what projective techniques presumably did for the psychodynamic therapist. If we are successful in our attempts, the questions a psychologist must ask about maladaptive behavior can be answered more quickly.

No matter how the answers to these questions are obtained they will tell the psychologist and hence the educator a great deal about what to do for a child in order to help him develop his behavior in a more adaptive direction. The answers are guides to action, not ways of classifying the child or ascertaining the etiology of his problem. Whether the result of a functional analysis of behavior represents a diagnosis depends on which dictionary definition one selects. If diagnosis means "analysis of the nature of a problem," or "a statement concerning the nature of a phenomenon," then a functional analysis leads to a diagnosis. If diagnosis means "the act of identifying a disease from its signs and symptoms," the far more common definition, then one had better not speak of diagnosis. My personal preference is to avoid that term because of its medical, disease-oriented connotations.

I have elsewhere (Ross, 1968) tabbed as the *Rumpelstiltskin Fixation* that preoccupation of psychologists with whether a given mentally retarded child is or is not brain-damaged. That question and related questions of etiology and classification often preoccupy psychological evaluations and staff conferences as if everything depended on that one answer. In the well-known fairy tale the chance for the princess to live her life happily ever after depends on her discovering the name of an ill-tempered dwarf. As a result she goes to great lengths to learn his name, and, upon doing so, earns her salvation. Many clinicians and educators seem to engage in similar fairy tale behavior. They act as if, could they but give the condition a name, the child would be saved. Hence: mild, moderate, severe, profound; cretin, idiot, imbecile, moron; retarded, subnormal, deficient, feebleminded; trainable, educable, exogenous, endogenous; familial, organic, genetic, brain-injured; neurotic, autistic, psychotic, symbiotic; not to mention garden variety and emotionally disturbed. These are but some of the names that have been tried on the dwarf—but he still has not disappeared. I would urge that psychology and education do away with these labels. We must rid ourselves at long last of the mistaken notion that one of our tasks is "identifying a disease from its signs and symptoms." We should instead get on with our job of training, teaching, and rehabilitating the children who have a limited behavioral repertoire and thus cannot cope successfully with aspects of their environment. The interrelated reasons they came to have this limited repertoire need not be our concern.

If we know that a six-year-old child cannot dress himself, does not use the toilet, speaks in monosyllables, hits out at other children, and will not remain in his seat, we know the areas where he needs help and we should get on with that job without wasting time trying to "explain" his condition by calling him a brain-injured, moderately retarded, aggressive child with an I.Q. of 42. Such a label not only provides no explanation; it, like all other labels used to date, tells us nothing about the steps we must take to help him learn bowel control and the other behaviors he needs in order to gain better adaptation to his environment.

The *Rumpelstiltskin Fixation* derives from the disease model which makes one look at maladaptive behavior as if it were the symptom of an underlying disease. Reasoning by analogy from physical illness, a low score on an intelligence test and hyperactive behavior come to be viewed like raised temperature and abdominal pain. This analogy then leads one to seek a disease in the mentally retarded child, and some clinicians seem to find comfort once they think they have diagnosed brain damage. We have come to question the disease model in the area of the so-called emotional disorders. It is good to know that some of the leading people in the area of mental retardation have also come to question the disease analogy, and the resulting preoccupation with etiology. As Gallagher (1957) so aptly pointed out, the educator who wants to help the individual child gains far more information from the fact that he is not responding appropriately to perceptual stimuli than from the fact that he is brain-injured.

More recently, Robinson and Robinson (1965) in their excellent text, *The Mentally Retarded Child,* pointed out that

> "Indicating the mere presence or absence of brain injury on the basis of psychological evaluation is usually limited in usefulness. Insofar as neurologic diagnosis and medical treatment are concerned it is the physician who is responsible. On the other hand, the psychologist is often best equipped to appraise the assets and liabilities and the unique behavioral patterns of the child who is to be helped. If perceptual difficulties are present, as they often are, their extent and nature need clarification. Intellectual ability, capacity for expressing ideas, ability to attend to tasks, and skill in understanding and in using abstract concepts all can be explored with the use of psychological tools [p. 246]."

To this one might add that the psychologist is uniquely prepared to determine and describe the approaches that must be used in order to help the child maximize his potential, provided he views assessment of the child's present condition as a starting point for training and teaching and not as the basis for speculations about etiology and labels.

Etiology is Irrelevant

So much for unsupported assertions of opinion that can be refuted by anyone with louder voice or sharper pen. I shall now offer some support for these opinions by citing research that has become available during the past few years. Some of this research was stimulated by the conceptual reorientation I have tried to outline. Thus, Herbert Birch and his colleagues (Birch, Belmont, Belmont, & Taft, 1967) sampled all educable mentally retarded children aged 8, 9, and 10 living in the city of Aberdeen, Scotland, administered the WISC, and compared the test pattern with independent evidence of central nervous system damage. Finding no association, they concluded that the existing psychometric evidence does not support the view that educable, mentally subnormal children can be designated "brain damaged," "garden variety," or "non-brain-damaged." They suggest that either the WISC is insensitive to these etiologic niceties or that all of the children examined had brain defects. The third possible explanation, that all of these children have had similar reinforcement histories so that their test behavior is similar, was apparently not considered. Regardless of which explanation is correct, it would not appear very productive to aim one's assessment efforts at establishing etiologic classification using the Wechsler scale.

A research effort undertaken from a more traditional point of view, thus making the negative results particularly significant, was the mammoth, seven-year-long Ability Structure Project directed by Johs Clausen (1966). Among the ambitious aims of this project was "To differentiate the mentally retarded into subgroups which are psychologically and behaviorally more homogeneous than those provided by current classification systems [p. 4]," and to relate the factors underlying these subgroupings "to etiology as presumed from medical and family history [p. 5]." In addition, Clausen proposed "To provide the raw materials which may make possible the development of new diagnostic tools and to provide new ways of combining results of existing tests to achieve maximum diagnostic power [p. 5]." The traditional orientation toward classificatory grouping, diagnosis, and the importance of etiology is apparent in these explicit aims.

The project used 388 children from six institutions who were tested on 33 tasks ranging from psychophysical measures, such as two-point threshold and brightness discrimination, to such intelligence tests as the Porteus Mazes and Thurstone's Test of Primary Mental Abilities. On the basis of their histories and medical records the children were classified into groups of familials, organics, mixed, mongoloids, unexplained, and not classifiable. All were given a neurological examination and an EEG. The data were then subjected to analysis of variance, correlational analysis, traditional factor analysis, inverse factor analysis, and a syndrome analysis. The published report on the project covers more than 200 pages.

In terms of its aims, the results of this massive effort were singularly disappointing. The relevant conclusions are summarized as follows: "The differentiation of the mentally retarded into subgroups . . . has not been particularly successful. The outline of some broad groups has been presented, but well defined, specific groups have not been encountered [p. 172]." "The finding of relationship between configuration of abilities and extent of central nervous system damage . . . has been only moderately successful [p. 173].""With limited success in defining homogeneous subgroups, the attempts to demonstrate relatonships between these groups and traditional etiological groups have not been very productive," and "It can hardly be said that new diagnostic tools have been developed . . . [p. 173]."

The results—or lack of results—of this ambitious project would seem to lend support to the contention that attempts to group mental retardates either in terms of ability or in terms of etiology are misdirected and unproductive. No currently available psychological test can differentiate among the traditional etiologic groupings, and new groupings do not emerge from sophisticated statistical analyses. Not even the much-used dichotomy of organic and familial held up in Clausen's study, leading him to conclude that "It is possible that mild organic impairment is of similar nature to the functional impairment of incomplete development which occurs in the familial retardate. The consequences of this would be that the etiological distinction into familials and organics, at least of the milder cases, has limited significance, as it does not reflect behavioral differences (p. 165f)." Could it be that children whose adaptive behavior is impaired (whatever the original reason) encounter such similar environmental experiences that the response repertoire they acquire makes them, as a group, more similar than different by the time they are tested at age 8, as was the case in the Clausen study?

Following this line of thought, it is perhaps significant that the key variables in Clausen's test battery that did differentiate the retarded from the normal subjects were pure tone threshold and such simple motor tasks as lower-arm movement and reaction time. Approaching these differences from the standpoint that leads investigators to search for a basic deficit common to all retardates, Clausen views his subjects' difficulties on these tests as reflecting impairment of such general factors as arousal, vigilance, effort, and response initiation.Neurologizing to yet a third level of inference, he then implicates the Ascending Reticular Activating System in the brain stem.

A far more parsimonious explanation for these children's lower performance on tasks requiring sustained attention (as does pure tone discrimination) and response initiation (as do the simple motor tasks) is offered by Zigler (1966) who suggests that such performance deficits reflect the children's learned "outer-directed response style."

According to Zigler (1966), this outer-directed style of problem solving is acquired in the oft-repeated situation where the child is selectively reinforced for careful attentiveness to external cues. When, on the other hand, he bases a response on his own meager cognitive resources, he almost invariably encounters negative consequences. He thus comes to acquire an overreliance on external cues, an outer-directness, as Zigler would have it. As this outer-directedness generalizes, the child would come to attend in rapid succession to a wide variety of stimuli. His behavior would then be characterized as "distractible," a characteristic that has often been attributed to the retarded child and has, in fact, been viewed by some as an inherent characteristic—a basic deficit—of the retarded.

While this learned behavioral characteristic tends to interfere with the problem-solving ability of retarded children because they attend to misleading and distracting cues (Achenbach & Zigler, 1968). Turnure and Zigler (1964) have shown that retarded children's problem solving can be enhanced when extraneous stimuli are task-relevant or if, as Zeaman and House (1963) have pointed out, these stimuli increase attention by introducing the collative variable of novelty.

From the point of view of assessment preparatory to training and teaching, an important behavioral dimension to investigate is, as these studies suggest, the child's ability to attend to a given stimulus or, conversely, his tendency to respond to extraneous, distracting, irrelevant stimuli. If distractibility or outer-directedness is a learned behavior, it should be possible to reduce this response tendency and to teach attentive behavior.

Intelligence Level is Unimportant

The research evidence mentioned so far supports the contention that the classification of the retarded in terms of presumed etiologies is neither feasible, using present-day psychological tools, nor necessary in terms of educational planning. As Birch et al. (1967) pointed out, the etiologic designation of brain damage does not lead to a clearly defined educational strategy so that "an evaluation of the individual educational capacities and incapacities of a child is more useful as the basis for a program of training (p. 256) "than knowing whether a child should be called brain-damaged, familial, mixed, or what-have-you.

Not only does it seem irrelevant to know the etiology of a child's maladaptive behavior, it also appears unnecessary to be too concerned with classification into intellectual catergories, that is by I.Q. test scores. Support for this statement can be found in the rapidly growing literature that shows that the basic principles of learning operate at all levels of intelligence.

From the point of view of the applicability of learning principles, there are no inherent differences between the normal and the retarded, regardless of degree of retardation. Certainly, genetic and physiologic conditions set limits on the ultimate response repertoire and the speed of acquisition, but learning can take place and does take place according to the same principles whether the learner be profoundly or mildly retarded.* As Ullman and Krasner (1969) have stated, not even the most severe defect rules out responses to the environment and alteration of behavior through training. From this point of view it makes no sense to differentiate between the trainable and the educable, a pseudoclassification which, we must remind ourselves, is simply another arbitrary cut-off on the continuum of intelligence test scores; it is no more valid than the discarded idiot, imbecile, moron trichotomy.

A demonstration of the applicability of principles of learning at even the profoundest level of retardation can be found in the work of Bailey and Meyerson (1969). These investigators worked with a 7-year-old boy who "was blind, at least partially deaf, had no speech or language, was not toilet trained, could not feed himself, and could not walk (p. 135)." Virtually his entire waking hours were taken up with such sterotyped behaviors as slapping his face, hitting himself on the chin, ears, and side of the head, sucking on his fingers or whole hand, and banging his head, teeth, or a foot against the bars of his crib. Having installed a leather-padded lever on the side of the boy's crib, Bailey and Meyerson recorded the frequency of lever pressing during a seven-day baseline period and found a mean of 135 responses per 24-hour day. Following this baseline period, vibration, produced by an apparatus mounted on the underside of the

---

*Kingsley (1968), for example, demonstrated that on an associative learning task a group of educable mentally retarded children performed in a qualitatively similar manner as other ability groups, while Morgan (1969) showed that there is no difference in responsiveness to stimulus complexity at different levels of intelligence.

crib, was made contingent on lever pressing, such that each lever press produced 6 seconds of vibration. During the 21 days when this condition obtained, the mean number of lever presses was more than 1000, ranging from 700 to 2000 per day. The responses were maintained on a steady rate for three weeks without decrement. When the vibration condition was discontinued, there was a striking decrease in lever pressing, with a drop to an average of 400 presses per day during the first week of this extinction phase.

When he was working the lever, the boy was observed "to press the lever lightly with his hand or kick it with his foot and then remain motionless or occasionally giggle while the vibrator was on. He would then press the lever again as soon as the vibration stopped (p. 137)." The data, together with this observation, indicate that this profoundly retarded boy had learned something and that the vibration was an effective reinforcer for lever pressing. While these authors do not report the relationship of the lever-pressing behavior to the self-stimulatory, injurious, stereotyped behavior the boy had displayed, it is possible that such behavior decreased while lever-pressing was emitted at a high rate. Furthermore, as Bailey and Meyerson point out, "a simple behavior generated with vibratory reinforcement might be considered a first approximation to enlarging a child's repertoire to include more complex and useful forms of behavior (p. 137)."

Operant behavior modification technique has been applied with other retarded children to establish toilet training and such basic self-help skills as feeding and dressing. Giles and Wolf (1966), for example, strengthened appropriate use of the toilet by five institutionalized, severely retarded males through the use of positive reinforcers. This study points to the importance of finding suitable reinforcers for each child. While candy is an effective reinforcer for many children, Giles and Wolf found one boy who refused candy but accepted baby food; for others a ride in a wheelchair, taking a shower, or being permitted to return to bed were rewarding consequences. Giles and Wolf also point out that training can be improved if, in addition to the positive reinforcement of desired responses, inappropriate behavior is followed by aversive stimuli. Where positive reinforcement alone produced no results, they introduced physical restraint, the removal of which, contingent on appropriate toileting behavior, came to serve as a negative reinforcer. With this combination of techniques, all subjects learned consistently to eliminate in the toilet.

Roos and Oliver (1969) studied the effectiveness of operant conditioning procedures using two control groups one of which, a placebo group, received more traditional special education training while the other received traditional institutional care. The results showed that the severely and profoundly retarded children in the experimental group made significantly greater progress in developing self-help skills than the two other groups. Beyond learning simple self-care skills, retarded children with I.Q. test scores as low as 30 have acquired appropriate classroom behavior (Birnbrauer, 1967), social skills (Baldwin, 1967), and academic subject matter (Birnbrauer, Bijou, Wolf, and Kidder, 1965).

The reason for referrring to these studies is not to stress the effectiveness of operant procedures but to emphasize that the same principles of learning apply regardless of the degree of a child's retardation and that establishing this degree in terms of test scores becomes a very secondary matter, more useful for administrative-damaged, familial, culturally deprived, schizophrenic, emotionally disturbed, or—normal. Studies supporting this point are too numerous to list and I have summarized them at length elsewhere (Ross, 1972). Suffice it to mention that the same operant principles that Giles and Wolf (1966) used with severe retardates were used by Wolf, Risley, and Mees (1964) to help an autistic child, are applied by Lovaas in teaching speech to schizophrenic children (Lovaas, Berberich, Perloff, and Schaeffer, 1966), have found application with a hyperactive, brain-damaged child (Patterson, 1965), are used to control problem behaviors in the home (Hawkins, Peterson, Schweid, and Bijou, 1966), have helped a culturally-deprived child to acquire reading skills (Staats & Butterfield, 1965), and are used every time a consistent mother tells her child, "Eat your beans; then you'll get your dessert."

Since the consequences of a response are powerful factors in determining whether this response will be weakened or strengthened, those who wish to modify the behavior of retarded children— or of any children for that matter, must, as we have said, first assess what conditions can serve as reinforcers. We are again indebted to Zigler (1966) for pointing to the differential effectiveness of reinforcers when retarded, and particularly institutionalized retarded, are compared with normal children. This difference can account for many of the performance deficits of retarded children. Zigler and deLabry (1962) showed that when the consequences of success on a concept-switching task were tangible reinforcers, the difference in performance between normal, lower-class children and retarded children disappeared. That is to say, when an effective reinforcer is introduced, the frequency of adaptive responses increases, bearing out the contention that it is at least as important to assess what constitutes an effective reinforcer for a given child as to count how many correct responses he can give on an intelligence test or, for that matter, what kind of a pattern his EEG tracing makes on a piece of paper.

Again, the stress must be on assessing the individual child. It would be folly to group all retarded children into one class and to assume, on the basis of the study just cited, that they will all do better under conditions of tangible reinforcement. A recent study by Byck (1968) is relevant here. He compared mongoloid children with familial retardates using a concept-switching task and found the mongoloids performing far worse than the familials, but this difference disappeared when the mongoloids were reinforced with affection and the familials with tangible objects.

Conclusion

Before closing, I wish to stress two points that might have been misunderstood. Knowing that a great variety of children, from the retarded to the delinquent, can be helped toward more adaptive behavior by the application of learning principles in no way permits us to draw conclusions as to how these children came to acquire their maladaptive or deficient behavior. Etiologic facts remain to be uncovered. *Post hoc, ergo propter hoc* reasoning is as fallacious here as elsewhere. The other point is related. Simply because available tests fail to differentiate between various groups of retarded children and simply because they can all be helped by the same basic techniques does not mean that these children are all alike. There are most probably differences in etiology and certainly differences in the degree of deficit. The point is that knowledge of these differences is unimportant from the point of view of training, teaching, and treatment. I have not said that the mongoloid and the culturally disadvantaged child are alike in any way other than they are both children.

To sum up: What mentally retarded children and, for that matter, all children with problems of maladaptive behavior need from psychology is not diagnosis and classification but the imaginative and bold application of known principles of behavior. The question is not "What should this child be called and how did he get this way?" but "What must he learn and how do we teach him?"

References

Achenbach, and Zigler, Cue-learning and problem-learning strategies in normal and retarded children. *Child Development*, 1968, *39*, 827-848.

Bailey, J., and Meyerson, L. Vibration as a reinforcer with a profoundly retarded child. *Journal of Applied Behavior Analysis*, 1969, *2*, 135-137.

Baldwin, V. L. Development of social skills in retardates as a function of three types of reinforcement programs. *Dissertation abstracts*, 1967, *27*, (9-A), 2865.

Bijou, S. W. A functional analysis of retarded behavior. In N. R. Ellis (Ed.) *International Review of Research in Mental Retardation*, Vol. 1. New York: Academic Press, 1966, 1-19.

Birch, H. G., Belmont, L., Belmont, I., and Taft, L. T. Brain damage and intelligence in educable mentally subnormal children. *Journal of Nervous & Mental Disease*, 1967, *144*, 247-257.

Birnbrauer, J. S. Preparing 'uncontrolable' retarded children for group instruction. Paper read at American Educational Research Association Convention, 1967.

Birnbrauer, J. S., Bijou, S. W. Wolf, M. M., & Kidder, J. D. Programmed instruction in the classroom. In Ullmann, L. P. , & Krasner, L. (Eds.) *Case studies in behavior modification*. New York: Holt, Rinehart & Winston, 1965.

Byck, M. Cognitive differences among diagnostic groups of retardates. *American Journal of Mental Deficiency*, 1968, 73, 97-101.

Clausen, J. *Ability structure and subgroups in mental retardation*. New York: Spartan Books, 1966.

Gallagher, J. J. A comparison of brain-injured and non-brain-injured children on several psychological variables. Monographs of the *Society for Research in Child Development*, 1957, *22*, #2.

Giles, D. K., & Wolf, M. M. Toilet training institutionalized severe retardates: An application of operant behavior modification techniques. *American Journal of Mental Deficiency, 1966, 70*, 766-780

Hawkins, R. P., Peterson, R.F., Schweid, E., & Bijou, S.W. Behavior therapy in the home: amelioration of problem parent-child relations with the parent in a therapeutic role. *Journal of Experimental Child Psychology*, 1966, *4*, 99-107.

Kingsley, R. F. Associative learning ability in educable mentally retarded children. *American Journal of Mental Deficiency*, 1968, *73*, 5-8.

Lovaas, O. I., Berberich, J. P.,Perloff, B. F., and Schaeffer, B. Acquisition of imitative speech by schizophrenic children. *Science*, 1966, *151*, 705-707.

Morgan, S. B. Responsiveness to stimulus novelty and complexity in mild, moderate and severe retardates. *American Journal of Mental Deficiency*, 1969, *74*, 32-38.

Patterson, G. R. An application of conditioning techniques to the control of a hyperactive child. In L. P. Ullmann and L. Krasner (Eds.), *Case studies in behavior modification.* New York: Holt, Rinehart & Winston, 1965.

Robinson, H. B., & Robinson, N. M. *The mentally retarded child: A psychological approach.* New York: McGraw-Hill, 1965.

Roos, P., & Oliver, M. Evaluation of operant conditioning with institutionalized retarded children. *American Journal of Mental Deficiency,* 1969, *74,* 325-330.

Ross, A. O. Conceptual issues in the evaluation of brain damage. In J. L. Khanna (Ed.), *Brain damage and mental retardation: A psychological evaluation.* Springfield, Ill.: Thomas, 1968.

Ross, A. O. Behavior therapy. In B. B. Wolman (Ed.) *Manual of child psychopathology.* New York: McGraw-Hill, 1972.

Staats, A. W., & Butterfield, W. H. Treatment of nonreading in a culturally deprived juvenile delinquent: An application of reinforcement principles. *Child Development,* 1965, *36,* 925-942.

Turnure, J., & Zigler, E. Outer-directedness in the problem solving of normal and retarded children. *Journal of Abnormal and Social Psychology,* 1964, *69,* 427-436.

Ullmann, L. P., & Krasner, L. *A psychological approach to abnormal behavior.* Englewood Cliffs, N. J.: Prentice-Hall, 1969.

Wahler, R. G. Oppositional children: A quest for parental reinforcement control. *Journal of Applied Behavior Analysis,* 1969, *2,* 159-170.

Zigler, E., & deLabry, T. Concept-switching in middle-class lower-class, ing procedures to the behaviour problems of an autistic child. *Behaviour Research and Therapy,* 1964, *1,* 305-312.

Zeaman, D., & Houx, B. J. In N. R. Ellis (Ed.) *Handbook of Mental Deficiency,* New York: McGraw Hill, 1963, 159-223.

Zigler, E. Research on personality structure of the retardate. In N. R. Ellis (Ed.) *International Review of Research on Mental Retardation.* Vol. 1, New York: Academic Press, 1966, 77-108.

Zigler, E. Developmental versus Difference theories of mental retardation and the problem of motivation. *American Journal of Mental Deficiency,* 1960, *73,* 536-556.

Zigler, E., & deLabry, T. Concept-switching in middle-class, lower-class, and retarded children. *Journal of Abnormal and Social Psychology,* 1962, *65,* 267-273.

8. Parents, Peers, and Child Patients Make the Best Therapists*

Paul W. Clement

Of all the people who could function as a therapeutic agent with a psychologically disturbed child, the professional child psychotherapist is in the poorest position to be of major help. Parents are usually in a better position to change their own child's behavior than is the professional therapist. As children grow older their peers may have even greater potential for bringing about therapeutic changes than have their parents. There are additional advantages in having a child's treatment consist of having him treat another child with a problem similar to his own. Finally, the ultimate child therapist is the child himself. This paper provides a rationale for the above propositions and outlines a number of psychological assessment and intervention skills which can be taught by clinical child psychologists to parents, peers, and child patients. All of the procedures which will be described have come from research in and clinical experiences with *behavior modification* with children.

The Goals of Child Psychotherapy

Different theoretical systems may appear to propose different goals for child psychotherapy, but ultimately all therapeutic goals fall into the following three categories: (a) to accelerate some behaviors, (b) to decelerate other behaviors, and (c) to maintain the remaining behaviors. Those behaviors which need acceleration are normally referred to as "behavioral deficits." Those behaviors which need deceleration are normally referred to as "behavioral excesses." When parents bring their children for professional help, their goals usually focus on changing the behavioral deficits and

*Preparation of this paper was partially supported by a grant (#MH 14395) from the National Institute of Mental Health and aided by the helpful comments of Richard McCrady and Jean McCrady.

81

excesses. Just as important however, is maintaining the child's behavioral assets. A particular behavior is considered to be an asset when it occurs with acceptable frequency, intensity, or at desired times.

Different child therapists have placed different amounts of emphasis on behavioral, emotional, and "mental" change. Ideally, the clinical child psychologist should be able to make precise therapeutic changes in all three; however, present technology only allows for precision therapy on the first two modes.

Assessing Behavior

Underlying the assessment approaches to be described below are a few important assumptions. First, the therapeutic agent (i.e., the person who will assess and treat the problems) must be able to observe the behaviors in order to modify them systematically. Second, behaviors which can be quantified and counted are easiest to change. The therapist needs to operationalize the target behaviors in terms of observables so that behavioral counting can take place. Third, problem behaviors which cannot be observed and counted are not likely to be changed by the therapeutic agent. Fourth, many psychological tests and assessment tools do not sample the behavior the therapist wants to change. The best way to predict how a child is going to behave tomorrow in a particular situation is to observe how he behaves in that situation today. Peterson (1968) and Mischel (1968) have provided extensive reviews of the issues underlying these assumptions.

The three basic approaches to a functional assessment of a child's behavior are interviewing, observation, and experimental manipulation. A new case normally begins with one or two hours of interviewing with the parents. The interviewer asks the following questions in order to help the parents establish their therapeutic goals:

What does your child do too often, too much, or at the wrong times that gets him into trouble? Tell me everything you can think of. We will label this category of problems as his *behavioral excesses*.

What does your child fail to do as often as you would like, as much as you would like, or when you would like? We will label this category of problems as his *behavioral deficits*. Tell me of any concerns you have about the way he thinks or feels.

What does your child do that you like? What does he do that

other people like? What do you consider to be his major *assets*?

What do you hope to accomplish as a result of consulting me? In particular let us consider what criteria we should use for deciding when to terminate treatment. What behaviors do you want to see changed, and how much must they change for you to be satisfied?

Now, which behavioral excess and which behavioral deficit do you most want to see changed? Under what conditions does the behavioral excess occur? At what times of day? Where? Who is usually present? What consequences follow the occurrence of the behavioral excess? Under what conditions does the low frequency behavior occur? When would you like it to occur? At the present time, what consequences follow the occurrence of the behavioral deficit?

At the end of the first interview, parents receive a Children's Reinforcement Survey (Clement & Richard, 1970). The Reinforcement Survey was designed to obtain information from parents, teachers, and children about the people, places, things, foods, and activities that can and/or do function as positive reinforcers for the target child.

Once the therapeutic priorities have been established, the psychologist asks the person who will function as the therapeutic agent to begin observing and counting all occurrences of the target behavior(s). Usually one of two general plans for data gathering is followed. The first option is the A-B-A-B design which has been used extensively by Skinnerians in the experimental analysis of behavior.

The second option for data gathering is the multiple baseline design. This approach requires the simultaneous tracking of two or more target behaviors. Baseline rates are established for all of the target behaviors, and intervention is then provided for one of the behaviors, all behaviors being continously observed and counted. Bijou, Peterson, Harris, Allen, and Johnston (1969) have provided a detailed description of procedures to follow when using either the A-B-A-B or multiple baseline design for observing the behavior of children in natural settings.

Regardless of who performs the behavioral observations, the more frequently the target behaviors are measured, the greater the possibility of making precise changes in those behaviors. The emphasis of "behavior modifiers" on day-by-day, hour-by-hour, and even minute-by-minute assessment of the behaviors being treated is probably their most significant contribution to the practice of clinical child psychology. This emphasis on measurement is probably more important than any intervention technique which has been used by behavior modifiers to date. In fact, once a parent or child learns to observe and track target behaviors, he is often able to develop a therapeutic intervention on his own. The systematic measurement allows him to assess the effectiveness of his intervention.

The first task in setting up a treatment program is to establish the client's goals. Once the goals have been identified, they are ranked according to the primary client's priorities. Whatever behaviors the client most wants to see changed usually become the focus of the first interventions, but he is not allowed to treat more than two target behaviors at any given time. Balanced against the proposition that treatment must begin with the most troublesome behaviors is the proposition that the client's first intervention attempts must be successful. Optimizing the chances for success is more important than beginning with the client's first choice, because he probably already has developed a set toward failing in dealing with the child in question. If he experiences failure at the beginning of the treatment program, such an experience is likely to reinforce a sense of hopelessness and helplessness which has caused the client to seek professional help in the first place.

Who Makes the Best Therapist?

In spite of all his training and sophistication, the clinical child psychologist (as well as all other professional child therapists) is not the best choice as the person who should treat a child whose behavior is disturbed and disturbing. When a professional therapist conducts the treatment in his office, that treatment is not conducive to generalization of therapeutic effects to "where the child lives."

By having parents treat their own children at home (e.g., Clement, 1970, 1971), generalization is virtually guaranteed because the behaviors are being changed in the very environment in which they have been and will be occurring.

Another problem confronting the clinical child psychologist who does psychotherapy in his office is the need to form a good relationship with the child *before* the primary treatment occurs. Building a strong, positive relationship often takes a great deal of time. Parents usually already have a strong relastionship with their children; hence, as therapeutic agents they are able to proceed directly and immediately to the primary treatment.

A third problem facing the professional is that he controls far fewer reinforcers for his child clients than do the parents. Those reinforces that the psychologist does control are usually weaker than many of those controlled by the parents; therefore, parents are usually in a position to have a more potent impact on their child's behavior than is the professional.

A fourth problem is cost. Even if parents were only as effective as the professional therapist, they would save substantial amounts of money by serving as the therapeutic agents. Much less professional time is needed to train and coach parents to treat their own child than is required for the psychologist to treat the child in his office.

Time constitutes a fifth problem area. There are far more children needing help than there are professionals available to deliver services. When the parents are trained, one professional can serve the whole family in contrast to the two professionals required in the classical child-guidance-clinic model. Also, most child problems require more than one 50-minute treatment a week, if the therapeutic goals are to be reached in the minimum possible time. In most of the treatment programs described later in this paper, there are daily administrations of treatment. In some cases the therapeutic interventions are delivered throughout the child's waking day. For a clinical child psychologist to devote so much time to a single case would be a highly inefficient use of the psychologist's skills as well as financially prohibitive for the family in most cases. Since daily treatment is often in the best interests of the child, ways need to be found for providing such services. Using parents as therapists is one such means.

A sixth problem area stems from the typical procedure in child guidance clinics of keeping parents relatively uninformed of what takes place in their child's therapy sessions. When parents are trained to treat their own children, the psychologist can avoid arousing parents' suspicions about what is being done to or with their child. Such suspiciousness quite naturally develops when parents are not fully informed of what treatments are being applied to their children, and when they receive interpretations *of* rather than answers *to* their questions.

Dissimilarities between the psychologist and the child constitute a seventh problem area. The therapeutic agent, professional or parent, provides a social model for the child to imitate. Other things being equal, the child will tend to imitate the behaviors of a model who is perceived as being most similar to himself (Bandura, 1969, pp. 171-172). The ''doctor'' is usually perceived as being quite dissimilar; therefore, he probably is not as effective a model as is the child's parents.

Finally, parents tend to seek professional assistance at a time when they are feeling helpless and hopeless. The attempts they have made to improve their child's behavior have failed to produce adequate changes. Although the thoughts are often not clearly verbalized, parents often communicate, ''Here he is, doctor. I've had it! You fix him up, and when he is all right, you can give him back to me.'' When the professional conducts the therapy himself, he may unintentionally be reinforcing the parents' set that they are not able to cope with their child. By being trained as therapists of their own child, the parents' competence and confidence to deal effectively with present and future problems are increased. The ultimate outcome of training parents to function as therapeutic agents is that they learn what creates, maintains, and eliminates behavioral problems in their children. Hence, the whole approach emphasizes *prevention* of future psychological difficulties.

Although having parents treat their own children solves the problems identified above, as children grow older their parents face increasing problems in functioning as therapeutic agents. As a child moves through the grades at school, peer relationships increasingly compete for allegiance with parent-child relationships. Also, as the child grows older, his parents control fewer and fewer of the reinforcing events in his life whereas his peers control increasingly more of them. Quantitatively, the child spends more and more time with his peers and less time with his parents. Finally peers are potent models regardless of the age of the child. Since using peers as therapists solves the same problems solved by using parents as therapists, plus solving the problems outlined above, peer-therapists seem to be an even better option for treating many children than parent-therapists.

Although there are advantages to using peer-therapists, there are also some problems with such a procedure. The more impaired the child patient, the less likely he may be to use ''normal'' peers as models. Another potential problem in the use of peers as therapists is that they may not always be motivated to function in such roles.

Another strategy is to have the target child treat someone else who has a problem similar to his own. This approach meets the above problems that are present when a professional, parents, or a peer is the therapist. If the target child's behavior changes in the process of treating the second child, the concepts of vicarious reinforcement and modeling seem to provide the best explanation for such changes. This approach removes any reason for the target child to struggle with the attempts of others to control his behavior. Although he was talking about neither a behavioral approach to therapy nor children, Riessman (1965) argued effectively that the best way to treat a person is to get him to treat someone else. He did not provide any experimental data to support this hypothesis, but rather presented a brief review of some relevant literature.

The biggest problem with the above strategy is that there are not always other children around with the same type of problem as that of the target child. Also, as with the peer therapist condition, both members of the pair may not be willing to participate in the therapeutic program.

If a child would benefit by treating another child who has a problem similar to his, how much more would he benefit by treating himself? When some other person is trying to modify a child's behavior, there is the possibility that the child will resist the person's efforts. When the child is his own behavior modifier, there is no reason to resist. This strategy handles all of the problems listed under the previous options. Having the patient become more responsible for himself is a major goal of most therapies, but they do not usually explicitly and specifically train the patient to be his own therapist. The present assumption is that children with disturbing behavior can be taught to regulate their own behavior in order to meet their needs better. They can follow a treatment plan provided by a behavioral consultant whose focus is not on changing them but on helping them to change themselves.

Specific Therapeutic Interventions

One of the distinctive features of the behavior modification approach is its emphasis on developing and identifying specific therapeutic packages which focus on specific target behaviors. Some techniques are designed primarily for increasing the frequency of certain behaviors. Some techniques are designed primarily for decreasing the frequency of other behaviors. Still other techniques are useful in simultaneously strengthening some behaviors and weakening others.

Some of the more common *acceleration techniques* of behavior modification are (a) goal setting, (b) education regarding the therapeutic strategies that will be used, (c) behavioral prescriptions, (d) behavioral rehearsal, (e) teaching children habits of emotional freedom, and (f) the conditioning treatment of enuresis.

Some of the more common *deceleration techniques* are (a) systematic desensitization, (b) implosive therapy (flooding), (c) massed (negative) practice, (d) thought stopping, and (e) covert sensitization.

Among those procedures which are just as often used for acceleration as deceleration are (a) contingency management, (b) self-administered behavioral tracking, (c) behavioral contracts, (d) audio and video feedback, (e) social modeling, (f) contact desensitization, (g) emotive imagery, and (h) time projection.

Detailed descriptions of and research on the above techniques can be found in the following journals: *Behavior Therapy, Behaviour Research and Therapy, Journal of Applied Behavior Analysis,* and *Journal of Behavior Therapy and Experimental Psychiatry.*

Training Parents to Treat Their Own Children

Once the psychologist and parents have completed a functional analysis of the child's behavior, the psychologist suggests interventions for the parents to use. When the interventions have been selected, the next step is to teach the parents the behavioral principles behind the procedures. It is helpful to provide the parents with reprints or descriptions of similar cases which have been treated with success. In addition, the psychologist will often find it helpful to model for the parents a specific therapeutic intervention which he expects them to perform. This may be done in the psychologist's office, in a clinic, or in the parents' own home. Normally the parents should be given an opportunity to practice interventions in the presence of the psychologist who can then provide them with social reinforcement for appropriate behaviors.

The *bug-in-the-ear,* a wireless transceiver system, is an especially useful device for providing feedback to parents or children in a treatment situation as they attempt new ways of behavior. The bug is worn by one person at a time, and only he can hear what the psychologist is saying from behind a one-way mirror. The psychologist is thereby able to deliver verbal prompts for what he wants the parent or child to do. As soon as the person wearing the bug exhibits an appropriate behavior, the psychologist can praise him. Thus, the bug provides for immediate social reinforcement and focused feedback to the subject who is interacting with other people.

Case Example

The case described below provides a good example of how a parent can be trained to treat even severe psychological problems in her own child. His teacher, his classmates, and the child himself were also involved in carrying out certain aspects of the treatment program.

Gilles de la Tourette's Syndrome. In the winter of 1969 a 9½-year-old boy considered to be the "number-one behavior problem" in his school district was referred for psychotherapy. Rich exhibited massive tics of the face, limbs, and vocal apparatus. The most disturbing tics of the limbs consisted of repeatedly "giving the finger" and making a grabbing movement toward the pelvis of other boys and men. The vocal tics consisted of a barking sound, obscene words and phrases, and bursts of "yes, no, yes, no, yes, no" in response to direct questions. At the time of the referral his teacher and mother estimated that he was using one obscenity about once every thirty seconds. The day before he was to have his first appointment he was expelled from public school.

Although the parents had not been given a label for Rich's problem, they had been told by a local psychologist and psychiatrist that Rich had a progressive disorder, and there was nothing they could do for him. They said that the only appropriate thing for the parents to do was to put the child in a residential treatment facility. The psychiatrist had tried several types of medication, but none seemed to alter his behavior. When Rich entered the treatment program described below, arrangements were made to have him placed on haloperidol, a tranquilizer, which he had not previously taken. The effects of this drug were, therefore, confounded with the effects of the behavioral treatment program.

In spite of his rather bizarre behavior, Rich was an attractive, outgoing child. The recommendations of Eysenck and Rachman (1965, p. 123) for the treatment of tics in extraverted people were followed in designing the interventions for Rich. The mother observed from behind a one-way mirror, while the psychologist gave Rich his first treatment. The treatment consisted of seating Rich in front of the therapist and telling him that every time the therapist tapped the table with a pencil, Rich was to say a designated obscene word. The therapist tapped the table at the rate of about two taps a second and kept this up for five minutes. Whenever Rich would begin to slow down, the therapist would repeat the obscenity and tell him to say it louder and more clearly. Within three minutes of the first five-minute trial, Rich seemed to develop marked tendencies to slow down and requested that the negative practice stop. The therapist persisted, however, and at the end of five minutes, he immediately had Rich lie down on the floor, close his eyes, and receive relaxation instructions for two minutes. Then Rich was up again in his chair for another five minutes of negative practice and down again for two minutes of relaxation on the floor with his eyes closed. These procedures required a total treatment period of fourteen minutes. Following this modeling session in the playroom, the therapist met with Rich, his mother, and a co-therapist who was helping consult with the mother. The four of them agreed that the mother would give Rich one full fourteen-minute treatment every two hours of each day, seven days aweek, from nine in the morning until seven at night.

Within three weeks the frequency of the primary vocal tic had dropped to less than once an hour. The mother gradually moved on to other words and phrases which Rich had emitted in tic-like fashion. In addition to administering the negative practice, the psychologist spent part of several sessions talking to Rich about the typical sexual interest and thoughts of boys his age. He was preoccupied with sexual thoughts, but nevertheless, he became very fidgety when sexual material was discussed. His mother also appeared uncomfortable in dealing with sexual themes. The therapist attempted to extinguish much of Rich's anxiety to sexual stimuli and also modeled for the mother how to talk to Rich about sexual topics. By playing a more active role in dealing with Rich, she seemed to implode herself on her own anxieties about sexual material.

Six months following the onset of treatment Rich was able to return to a regular classroom and spend a full day at school. All of his problems were not over, but there seemed to be no need for his parents or anyone else to give any consideration to placing him in a residential treatment center.

In the late fall of 1970, almost two years after Rich had received his first behavioral treatment, he had a major relapse of his tics. At the time of the relapse, he had not been to see the psychologist for a little more than a year. His parents did not call the psychologist for assistance until a month after the onset of the relapse, and by the time they came in, Rich's tics were occurring about as frequently as they were when he entered therapy two years earlier. He had just been suspended from school indefinitely at the time he returned to see the psychologist.

Since Rich had continued taking haloperidol throughout the two-year period, the relapse allowed a test of the effectiveness of the behavioral interventions without confounding their effects with those of the medication. In order to optimize therapeutic change, however, several behavioral interventions were applied to Rich's case. First, the mother and father reintroduced a systematic program of negative practice of the tics. Second, the mother kept track of the number of hours each day during which Rich emitted no tics. For each tic-free hour he received a point which could be traded for credit on bowling lessons. Introduction of these first two interventions was followed by a steady decline in the frequency of the tics. Rich had had a home teacher during the time he was suspended from school; he was allowed to return to school about three months after the interventions had been reinstated. For the third intervention his parents purchased a golf score counter which he wore to school on his wrist. He used it to keep track of the number of tics he emiteed each day at school. His parents provided back-up reinforcers to him at home for reducing his tic scores. Fourth, the teacher kept track of (a) the number of hours during which Rich emitted no audible tics and (b) the number of times the children in the class ignored Rich immediately following his emitting a tic. Both sets of points kept by the teacher could be traded by the whole class for extra art time each week. These interventions were accompanied by a reduction in the tic rate and the maintenance of acceptable classroom behavior from March through November, 1971 (the latter month being the time at which the present paper was completed).

Mothers as Child Group Therapists

For six years the present writer conducted research on child group therapy (Clement, 1968, 1971; Clement, Fazzone, & Goldstein, 1970; Clement & Milne, 1967; Clement, Roberts, & Lantz, 1970). For the first five years of the research program, most of the groups were led by professional child psychotherapists. In 1971, instead of using professionals, mothers and children were trained to function as group therapists. All children who participated in the research program had been referred because they exhibited shy, withdrawn behavior at school. They were from the second, third, or fourth grade. Each group consisted of four boys or four girls who received exactly sixteen one-hour sessions. While the children met in the playroom, their mothers met in another consultation room and received systematic training in the basic principles and strategies of behavior modification with children.

The mothers' groups followed a workshop format. Each week one mother from the mothers group joined the children in the playroom as "child therapist for a day." She wore the bug-in-the-ear and received coaching and verbal reinforcements from a research assistant who observed through a one-way mirror. The mothers took turns as child group therapists, with each mother functioning in that role once every four weeks. A mother only treated groups in which her own child was a member.

The mothers were taught how to use token reinforcement along with social reinforcements in leading the groups. Token reinforcement consisted of the delivery of brass tokens to the children for increasing levels of prosocial behaviors.

Training Children to Treat Each Other

There are two possibilities for the basic conditions under which a psychologist would want one child to treat another. In the first case, the child doing the treating would not be the focus of any treatment program. He would be a "normal" child who would be recruited to help in the treatment of the target child. The second possibility is that the person doing the treating is a target child himself whose treatment is to treat another child. A third possibility exists in which the first two approaches are combined so that the target child is treated by other children as well as acting as a therapeutic agent himself.

One way in which "normal" children can be used as therapeutic agents is to employ them as social models in a child psychotherapy program (e.g., Clement, Roberts, & Lantz, 1970). Another way is to have peers track the behaviors of a target child in the classroom. This has been done when teachers were unwilling or unable to do the behavioral tracking.

In all classroom management programs in which the behavior of the target child was the basis for special privileges for the entire class, the class became a therapeutic agent in the treatment of the target child. For example, one boy was being treated for excessive physical aggression on the playground and for a lack of age-appropriate, social play. He was earning points for reducing his physical aggression to below baseline levels and for increasing the number of five-minute intervals during which he was playing with someone constructively on the playground. His points were charted daily and the chart was placed on the wall in front of the whole class. The teacher had explained to the target child and to the entire class that his points could be cashed in for extra art time. The whole class had had a discussion at the beginning of the intervention period and had proposed to the teacher that the points be used to purchase the extra art time. Before the intervention had occurred, the target child had been a "social outcast" in his classroom. With the introduction of the intervention program, his status began to change. Children began to seek him out on the playground and they began to respond positively to him for his attempts to engage them in appropriate social interactions. Hence, the children provided increasingly higher levels of social reinforcement for appropriate social behaviors of the target child. Without realizing it, they were functioning as therapeutic agents in teaching the target child more effective ways of behaving and relating.

Although group play therapy is popular in a large number of child guidance clinics, and although I have been involved in the treatment of more than 30 children's groups, I no longer recommend group therapy in the clinic in which several strange children are brought together in order to treat their separate problems. Rather, at the present time, when a child seems to have socialization difficulties, we tailor-make a group for him. In such tailor-made therapy, the cooperation of some of his peers and/or friends from the neighborhood or his school is generally sought. The aim is to involve children with whom he will have contact outside the clinic. There is a wide range of possibilities for the specific nature of the interventions applied while the children are together in the child therapy room. It has often been the case that one of the parents functions as the explicit therapist under these circumstances, reinforcing the target child for appropriate social behaviors. In other cases, one of the peers is coached to behave in what is felt to be a therapeutic way.

Training Individual Children to Treat Themselves

The first time I explicitly used a self-regulation approach to child treatment, I did so out of necessity. I was working with Cynthia, a nine-year-old girl, and her foster mother. She was presenting a large number of behavior problems both at home and at school. The foster mother had been very cooperative and effective in carrying out a treatment program at home. However, Cynthia's teacher refused to take part in any systematic interventions at school, saying that she had repeatedly requested that the girl be removed from her class but that the principal had refused. All the teacher was willing to do was to keep her in class. Since there was no teacher aide in the room, and the foster mother did not have free time to spend in the classroom as a therapeutic aid, the therapist decided to train the child to treat herself. When the teacher had been interviewed, she said that the behavior she would like to see changed first was Cynthia's wandering about the room and bothering the rest of the children. Therefore, "sitting-in-seat" behavior was chosen as the target. The therapist saw Cynthia for 25 minutes each week. In the session just preceding the initiation of the self-regulation program, he and Cynthia made a verbal contract that she would keep track of the number of five-minute intervals she stayed in her seat through-out each school day. The therapist and Cynthia went to a local dime store and purchased a five-minute egg timer that Cynthia was to use in timing her intervals. The therapist also gave her a simple check sheet on which to keep score. They agreed that at the end of each school day, she would call the therapist's office and give his secre-tary the score for that day. The therapist wrote Cynthia's teacher a brief letter explaining what was happening and requesting that the teacher not allow the classmates to interfere with Cythia or her egg timer.

After two weeks on this self-regulation program the teacher reported a dramatic change for the better in Cynthia's in-seat behav-ior. Although the relationship between Cynthia and her teacher was far from perfect, Cynthia seemed to be much happier and more productive in the school situation for the remainder of the year than she had been up to that time. No back-up reinforcers had been provided to Cynthia for increasing her in-seat behavior. Merely keeping track and reporting her scores to her therapist seemed to be an effective intervention for her.

I have used self-treatment programs with a number of other children. To date the self-administered interventions have consisted primarily of various types of observing and counting one's behavior, e.g., number of times the child had a tantrum, the number of times the child emitted a vocal tic, or the number of five-minute intervals spent doing homework. In all cases in which I have used such procedures, the child, his parents, and/or his teacher have reported clear improvement.

During the 1960's, a large number of research papers were published dealing with self-reinforcement and other forms of self-regulation. Much of this research was stimulated by Skinner's dis-cussion of mechanisms of self-control (Skinner, 1953, pp. 227-241). Skinner described nine techniques which an individual can use to regulate his own behavior: (1) physical restraint and physical aid, (2) changing the stimulus, (3) depriving and satiating, (4) manipulating emotional conditions, (5) using aversive stimulations, (6) drugs, (7) operant conditioning, (8) punishment, and (9) "doing something else." Kanfer and Marston have systematically pursued some of Skinner's ideas by carrying out a long series of laboratory investiga-tions of self-reinforcement, self-control, and self-regulation (e.g.,

Kanfer and Marston, 1963; Marston, 1965, Duerfeldt, and le Page, 1969). Bandura and his colleagues carried out a series of studies of self-regulation in children under laboratory conditions. They identified four basic processes usually operating in a self-reinforcing event: (a) a self-described standard of behavior, (b) a comparison of one's own performance with that of other children, (c) reinforcers which are under the child's own control, and (d) the child, in fact, serves as his own reinforcing agent (Bandura and Perloff, 1967).

Systematic studies have not yet been performed to determine the degree to which child clinicians can substitute self-regulation programs for behavior modification programs administered by others on the target child.

Kanfer and Phillips (1970, pp. 426-454) provided a list of self-control procedures which have been applied to clinical problems. Most of these techniques, however, have not been systematically applied to children. The procedures are (a) covert sensitization, (b) contingency management, (c) self-punishment, (d) self-reinforcement, (e) contract management, (f) self-confrontation, (g) self-administered behavioral analysis, (h) self-monitoring, and (i) altering the discriminative stimuli for the target response. Kanfer and Phillips (p. 452) provided a set of guidelines which should be followed in setting up a self-regulation treatment program: (a) intervene early in the response sequence; (b) utilize environmental controls so that the burden of nonexecution of a symptomatic response does not come at a point where its potential pay-off and its response strength due to past experience are too great; (c) execute alternate behaviors that have a reasonably high potential for reinforcement; (d) practice controlling responses and expect that they will be reinforced by the social environment; (e) specify the desired terminal behaviors; and (f) obtain clear feedback during attempts to change.

A Final Word

Probably most systems of child psychotherapy would hold as an ultimate goal that the child should assume responsibility for his own behavior. However, the traditional systems have not provided much specific structure for training the child to be responsible for his own therapy. When a child is systematically taught how to function as his own therapeutic agent, it is believed that this will accelerate the process of his becoming responsible for himself. Also, for various reasons, it appears that self-administered behavior therapy is far less offensive to many psychologists than behavior modification strategies administered by someone other than the child himself. Self-regulation strategies in behavior modification with children may therefore provide a bridge between the behavior therapist and the more traditionally-oriented child therapist.

References

Bandura, A. *Principles of behavior modification*, New York: Holt, Rinehart & Winston, 1969.

Bandura, A., & Perloff, B. Relative efficacy of self-monitored and externally imposed reinforcement systems. *Journal of Personality & Social Psychology*, 1967, *7*, 111-116.

Bijou, S. W., Peterson, R. F., Harris, F. R., Allen, K. E., & Johnston, M. S. Methodology for experimental studies of young children in natural settings. *Psychological Record*, 1969, *19*, 177-210.

Clement, P.W. Operant conditioning in group psychotherapy with children. *Journal of School Health*, 1968, *38*, 271-278.

Clement, P.W. Elimination of sleepwalking in a seven-year-old boy. *Journal of Consulting & Clinical Psychology*, 1970, *34* (No. 1), 22-26.

Clement, P.W. Please, mother, I'd rather you did it yourself: Training parents to treat their own children. *Journal of School Health*, 1971, *41* (No. 2), 65-69.

Clement, P. W. Fazzone, R. A., & Goldstein, B. Tangible reinforcers and child group therapy. *Journal of the American Academy of Child Psychiatry*, 1970, *9*, 409-427.

Clements, P. W., & Milne, D. C. Group play therapy and tangible reinforcers used to modify the behavior of eight-year-old boys. *Behaviour Research & Therapy*, 1967, *5*, 301-312.

Clement, P. W., & Richard, R. C. *Children's reinforcement survey*. Pasadena, California: Child Development Center, 1970.

Clement, P. W., Roberts, P. V., & Lantz, C. E. Social models and token reinforcement in the treatment of shy, withdrawn boys. *Proceedings of the 78th Annual Convention of the American Psychological Association*. Washington, D.C.: APA, 1970, pp. 515-516.

Eysenck, H. J., & Rachman, S. *The causes and cures of neurosis*. San Diego: Knapp, 1965.

Kanfer, F. H., Duerfeldt, P. H., & le Page, A. L. Stability of patterns of self-reinforcement. *Psychological Reports*, 1969, *24*, 663-670.

Kanfer, F. H., & Marston, A. R. Determinants of self-reinforcement in human learning. *Journal of Experimental Psychology*, 1963, *66*, 245-254.

Kanfer, F. H., & Phillips, J. S. *Learning foundations of behavior therapy*. New York: John Wiley, 1970.

Marston, A. R. Imitation, self-reinforcement, and reinforcement of another person. *Journal of Personality & Social Psychology*, 1965, *2*, 255-261.

Mischel, W. *Personality and assessment*. New York: John Wiley, 1968.

Peterson, D. R. *The clinical study of social behavior*. New York: Appleton-Century-Crofts, 1968.

Riessman, R. The "helper" therapy principle. *Social Work,* 1965, *10* (No. 2), 27-32.

Skinner, B. F. *Science and human behavior*. New York: Macmillan, 1953.

9. The Journey Beyond Trips: Alternatives to Drugs*

Allan Y. Cohen

Interviewer: *Why do you use drugs?*
  User: *Why not?*
Interviewer: *How could someone convince you to stop?*
  User: *Show me something better.*

Of all the dialogues between clinical and research interviewers and their subjects, ones like the above, though terse, are incredibly significant.

Governments, social institutions and private individuals have been forced to respond to what is popularly known as "the drug epidemic." Total social response to the fact of drug use has been neither successful nor appropriate; one might say it has been badly botched. Intentions have been good, sometimes truly compassionate; but execution has missed the mark. But, "no blame"- the fault is due less to incompetance than to misconception.

It is the purpose of this paper, humbly conceived though opinionated, to outline some major misconceptions about the causes and solutions of the American drug problem, to offer a simple motivational model of drug use and to suggest a positive orientation which is relevant and applicable.

The Myths

Some obvious myths and stereotypes about drugs have been exposed adequately by previous commentators. Let us investigate more subtle myths, ones which have sprung up from initial public attitudes about drugs and "addicts," nurtured by well-intentioned

*Reprinted with permission from the *Journal of Psychedelic Drugs*, Vol. 3 (No. 2) Spring, 1971.

research and analysis, and rendered inappropriate by the phenomenal growth of drug experimentation. It is my contention that such questionable assumptions have implied strategies doomed to ineffectiveness in the control, treatment, prevention and amelioration of the drug crisis.

Those Weird Drug Users—One widespread notion is that drug "users" are a certain "breed" of people or social group. (To simplify language, "users" is taken to cover the broad range from "experimenters" to "drug dependers," unless specifically modified below.) Predictably, many studies have abounded with conclusions about personality and socio-cultural correlates of drug use. The object of such research, aside from pure science, is to understand "what makes drug users tick;" extrapolating the implications to prevention or to education.

But *is* there a certain type using drugs? Can one ever "predict" individuals predisposed to drug use? More importantly, does it help to talk in such terms . . . I think not. I say this because behind the common personality-social research lies an assumption which is now very suspect—that drug experimentation and use is a *minority* phenomenon, that study of this special group will generate practical insights.

On the contrary, the apparent survey and interview evidence suggests that drug use has become a majority phenomenon, not only among the young. Even excluding alcohol, coffee and cigarettes, it is now safe to estimate that over 50% of the total American population over 13 years of age has at least tried some powerful mind-altering drug via prescription or on the illicit market. Rare is the urban school using authentic survey data which reports that less than 50% of their secondary students have used amphetamines, psychedelics, barbiturates, cannabis products and like drugs within the last 12 months. No figures can be given on overall *regular* use, but scores of spot interviews indicate that the high school "dopers" peer culture is challenging the size of the "straights." In the adult world, one recent survey found that 25% of all American women over 30 were currently under prescription of amphetamines, barbiturates or tranquilizers, the percentage going up to 40% for ladies of higher income families.[1]

All things considered, it is my contention that drug use must now be admitted as the social *norm*. We must realize that our chemical culture has produced an atmosphere leading to the naturalness of using drugs—no matter what the underlying complaint or need. Failure to comprehend this cultural reality leads to dysfunctional priorities. Popular now is the notion that drug users are necessarily deviant or pathological. Drug use, too many surmise, indicates something terribly wrong with the person, either morally ("send 'em to jail") or psychologically ("send 'em to a mental hospital"). But we know better. Drug users may not necessarily show lack of morality or personality disturbance, at least not more than many non-users. Indeed, the non-user may be "deviant" in the purely statistical sense. It may well be that the primary question among youth presented with the opportunity for experimentation is no longer "Why?" but "Why not?" A basic inadequacy in this "deviance-minority" model is that it tends to focus emphasis on *symptoms* rather than *causes*. It produces a philosophy of social intervention which is essentially *reactive* and *negative*. Perhaps we might be able to come up with another kind of conceptual model, a more useful one, based on logic, common sense, and our accumulated knowledge of the drug scene.

The Motives

In this conceptual model, which leads to an ultimate emphasis on alternatives to drugs, we begin with a simple formulation of the most basic motivational forces leading to drug use.

Principle I —People take drugs because they want to.

Principle II—People *use* drugs to "feel better" or to "get high." Individuals *experiment* with drugs out of curiosity or hope that using drugs can make them feel better.

Principle III —People have been taught by cultural example, media, etc. that drugs *are* an effective way to make them feel better.

Principle IV —"Feeling better" encompasses a huge range of mood or consciousness change, including such aspects as oblivion-sleep, emotion shift, energy modification and vision of the Divine, etc.

Principle V —With many mind or mood-altering drugs, taken principally for that purpose, individuals may temporarily feel better. However, drugs have substantial short and long term disadvantages related to the motive for their use. These include possible physiological damage, psychological deterioration and cognitive breakdown. Drugs also tend to be temporary, relatively devoid of satisfying translation to the ordinary non-drug state of life, and siphon off energy for long term constructive growth.

Principle VI —Basically, individuals do not stop using drugs until they discover "something better."

Principle VII —The key to meeting problems of drug abuse is to focus on the "something better," and maximize opportunities for experiencing satisfying non-chemical alternatives. The same key can be used to discourage experimentation or, more likely, keep experimentation from progressing to dependency.

This model may seem simplistic, but I find it valuable. If I admit to the logic that people use drugs because they *want* to, I also have been forced to realize that people will only stop drug use *when* they *want* to.

The Alternatives

I shall call this kind of formulation the "Alternatives Model." While the above assumptions are most relevantly applied to the common psychotropic substances, they might even be extended to common medicinal drugs (i.e., if we gave as much attention to the natural prevention of the common cold as to cold remedies, we would all be healthier).

The Alternatives Model emphasizes *causes;* and mandates increased attention to the development and communication of alternative attitudes, strategies, techniques, institutional changes and life styles which could diminish the desire for using drugs to attain legitimate personal aspirations. "Alternative" is *not* just a synonym for "substitute" since it implies an orientation which is *more effective* than drugs for giving the person real satisfaction.

Considering its logical importance, the literature on alternatives to drug use is very sparse, although the situation seems to be improving.[2] Ironically, there is a huge store of literature and wisdom about possible alternatives, but this material has not been specifically applied to drug use education and research.

Once we presume that "alternatives" are important, we must expand the model to fit complex variables in all phases of the drug scene. We face questions like: "Which alternative for which drug?"— "Which alternative for which motive?"—"Which alternative for which person?" At this point, I wish to share a list of categories which has assisted me in thinking about applying alternatives. It was obvious to me that motives and relevant alternatives were intimately connected, and that one way of conceptualizing the relationship was in terms of different "levels of experience." Thus, as an illustration rather than an ultimate formulation, I have included Table 1. Each level of experience pertains to certain types of motives leading to drug use or experimentation, examples of which are listed in the Table. Across from each level-motive cate-

Level of Experience	Corresponding Motives (Examples)	Possible Alternatives (Examples)
Physical	Desire for physical satisfaction; physical relaxation; relief from sickness; desire for more energy; maintenance of physical dependency.	Athletics; dance; exercise; hiking diet; health training; carpentry or outdoor work.
Sensory	Desire to stimulate sight, sound, touch, taste; need for sensual-sexual stimulation; desire to magnify sensorium.	Sensory awareness training; sky diving; experiencing sensory beauty of nature.
Emotional	Relief from psychological pain; attempt to solve personal perplexities; relief from bad mood; escape from anxiety; desire for emotional insight; liberation of feeling; emotional relaxation.	Competent individual counseling; well-run group therapy; instruction in psychology of personal development.
Interpersonal	To gain peer acceptance; to break through interpersonal barriers; to "communicate," especially non-verbally; defiance of authority figures; cement two-person relationships; relaxation of interpersonal inhibition; solve interpersonal hangups.	Expertly managed sensitivity and encounter groups; well-run group therapy instruction in social customs; confidence training; social-interpersonal counseling; emphasis on assisting others in distress via education; marriage.
Social (Including Socio-Cultural & Environmental)	To promote social change; to find identifiable subculture; to tune out intolerable environmental conditions, e.g., poverty; changing awareness of the "masses."	Social service; community action in positive social change; helping the poor, aged infirm, young, tutoring handicapped ecology action.

Political	To promote political change; to identify with anti-establishment subgroup; to change drug legislation; out of desperation with the social-political order; to gain wealth or affluence or power.	Political service; political action; non-partisan projects such as ecological lobbying; field work with politicians and public officials.
Intellectual	To escape mental boredom; out of intellectual curiosity; to solve cognitive problems; to gain new understanding in the world of ideas; to study better; to research one's own awareness; for science.	Intellectual excitement through reading, through discussion; creative games and puzzles; self-hypnosis; training in concentration; synectics—training in intellectual breakthroughs; memory training.
Creative-Aesthetic	To improve creativity in the arts; to enhance enjoyment of art already produced, e.g., music; to enjoy imaginative mental productions.	Non-graded instruction in producing and/or appreciating art, music, drama, crafts, handiwork, cooking, sewing, gardening, writing, singing, etc.
Philosophical	To discover meaningful values; to grasp the nature of the universe; to find meaning in life; to help establish personal identity; to organize a belief structure.	Discussions, seminars, courses in the meaning of life; study of ethics, morality, the nature of reality; relevant philosophical literature; guided exploration of value systems.
Spiritual-Mystical	To transcend orthodox religion; to develop spiritual insights; to reach higher levels of consciousness; to have Divine Visions; to communicate with God; to augment yogic practices; to get a spiritual shortcut; to attain enlightenment; to attain spiritual powers.	Exposure to non-chemical methods of spiritual development; study of world religions; introduction to applied mysticism, meditation; yogic techniques.
Miscellaneous	Adventure, risk drama, "kicks," unexpressed motives; pro-drug general attitudes, etc.	"Outward Bound" survival training; combinations of alternatives above; pronaturalness attitudes; brain-wave training; meaningful employment, etc.

gory are examples of types of alternatives which might replace, ameliorate or prevent drug abuse. I expect the reader will come up with many more motives and an almost infinite addition of alternatives. Of course, there are other ways to conceptulalize the different kinds of alternatives—again, this Table is intended to serve only as an example and stimulant. Needless to say, several levels of experience may operate withing a particular individual or subgroup, so categories and motives may be related across levels and should not be taken as mutually exclusive.

There is one alternative not mentioned in the Table because it is so obvious. Yet it deserves some comment. A growing viable alternative to using drugs is *not to use drugs or to discontinue drug use*. Many long term users move away from drugs because they feel better *not* using them. For some, being "straight" or "clean" is a refreshing change in itself from being stoned or hooked. Often this response is out of negativity, e.g., fright from a bad trip, the agony of being strung out, the realization of personal self-destruction, the boredom of being stoned all the time, etc. The pre-experimenter who avoids drugs may also be acting from a flight from negativity— in this case, an avoidance of anticipated hurtful results. It may be, however, that most non-experimenters have already found an alternative so positive that there is no felt need for drugs or a reluctance to risk something preceived as valuable. Preliminary research[3] tends to confirm this supposition—that young non-users of common illicit drugs avoid them more because of satisfaction gained in exploring positive alternatives, rather than from a fear of consequent harm.

Thus, *not using drugs* only becomes a viable alternative in one of two cases: (1) when a drug user is suffering, and realizes the suffering is drug-related; or, (2) when a pre-user has so much going for him that perceived drug-related risks threaten present satisfaction.

Referring back to the Table, the Alternatives Model was originally developed around the issue of psychedelic drugs and cannabis. However, this type of categorization allows us to consider all types of psycho-pharmacological intervention, from the case of the heroin addict to the "housewife junkie" on diet pills; from the fourth grader sniffing airplane glue to the middle-aged alcoholic.

We are aware that an expressed motive may be different from the "real" underlying motive, and we should be alert to basic motives, no matter what is expressed. We should also remember that certain drugs may be most associated with certain kinds of motives. For example, heroin is likely to be more associated with the classic "escape" motives because of its consciousness-benumbing effect, whereas LSD might be used more to try to satisfy aspirations on the creative, philosophical or spiritual level of experience.

Implementing Alternatives: General Principles

The Alternatives Model can be very helpful in assigning priorities to social action for the control, treatment and prevention of drug abuse. Clearly, punitive control has severe limits upon its effectiveness because it does not respond with viable alternatives to the predisposing motives, and its fear-generating capacity is not an adequate deterrent.

In rehabilitation and treatment, sequences of intervention should parallel priorities in the level of experience category. For example, in treating heroin addiction, methadone represents a viable alternative to the physical component of the addict's needs, but the eventual treatment program must aim at providing more permanent fulfillment of deeper psycho-social needs. The existence or non-existence of these deeper aspirations will determine whether the addict can resist temptation after withdrawl from methadone. As a parallel case, the "Freak-out" victim of strong psychedelics is best first treated on the emotional and perhaps interpersonal levels to return him to ordinary consciousness. But, after that, adequate rehabilitation programs must respond to the things which got him hung up in the first place.

Perhaps the most powerful application of the Alternative Model lies in the field of drug education. There is still a powerful premise circulating among educators that individuals, especially children, can be *frightened* away from drugs with "proper information about dangers." In all frankness, this hope is a utopian fantasy. Before anyone gets optimistically excited about "dynamic, hard-hitting facts" in a drug abuse curriculum, he should give careful thought to the remarkable staying power of cigarettes in the mature adult population. The case against smoking cigarettes could hardly be much stronger (in view of the demonstrated dangers) and yet wide-spread anti-smoking publicity has made only a remarkably small dent in the smoking habits of those most "responsible" citizens.

In view of such a fact, does it seem reasonable to expect a "scare" campaign to be decisive? Of course not. The young are more non-rational, risk-oriented and unbelieving. Further, the effects of the most used drugs have not been accurately delineated and the credibility of authority figures is very strained. (One young pothead told me that he would not believe any research unless the study was conducted in Switzerland! Neutrality equals objectivity he guessed.)

Reliance on fear motivation can produce the instructor's ultimate frustration in the older age groups. He succeeds in persuading students that drugs have bad effects. But the students reason that they live in a dangerous world (bad air, chemicals in food, possiblity of war, etc.) and that the dangers of drugs do not outweigh the pleasure they can give in return. Once again, the educator has paid the price of the "deviance" theory, i.e., that reasonable people will not want to use drugs, and that education regarding the dangers will weed out all those pre-experimenters except the mentally ill or criminally inclined.

I do not wish to downgrade the real value of accurate information about drug effects—such information can be a significant help in the decision-making process. Further, it may serve to bolster the intuitive guess that drugs are harmful and may help some youths to justify to their peers the adoption of non-chemical alternatives. Educational honesty and credibility must be maximized in the same way that legislators should make drug use a public health and not a criminal concern. But the real promise in education would seem to involve educating about alternatives. There is no higher priority; and there are few other ways to give such a powerful assist to the minimization of drug abuse.

It is my contention that education about non-chemical alternatives for each level of experience is the best mode of "prevention." It is also the method of choice for moderate experimenters. And finally, the Alternatives Model is the treatment of choice for heavy users (here much stress would be put on the alternative of not using). In the application of the Alternatives Model, it must be realized that there is no one pat alternative for everyone, just as there is no one motive responsible for all drug use. Also, it should be noted that the alternatives of best application are those which are *incompatible* with being high. For example, "listening to recorded music" is not an alternative unless it precludes being stoned while listening. In this particular case, techniques or ways of listening must be sufficiently taught so that chemically-altered awareness gets in the way of the experience. In general, extremely *passive* alternatives must be utilized with a bit more care that alternatives necessitating *action* or work with one's resources. The more active and demanding alternatives are those which clearly interfere with a drug-taking life-style.

Implementation of Alternatives:
A Specific Example

To give one small specific instance in which the Alternatives Model may be applied to institutional action, let us take the case of the public schools, It has been argued that many of our public school systems through rigidity, misassessed priorities and lack of relevance, have contributed to the disatisfactions which lead children toward drugs. It seems indisputable that the "Art of Living" has become a critically important skill for young people, one not reflected in course curricula. The schools have become expert at transmitting information and training intellectual skills, but this is partially lost if the young are preoccupied and are not motivated to learn what the schools want them to learn.

The issue of educational reform is far too broad to treat in this paper, but let us offer one small suggestion based on the Alternatives Model. Most schools offer course experiences in non-intellective areas, but emasculate anti-chemical possibilities by assigning grades to such courses. I am referring to subjects like music, art homemaking, drama, physical education, manual training, family life education and the like. All of these subject areas *could* pertain to the motive levels discussed previously. They *could* get children so personally involved that drugs would not be so inviting. Usually they do not. The arbitrary grading process infuses anxiety and competition into just those areas which might provide creative relief. Students deliberately avoid electives in alternative areas for fear of lowering their academic average. Only the best students in really non-intellective areas are really encouraged to go on developing non-intellective resources, and even they are prey to "evaluation anxiety"—that fear of failure which makes neurotics out of prospective artists.

The abolition of grades in alternatives subjects would be a powerful stroke in turning the kids on to a "natural high", with little or any monetary outflow. Parents might object to a lack of competitive evaluation, but they should be reminded that one of the pulls to the drug scene is that no one gets an "F" for turning on. Logically related steps could include the expansion of subject hours in alternatives areas, invitations to community members who could share what turns them on nonchemically, time outside the walls to taste social involvement and service, a philosophical admission of the importance of interpersonal as well as intellectual skills. These are the kinds of steps which might come to mind when focusing on the necessity of alternatives.

Toward a Newer Humanity

When proposing a large scale turn towards the Alternatives Model, some might respond skeptically and ask for reseach findings which have demonstrated the model's effectivness. Long-term research simply has not yet been done in the alternatives area. However, survey and interview studies have amply suggested that most users stop (or would stop) because of a pereferable alternative.[4]

Perhaps the most exciting aspect of the Alternatives Models is that it can be applied to any level of action or reaction to drug use. It is limited only by the imagination and wisdom of the implementor. The positive possibilities seem limitless; while obsession with drug-related symptoms and dangers appears an endless pit of futility.

There are other advantages to the Alternatives Model. Application of provided alternatives to drug use simultaneously provides alternatives to other forms of human difficulties. After all, truly effective solutions to the "problem of drugs" are the "problem of life." Very possibly, deterioration may be shifted to harmony. Those solutions, applied to every level of experience could make man's abuse of himself and others fade into an historical rememberance of a tankfully transcended cultural psychosis.

References

1. Data relayed in a 1970 speech by Professor Joseph Maloney, University of Kentucky.
2. Articles: Dohner, A. V. "Mood-Altering Agent Use in America: Why Drugs?" Rocky Mountain Med. J. (February, 1970): Chanin, A. "Understanding Teenagers: Alternatives to Drug Abuse." Clin. Pediat. Vol. 8: 6-10. (January, 1969)' Townshend. P. "In Love with Meher Baba." Rolling Stone. No. 71: 25-27. (26 November, 1970). Books: Gustatis, R. Turning On. (New York: Macmillian, 1969); Needleman, J. The New Religions. (New York: Doubleday, 1970); Marin, P. & Cohen, A. Y. Understanding Drug Use: An Adult's Guide to Drugs and the Young. (New York: Harper & Row, 1971); Payne, B. Getting There Without Drugs. (New York: Viking Press, In Press).
3. Survey conducted by students, Pacific High School, San Leandro, California. In response to an essay question: "If you do not use drugs, what has been the biggest deterrent for not using them?",

39.8% said there was "no need' (or "life is fine, I'm happy," "turn on other ways," etc.). This contrast with 7.1% who mentioned laws or "getting busted," (study conducted in 1968-1969).
4. Cohen, A. Y. "Relieving Acid Indigestion: Psychological and Social Dynamics Related to Hallucinogenic Drug Abuse," Final report submitted to the Bureau of Drug Abuse Control under Research Contract 67-25. (1968). (Now possibly available through the Bureau of Narcotics and Dangerous Drugs, Washington, D.C.)

10. Psychologist and Pediatrician: A Mental Health Team in the Prevention and Early Diagnosis of Mental Disorders

Lee Salk

Today, perhaps as never before, the pediatrician more than any other professional holds a most influential role for the mental health of future generations. Only recently has it become known how profound the effects of early experience on later behavior can be. We know that newborn infants are selective in some of their responses, habituate to various stimuli, and can show conditioned responses. Sociologists, anthropologists, biologists, and educators along with the psychologists have shown how early environmental conditions can help shape personality, learning ability, and capacity to tolerate stress and can effect structural and biochemical alterations of the body.[1,3] These effects during early development are very profound and are often extremely difficult to change later on.

The pediatrician sees more human beings during their most critical phases of development than any other professional person. Often he detects developmental and psychological problems and is in a position to recommend further study of the problems and methods for dealing with them, or to refer to another professional for treatment. Although the pediatrician, logistically, is in a position for early detection of psychological and developmental disorders, he is often unable to do so because he is not trained or skilled in the methods of detecting these disorders. Moreover, he is most likely overwhelmed by medical problems so that little time is available to him even if his training skills were sufficient for the early diagnosis of psychological problems.

The pediatrician's potential for identifying early developmental and psychological problems represents one important aspect of his mental health role but perhaps even more important is his vast influence on the attitudes of many parents towards child-rearing practices. Usually it is the pediatrician who tells a parent when the child cries to "pick it up" or "let him cry it out," when he soils his pants at age three to "punish him" or "ignore it." Such contradictory advice is not uncommon among pediatricians and is ofter founded only on their personal preference and not on any logical theory or body of scientific data.

This is not meant to be in any way derogatory towards the pediatrician but merely to focus on the dilemma of the pediatrician, who is looked upon as an expert in child-rearing practices, but, more often than not, lacks the knowledge and training required for such a role. Part of the reason for this gap in pediatric training lies in the fact that medical centers rely on psychiatry for training in human behavior rather than on the broader behavioral sciences that focus more on psychological theory and social organization.[2] Traditionally, it has been the psychiatrist whom the pediatrician is expected to turn to for his knowledge of human behavior, and very often the problems the pediatrician is concerned with do not require the traditional psychiatric approach but require a broader knowledge of psychological theory. In view of the fact that the pediatrician holds an important mental health role, it is somewhat paradoxical to find that this same individual receives little preparation for this role.

Since progress often begins with the recognition of what we do not know and since change is often initiated with the recognition that existing practices are no longer functional, we have no alternative but to make certain recommendations if the pediatrician is to adopt his role effectively in preventing psychological problems and promoting mental health.

Clearly, pediatricians must receive more and intensive training in the behavioral sciences and, in particular, personality growth and development. Furthermore, the pediatrician should have available a consultant trained in the behavioral sciences and equipped to screen, diagnose, and advise on problems pertaining to development, learning, behavior disorders, nervous system dysfunction, and patient management as well as on child-rearing practices. This psychological consultant should be available to pediatricians without delay so that they can continue to assume responsibility for their patients without loss of continuity, and can become more sensitized to psychological factors, and more adept in "feeling out" potential problems. By working closely with such a consultant, pediatricians will be able to deal with patients medically without loss of time or unnecessary involvement while offering good mental health service. What is fast becoming a new specialty in psychology—pediatric psychology[7]—has grown out of the need on the part of the pediatrician for such a consultant.

This need has been recognized by the American Psychological Association which has, under the sponsorship of the Section on Clinical Child Psychology, supported the development of the Society of Pediatric Psychology. Clearer definitions of pediatric psychology as a specialty group are evolving. New training requirements are being considered as well as the parameters of operation and their relationship to other professional groups.

I would like to focus now on the purposes and functions of the pediatric psychologist as they have evolved from the development of our Division of Pediatric Psychology at The New York Hospital-Cornell Medical Center, but first I would like to quote some remarks by William Scofield[6] that serve as a backdrop for the ideas put forth in this paper. Scofield presents a very enlightening view that embraces the specifics of how psychologists contribute to the delivery of health services. He says:

"Thus far, only a smattering of psychologists have interested themselves in clearly medical nonpsychiatric problems. . . . The potential for psychology to contribute to health services outside of the mental health area is not likely to be realized unless the current pattern for the training of the scientist-clinician undergoes a very marked correction of its rather exclusive focusing on psychiatric illness, psychiatric patients, and psychiatric services. There will be a continuing need for psychologists trained with this emphasis. It would be well, however, for a few centers to explore modifications of their training programs, especially in regard to minor studies and internship, so as to produce a desirable variant, the medical psychologist. He would be a scientist-clinician like his more common prototype, but with a particular sophistication in physical illness, equipped to research and consult with regard to the psychological concomitants of physical disease."

These remarks by Scofield exemplify much of the approach and thinking we have undertaken in establishing our Division of Pediatric Psychology.

The pediatric psychologist in this agency is a scientist-clinician who serves as a consultant to the pediatric staff on matters concerning mental health needs as they arise in pediatric practice. Because our division of Pediatric Psychology is administratively and clinically part of the Department of Pediatrics, our psychologists work directly with the pediatric staff and not indirectly through a psychiatric facility. The medical responsibility for patient care, therefore, rests with the physician in charge of the patient, the pediatrician. This is a very sensible approach for everyone involved, particularly the patient. Moreover, it increases the efficiency of the psychologist, not only in his role as a clinician, but in his role in medical education as well. This point will become more apparent as I describe our functions and procedures.

I want to emphasize the importance of having the pediatric psychologist function as a *consultant* and not as a technician. In his role as a consultant, he deals with problems concerning human behavior. As a technician he becomes technique-oriented and is busy doing what is commonly referred to as "psychologicals," "routine psychological testing," "a battery of tests," "psychometrics," and "projectives." This tradition commonly results in long waiting periods for these time-consuming procedures to be administered; also, they are usually requested without the benefit of a conference between the referring physician and the psychologist. Furthermore, as a result, many patients are over-examined, some who do not really require testing are examined, and often the outcome is an unnecessarily long report that might not provide the physician with the information he wanted in the first place. This technique-oriented procedure of "routine psychologicals" usually overtaxes the already burdened psychological services and interfers with the efficient delivery of greatly needed mental health services.

A long delay between the referral for psychological help and its implementation usually results not only in many patients failing to keep their appointments, but it can interfere with the total workup of a patient's problems which in a medical setting requires greater speed. In teaching centers, medical students, interns, and residents would probably have rotated to a different location by the time the psychologist has completed his task and would miss out on the opportunity of learning about the behavioral implications of the patient's problems. This lag has done much damage to the image of our profession and has understandably caused many physicians to place little value on psychological help.

Technique-oriented service places very great stress on administrative, secretarial, and professional efforts and very often occurs in a setting that engages in other routine, time-consuming procedures such as intake interviews and intake conferences requiring a patient to unburden to a number of people before help is offered. At The New York Hospital-Cornell Medical Center we have eliminated the problems I have enumerated by adopting the following orientation in the performance of pediatric psychological services. These services include (1) diagnostic evaluation, (2) assistance in patient management, and (3) behavior modification or psychological therapy.

When assistance in these areas is required, the request for a *psychological consultation* is made by the physician in charge of the patient, and not by anyone else, in the form of questions or problems that the pediatrician has concerning this patient and *not* as a request for a particular technique to be administered. The consultation request is made by telephone at the time the physician is with the patient and, generally, a meeting is arranged within one hours. This we call an "on-the-spot consultation" which provides an opportunity for discussion about the patient immediately and in the presence of nurses, medical students, interns, and other staff concerned with that patient. It enables clarification of the problem and offers the psychologist the opportunity of doing his own screening and, in particular, the chance to screen out the inappropriate referrals right away without putting the patients' names on a waiting list. Moreover, it eliminates the time-consuming job of wading through charts since the referring physician can summarize the relevant information verbally, and it facilitates referral of the patient to other resources, if appropriate, without further delay. Most important, it enables the psychologist to see the patient immediately for a diagnostic evaluation if that is necessary or to arrange an appointment directly with the patient if it is not possible for the patient to be seen at that time.

When a diagnostic evaluation is conducted, the procedures employed are determined by the questions about the patient which the pediatrician and psychologist have arrived at in their discussion. Very often the answers to these questions can be obtained within a short period of time. By focusing on the question or the problem we avoid over-examination of the patient; consequently, we are not burdened by the time-consuming routine battery of tests and can see more patients with very little, if any, delay. The efficiency of this method of operation for patient care is clearly implied by its immediacy. We have been able to operate on this basis for a considerable period of time now, with a relatively small staff, without accumulating any waiting list. Before this procedure was instituted, a six-month waiting list had been accumulated. A monumental effort was required to clear that list while handling all new consultation requests "on the spot."

These procedures have been very helpful to our pediatric staff who now view psychology in the most positive way. They turn to us frequently, thus allowing us to share our knowledge about human behavior, which has resulted in a heightened respect for the psychological aspects of pediatric practice and has gained us their recognition as valuable behavioral scientist-clinicians.

Through the development of this new orientation, where the psychologist is a consultant rather than a technician, where he directs his focus on probelms and questions rather than techniques, and where he does his own screening "on the spot," a very efficient mental health service has been developed. It provides:

1) Immediate screening so that little delay occurs for other disposition.

2) Early diagnosis of learning, developmental, and emotional problems.

3) Transmission of the most current knowledge from the behavioral sciences to the pediatric staff.

4) Knowledge of child-rearing practices towards the development of greater emotional strength.

5) Sensitization of the pediatric staff to the emotional needs of children and help in decreasing the traumatic nature of medical procedures and hospitalization.

   With the psychologist directly available to the pediatrician in the manner I have outlined, the pediatrician can exercise his potentially strong position in the early diagnosis and prevention of mental disturbances.

References

1. New Issues in Infant Development. *Annals of the New York Academy of Sciences*, 1965, Vol. 118.
2. Brown, J.H.U. Behavioral sciences and the medical school. *Science*, 1969, *163*, 964-967.
3. Dubos, R., Savage, D., and Schaedler, R. Biological Freudianism—lasting effects of early environmental influences. *Pediatrics,* 1966, *38*, No. 5, 789-800.
4. Salk, L. The pediatrician's mental health role: A psychologist's view. *Pediatric Psychology Bulletin*, 1969, *1*, No. 1.
5. Salk, L. Psychologist in a pediatric setting. *Professional Psychology*, 1970, *1*, No. 4, 395-397.
6. Scofield, W. The role of psychology in the delivery of health services. *The American Psychologist*, 1969, *24*, No. 6, 565-584.
7. Wright, L. The pediatric psychologist: A role model. *The American Psychologist*, 1967, *22*, 323-325.

Part Three

FROM RESEARCH IN
CHILD DEVELOPMENT
TO DEVELOPMENTAL CHILD CARE

The research of child psychologists has provided the impetus for what is now a massive child care movement. The struggle to implement the knowledge that will benefit young children has forced the clinical child psychologist into the arena of vested interests, community control, and power politics. The struggle continues as we enter an era of innovative intervention on behalf of young children.

11. Psychological Assessment, Developmental Plasticity, and Heredity, with Implications for Early Education*

J. McV. Hunt

Evidence from comparative linguistics convinced Benjamin Whorf (1956) that language does a great deal to shape throught and understanding. Although our topic is cognitive development, the concern is with what in these days we term *mental retardation*. This term seems to indicate that something in the mind has slowed or lagged. It makes time *per se* the central factor in the development of mind. It was not ever thus. When I was taking graduate courses instead of teaching them, the prevailing term for the set of conditions now subsumed under *mental retardation* was *feeble-minded*, or if one wished a fancy term with Greek roots, *oligophrenia*, which also means weak-minded.

Euphemisms are the rule in the semantics of behavioral defects. While in the end both "weakness" and "retardation" imply defect, this shift in terminology, for which we psychologists are in large measure responsible, carries a substantial shift in conception which influences behavior. I suppose the empirical grounds for this shift were laid by Binet and Simon when they first noted a rough correlation of competence on their tests of judgment, comprehension, and reasoning with age. From this rough correlation came their term *mental age*. This shift in emphasis from weakness of mind to delay in development got further support in 1912 when Wilhelm Stern suggested dividing mental age by chronological age to get the intelligence quotient (IQ). Stern made this suggestion on the assumption that the rate of development is a fundamental trait in which individuals differ. This shift in emphasis got fixed in our culture when, in the 1920s and '30s, IQs and mental ages based on Ter-

---

man's 1916 revision and standardization of the Binet scales came to provide the legal limits for what had theretofore been loosely defined terms: *moron* (IQ: 50-75, or MA: 8-12), *imbecile* (IQ: 12-49, or MA: 2-7), and *idiot* (IQ less than 20, or MA less than 2 years). When Arnold Gesell's descriptions of the behavior typical of successive ages got widely disseminated, they habituated the notion that development comes more or less automatically with age. Despite the controversy over the developmental constancy of the IQ, this habit of thought about the role of time in development and about the longitudinal predictive value of IQs has become strong and persistent.

During the past decade we have been encountering some unhappy consequences of this habit of thought. Outside professional circles of psychology and education, people in various minority groups have rebelled against the implication that an hour's performance in an artificial testing situation could demonstrate and prove the inevitable and permanent retarded inferiority of their children. They have made their rebellion felt. Within the profession, moreover, habits of thought about the IQ have led to disappointment and confusion when gains in IQ from special educational programs shortly disappear after the gainers were returned to the home and school environments from whence they had come.

Such obviously unhappy consequences are, I believe, but the visible portion of an iceberg of misconception. Unobvious but perhaps more unfortunate are other consequences. Exceedingly unfortunate are the fates of those children whose low scores on IQ tests have led their teachers to expect from them little learning and therefore to use little teaching ingenuity in their behalf. Just as unfortunate is the failure of tests of intelligence to provide information of use in selecting curricular materials to promote development and learning. Most unfortunate of all, perhaps, is the false confidence in a view of intelligence as a kind of power in which individuals differ consistently regardless of the circumstances of their lives. The process of measuring this power by comparing the test scores of individuals, moreover, has probably greatly increased the tendency toward competitiveness in our society. Comparative rankings and competitiveness are probably inevitable in human affairs. A degree of competitiveness is highly desirable, but assessing development by way of individual differences has exaggerated this proneness to competitiveness and distracted both parents and teachers from focusing on what is to be learned and on the task of encouraging the development of the young. Moreover, this comparative approach to assessment has tended to prevent educators and psychologists from concerning themselves with the concrete nature of the intelligence and motivation underlying competence as a hierarchy of learning sets, of strategies for processing information, of concepts, and of skills built up sequentially in ordinal fashion. The false confidence in a view of intelligence as a kind of faculty-like power, moreover, has stood in the way of investigating the implications of this hierarchical view. Thus, if the obviously unhappy consequences of what has become our traditional habit of thought in this domain call forth a conceptual revision, that will be splendid. This revision should lead, I believe, to a new strategy in the assessment or measurement of psychological development and of competence which, hopefully, will encourage rather than discourage ingenuity in teaching.

Toward a Revised Conception of Intelligence

A decade ago, in *Intelligence and Experience* (Hunt, 1961), I tried to alter our habits of thought about cognitive development and intelligence with both argument and evidence. On the side of argument, I contended that IQ scores on tests of intelligence are valid only as an assessment of past acquisitions, that they have very little validity as predictors of future IQs or performances without knowledge of the circumstances to be encountered. I suggested that we should think of psychological development and of intelligence as a hierarchy of learning sets, strategies of information processing, concepts, motivational systems, and skills acquired in the course of each child's on-going interactions, and especially informational interaction, with his environmental circumstances. On the side of evidence, I reviewed a substantial body of investigative results indicating a great deal of plasticity in psychological development. From these several lines of evidence and argument, I suggested that readiness is no mere matter of maturation that takes place automatically with living to a given age. Rather, it is a matter of information stored, of concepts, strategies, and motivational systems achieved, and of skills acquired. There I also introduced what I like to call *"the problem of the match"* which I later elaborated (Hunt, 1963a, 1965, 1966). This is a problem especially for parents and teachers and for all those who wish to foster psychological development in the young. The nature of the problem is based on the view that adaptive growth takes place only, or at least chiefly, in situations which contain for any given infant or child information and models just discrepant enough from those already stored and mastered to produce interest or challenge and to call for adaptive modifications in the structure of his intellectural coping, his beliefs about the world, and his motor patterns which are not beyond his adaptive capacity at the time.

Theorizing and investigating relevant to these views coming during the past decade have served both to strengthen them and to suggest elaborations. Let me mention a few of these theoretical developments and bits of evidence.

The decade brought Humphreys' (1962a) demonstration-argument that tests of intelligence are basically like tests of achievement in that both call upon previously acquired percepts, concepts, motives, and skills. The fact that the tests of intelligence call for older acquisitions for which the learning situations are more difficult to specify than do achievement tests does not destroy the basic similarity. Moreover, Humphreys (1962b) has extended Ferguson's (1956, 1959) explanation of the ability factors derived from factor analysis in terms of positive transfer of training by showing how the experimental manipulations which have traditionally been used to study the transfer of training can account for the obtained nodes of intercorrelation among abilities. While these analyses provide a clear theoretical basis for an important role of experience in the development of intelligence as it has been traditionally measured and analyzed, they provide parents and teachers with little in the way of guidance concerning how interests and abilities build dynamically one upon another, and they are of little use in choosing the circumstances best calculated to foster the development of new levels of ability in children.

My notion of the "problem of the match" and its later elaborations (Hunt, 1963a, 1965, 1966) make cognitive acquisitions of central importance for development in other domains and especially for motivation. This notion has received considerable support. Several studies of attentional preference in very young infants, done by my own group, have lent support to the view that emerging recognitive familiarity motivates the maintenance of perceptual contact with whatever is becoming perceptually recognizable (Hunt, 1970; Uzgiris & Hunt, 1970; Greenberg, Uzgiris, & Hunt, 1970; Weizmann, Cohen, & Pratt, 1971). The motivational import of what is becoming recognitively familiar is less a stage of psychological development, however, than a phase in the course of information processing. This is suggested by a still tentative finding that when infants nearly a year old are presented regularly in tests of four minutes with pairs of patterns, one of which is presented regularly test after test and the other intermittently every seventh test, they come to look longer at the regularly presented patterns before (i.e., after fewer tests than) they come to look longer at the intermittently presented patterns (Hunt & Paraskevopoulos, in preparation). Other observational evidence came in the course of developing our ordinal scale of imitation (Uzgiris & Hunt, 1966, 1968). Our observation that infants regularly showed pseudo-imitation of highly familiar gestural and vocal patterns before they imitate unfamiliar ones suggests this same course of development. Moreover, our observations indicated great motivational importance for the match between the model presented and the previous achievements of the infant. Infants are strongly motivated to imitate only models which challenge to a proper degree their perceptual and cognitive grasp or their motor skills. They withdraw from models too "old hat" or simple out of apparent boredom. They become distressed and angry with models which call for either cognitive or motor adaptations beyond them. I believe one can say that an infant will imitate only what he can understand. Thus, what he does toward imitating a given model often serves to show what he understands of that model or how he views the model

Other bits of evidence supporting this view that cognitive developments are of importance to development in various other domains such as emotion and motivation have come from investigations in other laboratories. The role of cognitive achievement in behavior indicative of emotion is illustrated in a very recent study by Schultz and Zigler (1971). On the assumption that a clown presented in a stationary condition would be easier to assimilate perceptually than the same clown in motion, due to difficulty in following contours, they predicted that such expressions of pleasure as visual fixation, smiling, and nonstressful vocalizing would occur earlier for the stationary than for the moving condition. The findings clearly confirmed this prediction. The role of cognitive achievement in motivation is illustrated in the finding by Zigler, Levine, and Gould (1967) that children of school age appreciate and prefer cartoons near the upper limit of their comprehension. In my own theorizing (Hunt, 1965), I have suggested that the self-concept, and especially the ideal self-concept, may well be the most important cognitive construct for the motivation of achievement and social behavior. It was especially interesting, therefore, to find Katz and Zigler (1967) suggesting that the disparity between the concepts of self and ideal self should be related to developmental maturity because such maturity involves capacity for cognitive differentiation. Their finding of positive associations of both chronological age and IQ with the size of the disparities between the self and the ideal self lend support to this contention that cognitive development is important in other domains, and especially in motivation. In this same vein, Kohlberg and Zigler (1967) have suggested that a child's concept of his sex role results largely from having categorized himself as either male or female early in development. Inasmuch as cognitive development involves transformations of the mental constructions of a child's environment, they reason that both mental age and IQ should be positively correlated with maturity of social development, and they found mature trends in social development coming earlier in children with IQs above average than in children of average IQ.

The Issue of Motivational Autonomy

While these findings lend support to the contention that developments within the cognitive domain are of importance for development in other domains of psychological development, they also raise questions. All too seldom do the gains on tests of intelligence and achievement from various systems of compensatory education persist once the children are returned to the environments of their homes and standard schools. From the traditional view of essentially predetermined maturation and development, one would argue that these gains have been obtained only in the limited cognitive skills assessed and that development in the other domains awaits maturation of the organism as a whole. Inasmuch as the evidence which I shall shortly synopsize suggests that maturation itself shows considerable plasticity, I question seriously such an explanation. I suspect that the failure of the gains from so many systems of compensatory education to persist resides rather in their failure to provide experiences calculated to inculcate ideal self-concepts which include professed ability to learn readily along with pride in such learning which yield autonomous striving.

It is likely that such motivational systems have their developmental beginnings very early. Burton White (1971) has found that the behavioral patterns of outstanding over-all competence are already present in children by age three. He is now emphasizing the importance of the period between ages 10 months and three years in early home-based education. Inasmuch as evidence of great plasticity exists in various lines of development during the first year, however, this finding is probably based on cultural practices of child-rearing during the first year which differ relatively little from home to home and class to class. It is rather during the period from 10 months to 3 years in age when the burgeoning capacities of infants for manipulation and locomotion put considerable stress on mothers that the child-rearing across homes probably differs enough to show prominently in the competence of the young by age three. Observations of the joy which infants of only two months show in connection with making a mobile sway by shaking themselves (Hunt & Uzgiris, 1964; Uzgiris & Hunt, 1970) and similar observations by Watson (1966, 1967) suggest that the beginnings of the motivation to act upon the world to achieve ends anticipated by the infant begins very early indeed. Robert White (1959) has characterized such motivation by the term *competence* and contended that it is an associated emotion which he calls *effectance*. I have attempted to describe a mechanism for such motivation inherent in information processing and action (Hunt, 1960, 1963b, 1965, 1971a, 1971b).

The importance of perceptual feedback to action in such early development has been illustrated in a study reported by Yarrow, Rubenstein, and Pedersen (1971) at the Society for Research in Child Development. This system of motivation (there called goal orientation) was assessed in infants at six months of age by a cluster of six items on the Bayley Scales which included some persistent and purposeful attempts to secure objects out of reach. Highly consonant with the view I have described is the fact that the measure of goal orientation correlated $+.38$ infants' with maternal responsiveness to their infants' expressions of distress. According to standard operant theory with its emphasis upon overt behavior, the contingency of maternal response to such distress behaviors as crying should reinforce those overt behaviors. It did not. In such young infants, apparently, the contingency of maternal response to distressful vocalization reinforces hope of change in the circumstances and contributes toward a general level of confidence on the part of the infant that he can control his circumstances. Such is the epigenesis of early development that later, however, such a contingency would reinforce the overt crying. Out of such experiences of being able to change conditions comes gradually, I suspect, a kind of learning set which we (not the infant) might verbalize as: "If I act, I can get what I want and make interesting things happen." I contend that this learning set is basically cognitive in character. It is knowledge of infant self in relation to the world. If the child has tried and tried to no avail, he derives another kind of learning set which must be corrected if he is ever to achieve confidence and hope that he can achieve his ends and to develop the pride in achievement that leads to the achievement of excellence in performance.

We know all too little about the successive landmarks in the development of these learning sets and concepts with motivational significance. Because we have thought of cognition largely in terms of such school skills as language, or reading, or numbering, our various systems of compensatory education have omitted even any attempt to provide corrective experiences of significance for motivation. Years ago, Andras Angyal (1941) described and emphasized a general dynamic trend toward increasing autonomy in psychological development. We need to know more about fostering such motivational autonomy and more about how long it takes.

Maturation and Experience

In our various conceptions of development, learning and maturation have been as separate conceptually, and presumable in actuality, as Kipling's east and west. The decade just past, however, has brought clear evidence that informational interaction, or especially encounters with circumstances through the eyes, influences maturation within the central nervous system. Studies of the effects of early perceptual experience on maze learning in rats and dogs, inspired by Hebb's (1949) theorizing, go back to the decade of the '50s (see Hunt, 1961, pp. 100-106). Riesen, also inspired by Hebb's theorizing, first reported even earlier (Riesen, 1947, 1958) the effects of rearing chimpanzees in the dark on the number of nerve cells and glial cells in their retinal ganglia as adults. And Brattgard (1952), inspired by the biochemical theorizing of Helgar Hyden, had reported that rearing rabbits in the dark caused a paucity of RNA production of their retinal ganglia as adults. Since then, the California group has reported that thickness of the cerebral cortex and the level of total acetylcholinesterase activity of the cortex as well as rate of adult maze—learning are a function of the complexity of the environment during early life (Bennett, Diamond, Krech, & Rosenzweig, 1964; Krech, Rosenzweig, & Bennett, 1966). Moreover, studies of the effects of dark-rearing during early life have been extended up the visual system. Such dark-rearing produces a paucity of both cells and glial fibers in the lateral geniculate body of the thalamus (Wiesel & Hubel, 1963). And, as the Spanish investigator Valverde has shown, dark-rearing also decreases both dendritic branching and the number of spines which develop on the dendritic processes of the large apical cells of the striate area in the occipital lobes of mice (Valverde, 1967, 1968; Valverde & Esteban, 1968). Calmerde's approach should now be extended to the coordination of the visual system with other systems. Such evidence strongly suggests considerable plasticity in the maturation of the neuroanatical equipment for information processing.

Spurious Factors in Longitudinal Validity

Intelligence testing has assumed approximately equal opportunity for learning, at least in typical families. This past decade has yielded evidence of vast variations in the opportunities which present themselves for acquisition of cognitive skills, motivational systems for competence, and values and standards of conduct required by a complex organized society (see Hunt, 1969, pp. 202-214). Such opportunities are lacking most often for children of the poor, but Burton White (1917) has found some of the mothers who are most effective as infant teachers within the poverty sector of Aid to Dependent Children. Moreover, we all know examples of children in middle-class families whose opportunities are limited in various ways by ineffective mothering.

Results from other recent studies have raised other methodological issues which depress the traditional import of longitudinal validity coefficient at least to me, yet both psychologists and educators ask almost regularly about the predictive value of the measures of development from the ordinal scales which Uzgiris and I have developed. It seems likely that the failure of the evidence for plasticity to be more widely convincing resides in the longitudinal validity correlations between the IQs from testing widely separated in time. Bloom (1964) based much of his discussion of stability and change on such evidence. It has been presumed generally that the basis for the existence of such correlations resides within the individual differences in the rates of development for the tested individuals. This is, to be sure, one source of the obtained coefficients, but there are, I believe, at least two other sources which are spurious for such an interpretation.

If tests of intelligence measure achievement, as I believe Humphreys (1962a) has demonstrated, then the correlation between successive testings involves part-whole relationships in which the size of the part in the first testing approaches the size of the whole in the latter testing as the time between the testings decreases (Humphreys, 1962b). The portion of a longitudinal validity coefficient deriving from this part-whole relationship is completely irrelevant to any assumption of inherent stability in rates of individual development.

The second spurious factor in these longitudinal correlations is to be found in consistency of developmental impact of home and neighborhood environments. The recent investigation by Yarrow, *et al.* (1971) is relevant here. On his team Pedersen reports that measures of home environments—social and inanimate—which were based on two three-hour time samplings taken a week apart show correlations with various measures of performance from the Bayley Scales ranging to above .5, thereby accounting for 25% of the variance in the measures of infant performance at age 6 months. If merely two three-hour samples a week apart can represent the impact of environmental circumstances for the first half year of the lives of infants sufficiently well to account for 25% of the variance in any of their performances at 6 months, then the consistency in the developmental impact of home environments is much greater than we have ever conceived such consistency to be. Whatever portion of the longitudinal validity-coefficient derives from this consistency in the developmental impact of home environments is entirely spurious as an indicator of inherent individual differences in rate of maturation. These spurious contributions from the part-whole relationship and from the consistency in the developmental impact in the environment subtracts substantially from the traditional import of the longitudinal validity-coefficients for the IQ.

Revised Strategies of Measurement

In his lectures *On Understanding Science,* Conant (1947, p. 48) "put down as one of the principles learned from the history of science that a theory is only overthrown by a better theory, never merely by contradictory facts." I believe Conant might have added that whenever a strategy and technology of measurement is imbedded in a prevailing conceptual scheme, it becomes additionally difficult to revise that conceptual scheme with a combination of both evidence dissonant with it and new conceptual alternatives. The tests of intelligence are generally recognized as one of the great monuments of achievement by modern psychology. Yet, as I have already pointed out, they have left many problems in psychological development unsolved and have even distracted attention from them. For three-quarters of a century they have focused attention on comparative measures of individual differences in a power (the IQ or Spearman's g) or a multiplicity of powers (Thurstone, 1938; Guilford, 1967). I believe this focus has distracted investigators from seeing how in the various lines of psychological development the actual landmarks of ability and of motivation build one upon another. I believe this focus has also distracted investigators from investigating the nature of the successive learning sets which enable and motivate a child to process information and to solve problems at successive levels of complexity. Instead of helping to tell teachers how to prepare the curricular environment to foster the development of any given child, the scores from the tests have tended to destroy the motivation for ingenuity in teaching by explaining poor pupil performance as "to be expected." Forunately, the beginnings of new strategies for the measurement of learning and development are appearing.

One of these consists of criterion-referenced tests (Glaser, 1963). This strategy derives from the hierarchical conception of intelligence suggested by Gagne's studies of adult problem-solving (Gagne & Paradise, 1961). In this strategy, Glaser (Glaser, 1963; Glaser & Nitko, 1971) contrasts the *criterion-reference* with the *norm-reference* which is characteristic of the standard test-batteries for both intelligence and achievement. In the case of traditional norm-referenced tests, the performance of an individual acquires its meaning from some index of its comparative rank among the scores describing the performances of the various individuals in the representative group on which the norms for the test are based. In the case of criterion-referenced tests, on the other hand, the meaning of any individual's performance derives directly from the behavioral goal of the educational experience which has been provided for him. It is this behavioral goal which defines the performance desired of the tested subject, and his performance in turn determines the criterion of success for the educational effort. This strategy of criterion-referencing gives new meaning to the standard concepts of reliability and validity for test scores (Popham & Husek, 1969). Reliability derives from examiner agreement and validity is inherent in the relationship between the examinee's performance and the educational goal. Thus, this strategy also has the very considerable advantage of focusing the attention and effort of both teacher and student upon the goal of the educational effort and of avoiding the distraction which is almost inevitable from the interpersonal comparisons involved in norm-referencing. Missing from such a strategy, however, is any developmental frame of reference which can help explain failure and help guide a teacher's choice of learning experiences. It might also be noted that age and time figure not at all in this strategy of measurement.

The second new strategy consists of ordinal scales of psychological development. This strategy is at least illustrated by our own ordinal scales of development in infancy (Uzgiris & Hunt, 1966, 1968). These scales, inspired by Piaget's (1936, 1937) observations of his own three children, consist of sequentially ordinal landmarks for six overlapping lines of development through what Piaget has termed the sensorimotor phase. Each landmark consists of specified behavior elicited by a specified situation. Inter-observer agreement on the criterion behaviors is typically above 95%. Test-retest consistency for examinations conducted within 48 hours is typically above 85%, and the great majority of the changes which occur are upward on the scales. The ordinality of the steps on the various scales as indicated by Green's (1956) index of consistency range from a low of .802, for the scale on the development of relating to objects, to a high of .991, for the scale on the construction of operational causality. For all but two of our six scales, Green's index of consistency is well above .9. In some instances, the invariance in sequence is logically built in, but contrary to the argument of Mary Shirley (1931) such invariance of sequence need logically imply no predetermined maturation. It is basically a function of the infant's informational interactions with his environment. These interactions produce developments which permit other, higher-order forms of information interaction.

The sequential ordinality of steps in these scales provides a novel strategy for the measurement of psychological development. One can compare the development of two infants, regardless of their ages, in terms of their positions on each of the scales. This ordinality permits one to reverse the traditional strategy of measuring psychological development. It permits making age the dependent variable which varies as a function of kind of experience instead of the independent variable implied in our traditional concept of the IQ and in the normative descriptions of Arnold Gesell, et al. (1940). These sequentially ordinal landmarks permit one to define successive levels of development in terms of success on lower landmarks on the scale and failure on those above. One then can compare the means and variances of age for infants who have lived from birth under differing kinds of circumstances. These variations in age permit one to compare the educational, or development-fostering, quality of these differing circumstances. Such measures based on ordinals scales may have the additional value of referring only to past experience and making no claims of persistence in the rate of development.

Ordinal landmarks in development need imply no position on the issue concerning whether psychological development is continuous or stepwise. We have identified more landmarks than the six sensorimotor stages described by Piaget. Our scale of object permanence, for instance, consists of 14 sequentially ordinal landmarks. From the evidence with which I am now acquainted, I believe that psychological development is continuous and that high consistency values for measures of sequential ordinality are a function of selecting behavioral landmarks with sufficient distance between them. This domain is wide open for investigation. The landmarks which we have selected are little more than first approximations of what can ultimately derive from exploring behavioral development with such a strategy. If we are ever to have the basis for guiding the learning of the young in what Piaget has termed the pre-conceptual phase, I believe this strategy must be extended through this phase. I suspect that investigations might be especially fruitful in providing the evidences of effectiveness for new educational efforts with pathologically retarded children.

It should be noted that the examining operations which define the sequentially achieved landmarks in development resemble criterion-referenced tests. In neither case does the meaning of an individual child's performance derive from comparison with the performance of others. In ordinal scales of psychological development, however, there is no educational experience with a behavioral goal to give meaning to the performance. Once the sequentially achieved landmarks have been identified, the meaning of any child's performance derives from where the performance places him along the sequentially ordinal scale.

New Evidence of Plasticity

The ordinal strategy of assessing psychological development is beginning to yield new evidence of plasticity. Elsewhere (Hunt, 1971c), I have called attention to the finding that providing very young infants with stabile patterns over their cribs to look at for at least half an hour each day has served to reduce the age at which the blink response appears by somewhat more than 3 weeks, (Greenberg, Uzgiris, & Hunt, 1968). There I have also called attention to White's (1967) experimental demonstration that experimental enrichments in which the chief factor appears to have been the opportunity to view stabiles of complexity adjusted to the infant's level of development served to reduce very substantially median ages for "fisted swiping" and "mature reaching" which are two of

the outstanding landmarks in the development of eye-hand coordination. For "mature reaching" the change in median age was from
145 days to 89 days. This result implies that what geneticists, since
the days of Waltereck (see Dunn, 1965), have termed the *norm of
reaction* for the age at which this landmark appears must be at least
the 56 days by which these two medians differ.

Neither the blink response nor eye-hand coordination are very
general or instrumental to later development. Neither are they
within the domain of what we usually think of as cognitive. On the
other hand, I believe that object construction is all three and I
believe that imitation is within the domain of cognition and that it is
motivationally instrumental to later development. We have recently
had examined with the scales of object permanence and both gestural and vocal imitation all of the children aged between 5 months
and 5 years who have lived from birth in two Athenian orphanages
with differing regimes of child-rearing (Paraskevopoulos & Hunt,
1971). The difference between the regimes of child-rearing can most
easily be specified in terms of the child-caretaker ratio. In the
Municipal Orphanage, this ratio is of the order of 10/1. In the other,
the Metera Baby Centre which attempts to be a model institution for
children, this ratio is on the average through the day approximately
3/1 or 4/1. We also had examined some 94 home-reared children
from working-class families. The mean ages for the children of the
Municipal Orphanage lagged progressively for those at successive
levels of object permanence. Let me take, for example, that level at
which children follow an object through one hidden displacement
but not through a series of such displacements. The mean ages of the
children at this level in the Municipal Orphanage was 33.2 months,
of those at Metera, 21.8 months, and those home-reared 20.3
months. The mean for the children at the Municipal Orphanage
differs significantly from both those at Metera and those
homereared. As an empirical estimate of the age norm of reaction
for this level of object permanence, these mean ages for infants in
these two orphanages are but a part of the picture. David Schickedanz has been following the development of infants in the
Parent-and-Child Center at Mt. Carmel, Illinois. Six successive
infants from parents of poverty who have been developing under the
regime there, which I shall characterize shortly, have achieved this
level of following an object through one hidden displacement before
they were a year old. Their average age would be approximately
11.5 months. Thus, the norm of reaction of this level of object construction must be at least of the order of 21 months. Similar norms of

reaction exist for the ages at which children achieve the upper levels of vocal imitation. Clearly the circumstances encountered by children can make a very substantial difference in the ages at which such early intellectual and notivational landmarks are achieved. How important various degrees of lag in such early development are for future development remains for investigation. Perhaps I should note here also that, unless my clinical hunch is far afield, language development demands having achieved both object construction through hidden displacements and the development of an interest in imitating unfamiliar vocal patterns. In order to disabuse myself as soon as possible of a mistaken hypothesis, I am now looking for children who have begun to speak who lack one or the other of these achievements. How object construction and language are related in blind children deserves special scrutiny in this connection. I should also note in passing that it is hard not to view social-class differences in ability to communicate to be related to those very conditions of social interaction in which the childrearing of the social class have been shown to differ most, at least on the average (Hunt, 1969, Ch. 7).

A methodological implication should be mentioned here. Neither the traditional cross-sectional strategy of assessing development in differing groups nor traditional longitudinal investigation which follows the development of individuals within a given ecological niche can yield the kinds of information we need about the relation of psychological development to environmental encounters for purposes of childrearing and education. What we need is to combine the longitudinal approach with the experimental, or quasi-experimental, by following longitudinally the development of comparable groups of genotypes developing under differing conditions. In this connection, simultaneously contemporary experimental and control groups are probably unfeasible, but one can use wave design with successive groups developing under progressively enriched conditions.

Plasticity and Heredity

I have been using here the genetic concept of the "norm of reaction." This concept should be more familiar to educators and psychologists who are typically so concerned with the pseudo-issue of whether environment or heredity is more important that they make two common conceptual errors. First, as Hirsch (1970), the behavioral geneticist, has pointed out, they typically test groups of individuals at a single time of life. The resulting proportions of the variance assigned to environment and to heredity concern the relative amounts of variance among individuals developing within a given range of variation in circumstances. Such assessments of variance are then applied quite incorrectly to individuals. Secondly, these assessments of variance among individuals or comparable statistical indices of heritability are used to make inferences about the educability of individuals. The educability of an individual calls for solid evidence about the norm of reaction. But a statistical index of heritability, to quote Hirsch (1970, p. 101) "provides no information about the norm of reaction."

Concern with this pseudo-issue of whether environment or heredity is more important gets those who find and point out the evidence of plasticity in phenotypic measures of intellectual and motivation development tarred with the opprobrious semantic brush of environmentalism. I wish to point out that evidence of plasticity are not dissonant with a primary role for heredity. Heredity is always primary. The genotype in the fertilized ovum constitutes the starting point for an individual. The DNA in the genes contains information which set the main lines of development throughout life. Yet this information goes nowhere in an environmental vacuum and gets modified by variations in various environmental conditions. This DNA is far from totally predetermining. Development comes dynamically in the course of a continuing process of interaction between the individual at any given time and its environmental circumstances at that given time. The resulting norm or range of reaction for most of the traits in which educators and psychologists are interested is great. Even so, heredity remains primary in determining the size of the difference between phenotypic measures which will come from any two sets of differing circumstances. One might put this principle more simply by saying that the genotype determines the norm of reaction. Unfortunately such a statement is scientifically meaningless because neither the genotype nor the ultimate norm of reaction is measureable and knowable.

One can best illustrate this principle concretely. Suppose, for example, the existence of two pairs of identical twins, one pair typical or normal, the other mongoloid. Suppose one of each pair were reared from birth in the Municipal Orphanage of Athens where neither becomes a pet of the caretaker. Suppose the other is reared in Metera under the carefully supervised regime there. Which pair would show the greater difference in age of achieving that level of object construction in which it follows an object through one hidden displacement but not several? I believe you will agree that the difference in age to be expected for the normal pair will be greater than that for the mongoloid pair. I have designated one pair as mongoloid here in order to permit recognition of the limitation on genotype potential at birth. In principle, the same prediction should hold for pairs which differ in potential within the normal range. Thus, hypothetically at least, the genotype determines the amount of the effect on a phenotype measure which on-going interaction in two differing environments can have. The threshold conception of environmental influence, epitomized as "normal environmental conditions" in which this hypothetical threshold is regularly achieved in typical families, is likely to be very far from true. Evidence from the study by Paraskevopoulos and Hunt (1971), already cited, calls this view into serious question. This evidence derives from the standard deviations of the ages for the children at the higher levels of object construction and vocal imitation. As might be expected, the standard deviations for children who follow an object through one or more hidden displacements are smallest (approximately 2.5 months) for those children at Metera where conditions of rearing are relatively standardized. At the Municipal Orphanage, where the child-caretaker ratio of 10/1 inevitably results in combinations of pets and neglected children, the standard deviations of ages for children at this same pair of levels are of the order of 7 months; for home-reared children the standard deviations at these levels are even larger, through not significantly larger, than those for the Municipal Orphanage. Moreover, these large standard deviations come not from distributions composed of a cluster of cases at the lower end of the distribution with a single case or two at the high end as would be expected if the environment operates in threshold fashion.

Implications for the Mentally Retarded

The implications for the mentally retarded from the conceptual revisions and evidence I have outlined come in two categories. One category consists of suggestions for fostering their intellectual and motivational development. The other category is methodological, namely, that we utilize the interest which exists in those mentally retarded to get a better understanding of the nature of psychological development.

The fact that the babies of parents from the poverty sector of the Parent-and-Child Center in Mt. Carmel, Illinois, are developing rapidly, as evidenced by the early ages at which they are achieving the successive landmarks on our Ordinal Scales, and also happily, suggests that what the caretaker-mothers of these children are being taught about child-rearing is on at least a promising track. What they

are being taught by Mrs. Earladeen Badger (1971, 1972) is conceptually quite simple. First, the mothers, who are also the caretakers
in this Parent-and-Child Center, are encouraged strongly to believe
that how they interact with and treat their babies will make an
important difference in their future. Second, they are encouraged,
while their babies are very young, to be responsive to their behavioral indicators of distress. Third, they are taught to observe their
infants in their interaction with models and play materials for behavioral indications of interest and surprise, of boredom, and of the distressful frustration that comes with situations with which the infant
cannot cope. Fourth, they are encouraged to provide their infants
with materials and models which bring forth the behavioral signs of
interest, and to remove those which appear to be either boring or
threatening. Finally, they are shown something about the sequences
of developing abilities and interests to help them choose materials
which will interest their infants.

In the course of her own teaching of mothers and observing of
children, Mrs. Badger is gleaning a number of clinical suggestions
about these developmental sequences extending beyond the sensorimotor into the preconceptual phase. For instance, once infants
in their play with a shape-box have achieved the level where they
put the blocks of varying shapes in holes with appropriate shapes
without active experimentation but merely from visual inspection,
they can be happily interested in picture-matching games. On the
other hand, while they are still struggling with a rectangular block in
a square hole, and a square block in he circular hole, any attempt to
introduce picture-matching games is a source of threat and distress.
Such procedures should be helpful in devising and testing educational strategies for fostering the psychological development of
chilren with mental retardation based upon pathological herdity.

In the methodological category, if we once take seriously the concept of psychological development as a hierarchy of learning sets,
strategies of information processing, and skills, built one upon
another in ordinal fashion, we must face the fact that our ignorance
of the details of its nature is abysmal. Two aspects of mental retardation suggest that mentally retarded children may be enabled to
gain something while simultaneously helping us to reduce our ignorance. Genotypically based difficulties in learning may actually be
helpful in uncovering the nature of the hierarchy of learning sets and
the special kinds of experience which foster their acquisition. In
1930, I spent nearly a half an hour a day throughout the summer
attempting unsuccessfully to teach an 8-year-old imbecile to count.

Following suggestions derived from the writings of Fernald, my method was to attempt through repetition to get this boy to coordinate in time saying the successive numbers and pointing to one object after another. It failed. I suspect that I failed because I had not considered providing him with experiences which then would have seemed quite irrelevant to the learning task. It did not then occur to me to consider or look for understandings and skills propaedeutic to such a coordination as that between saying numbers and pointing to objects. Neither did I think of ways to make that coordination meaningful and important. Today, in both cases, these are things I would consider although I confess that the search might be difficult.

Secondly, the new-found and growing interest in mental retardation promises to provide the support for investigators interested in utilizing the educational process to investigate the nature of the hierarchical structure of competence in mentally retarded infants and young children. A decade of taking seriously the hierarchical conception of learning sets in psychological development and investigating its concrete nature will almost certainly yield knowledge that will greatly improve our technology of early education. After such a decade, time *per se* will no longer loom so large as a cause of development. Perhaps, we shall then have new terminology for what we now call mental retardation.

References

Angyal, A. 1941. *Foundations for a science of personality.* New York: Commonwealth Fund.

Badger, Earladeen D. 1971. A Mother's training program—the road to a purposeful existence. *Children, 18* (No. 5), 168-173.

Badger, Earladeen D. 1972. The Mother's training program—Implementing a home start model in Parent-and-Child Centers. *Children,* (scheduled for March-April).

Bennett, E. L., Diamond, Marian C., Krech, D., & Rosenzweig, M. R. 1964. Chemical and anatomical plasticity of the brain. *Science, 146,* (No. 3644), 610-619.

Bloom, B. S. 1964. *Stability and change in human characteristics.* New York: Wiley.

Brattgard, S. O. 1952. The importance of adequate stimulation for the chemical composition of retinal ganglion cells during early post-natal development. *Acta Radiologica,* Stockholm, Suppl. 96, 1-80.

Conant, J. B. 1947. *On understanding science.* New Haven: Yale Univer. Press [Mentor Books, No. 68, 1951].

Dunn, L. C. 1965. *A short history of genetics.* New York: McGraw-Hill.

Ferguson, G. A. 1956. On transfer and the abilities of man. *Canadian Journal of Psychology, 10,* 121-131.

Ferguson, G. A. 1959. Learning and human ability: A theoretical approach. In P. H. DuBois, W. H. Manning, & C. J. Spies (Eds.), *Factor analysis and related techniques in the study of learning.* Technical Report No. 7, Office of Naval Research Contract No. Nonr 816 (02). Pp. 174-182.

Gagne, R. M., & Paradise, N. E. 1961. Abilities and learning sets in knowledge acquisition. *Psychological Monographs, 75,* No. 14 (Whole No. 518.)

Gesell, A., Halverson, H. M., Thompson, Helen, Ilg, Frances L., Castner, B. M., & Bates, Louise. 1940. *The first five years of life.* New York: Harper.

Glaser, R. 1963. Instructional technology and the measurement of learning outcomes: Some questions. *American Psychologist, 18,* 519-521.

Glaser, R., & Nitko, A. J. 1971. In R. L. Thorndike (Ed.), *Educational Measurement.* 2nd ed. Washington D. C.: American Council on Education.

Green, B. F. 1956. A method of scalogram analysis using summary statistics. *Psychometrika, 21,* 79-88.

Greenberg, D., Uzgiris, Ina C., & Hunt, J. McV. 1968. Hastening the development of the blink-response with looking. *Journal of Genetic Psychology, 113,* 167-176.

Greenberg, D. J., Uzgiris, Ina C., & Hunt, J. McV. 1970. Attentional preference and experience: III. Visual familiarity and looking time. *Journal of Genetic Psychology*, 117, 123-135.

Guilford, J. P. 1967. *The nature of human intelligence.* New York: McGraw-Hill.

Hebb, D. O. 1949. *The organization of behavior.* New York: Wiley.

Hirsch, J. 1970. Behavior-genetic analysis and its biosocial consequences. *Seminars in Psychiatry, 2,* 89-105.

Humphreys, L. G. 1962a. The nature and organization of human abilities. In M. Katz (Ed.), *The 19th Yearbook of the National Council on Measurement in Education.* Ames, Iowa. Pp. 39-45.

Humphreys, L. G. 1962b. The organization of human abilities. *American Psychologist, 17,* 475-483.

Hunt, J. McV. 1960. Experience and the development of motivation: Some reinterpretations. *Child Development, 31,* 489-504.

Hunt, J. McV. 1961. *Intelligence and experience.* New York: Ronald Press.

Hunt, J. McV. 1963a. Piaget's observations as a source of hypotheses concerning motivation. *Merrill-Palmer Quarterly, 9,* 263-275.

Hunt, J. McV. 1963b. Motivation inherent in information processing and action. In O. J. Harvey (Ed.), *Motivation and social interaction: The cognitive determinants.* New York: Ronald Press. Pp. 35-94.

Hunt, J. McV. 1965. Intrinsic motivation and its role in psychological development. In D. Levine (Ed.), *Nebraska Symposium on Motivation, 13,* 189-282. Lincoln: University of Nebraska Press.

Hunt, J. McV. 1966. Toward a theory of guided learning in development. In R. H. Ojemann & Karen Pritchett (Eds.), *Giving emphasis to guided learning.* Cleveland, Ohio: Educational Research Council. Pp. 98-160.

Hunt, J. McV. 1969. *The challenge of incompetence and poverty: Papers on the role of early education.* Urbana: University of Illinois Press.

Hunt, J. McV. 1970. Attentional preference and experience: I. Introduction. *Journal of Genetic Psychology, 117,* 99-107.

Hunt, J. McV. 1971a. Intrinsic motivation: Information and circumstance. In H. M. Schroder & P. Suedfeld, (Eds.), *Personality theory and information processing* New York: Ronald Press. (Ch. 4).

Hunt, J. McV. 1971b. Intrinsic motivation and pyschological development. In H. M. Schroder & P. Suedfeld, (Eds.), *Personality theory and information processing.* New York: Rona'd Press.(Ch. 5).

Hunt, J. McV. 1971c. Parent and child centers: Their basis in the behavioral and educational sciences. *American Journal of Orthopsychiatry, 41,* (1), 13-38.

Hunt, J. McV., & Uzgiris, Ina C. 1964. Cathexis from recognitive familiarity: An exploratory study. Paper presented at the Symposium to Honor J. P. Guilford, Convention of the American Psychological Association, September. To be published in P. R. Merrifield (Ed.), *Experimental and factor-analytic measurement of personality: Contributions by students of J. P. Guilford.* Kent, Ohio: Kent State University Press.

Katz, P., & Zigler, E. 1967. Self-image disparity: A developmental approach. *Journal of Personality and Social Psychology, 5,* 186-195.

Kohlberg, L., & Zigler, E. 1967. The impact of cognitive maturity on the development of sex-role attitudes in the years 4 to 8. *Genetic Psychology Monographs, 75,* 89-165.

Krech, D., Rosenzweig, M. R., & Bennett, E. L. 1966. Environmental impovishment, social isolation, and changes in brain chemistry and anatomy. *Physiology and Behavior, 1,* 99-104 (Pergamon Press, Great Britain).

Paraskevopoulos, J., & Hunt, J. McV. 1971. Object construction and imitation under differing conditions of rearing. *Journal of Genetic Psychology,* December, 1971.

Piaget, J. 1936. *The origins of intelligence in children.* (Margaret Cook, Transl.) New York: International Universities Press, 1952.

Piaget, J. 1937. *The construction of reality in the child.* (Margaret Cook, Transl.) New York: Basic Books, 1954.

Popham, W. J., & Husek, T. R. 1969. Implications of criterion-referenced measurement. *Journal of Educational Measurement, 6* (No. 1), 1-9.

Riesen, A. H. 1947. The development of visual perception in man and chimpanzee. *Science, 106,* 107-108.

Riesen, A. H. 1958. Plasticity of behavior: Psychological aspects. In H. F. Harlow & C. N. Woolsey (Eds.), *Biological and biochemical bases of behavior*. Madison: Univ. of Wisconsin Press. Pp. 425-450.

Schultz, T. R., & Zigler, E. 1971. Emotional concomitants of visual mastery in infants: The effects of stimulus movement on smiling and vocalizing. *Journal of Experimental Psychology, 10,* 390-403.

Shirley, Mary M. 1931. A motor sequence favors the maturation theory. *Psychological Bulletin, 28,* 204-205.

Thurstone, L. L. 1938. *Primary mental abilities.* Chicago: University of Chicago Press.

Uzgiris, Ina C., & Hunt, J. McV. 1966. An instrument for assessing infant psychological development. Mimeographed paper, Psychological Development Lab, Univer. of Illinois.

Uzgiris, Ina C., & Hunt, J. McV. 1968. Ordinal scales of infant psychological development: Information concerning six demonstration films. Mimeographed paper, University of Illinois, Psychological Development Laboratory.

Uzgiris, Ina C., & Hunt, J. McV. 1970. Attentional preference and experience: II. An exploratory longitudinal study of the effects of visual familiarity and responsiveness. *Journal of Genetic Psychology,* in press.

Valverde, F. 1967. Apical dendritic spines of the visual cortex and light deprivation in the mouse. *Experimental Brain Research, 3,* 337-352.

Valverde, F. 1968. Structural changes in the area striata of the mouse after enucleation. *Experimental Brain Research, 5,* 274-292.

Valverde, F., & Esteban, M. E. 1968. Peristriate cortex of mouse: Location and the effects of enucleation on the number of dendritic spines. *Brain Research, 9,* 145-148.

Watson, J. S. 1966. The development and generalization of "contingency awareness" in early infancy: Some hypotheses. *Merrill-Palmer Quarterly of Behavior and Development, 12* (no. 2), 123-135.

Watson, J. S. 1967. Memory and "contingency analysis" in infant learning. *Merrill: Palmer Quarterly of Behavior and Development, 13* (No. 1), 55-76.

Weizmann, F., Cohen, L., & Pratt, Jeanine. 1971. Novelty, familiarity, and the development of infant attention. *Developmental Psychology, 4* (No. 2), 149-154.

White, B. L. 1967. An experimental approach to the effects of experience on early human development. In J. P. Hill (Ed.), *Minnesota Symposia on Child Development*. Minneapolis: University of Minnesota Press. Pp. 201-226.

White, B. L. 1971. An analysis of excellent early educational practices: Preliminary report. *Interchange, 2* (2), 71-88.

White, R. W. 1959. Motivation reconsidered: The concept of competence. *Psychological Review, 66,* 297-333.

Whorf, B. L. 1956. *Language, thought, and reality.* New York: Wiley.

Wiesel, T. N., & Hubel, D. H. 1963. Effects of visual deprivation on morphology and physicology of cells in the cat's lateral geniculate body. *Journal of Neurophysiology, 26,* 978-993.

Yarrow, L. J., Rubenstein, Judith L., & Pedersen, F. A. 1971. Dimensions of early stimulation: Differential effects on infant development. Paper presented at the meetings of the Society for Research in Child Development, Minneapolis, Minn. 4 April 1971.

Zigler, E., Levine, J., & Gould, L. 1967. Cognitive challenge as a factor in children's humor appreciation. *Journal of Personality and Social Psychology, 6,* 332-336.

12. Infant Development Projects: Problems in Intervention*

Alice S. Honig

For those who are or will be involved in the growing variety of programs for infants and their families, it is instructive to consider the spectrum of possible problems associated with establishing, operating, and evaluating projects in infant intervention. At each choice point where problems can arise, we shall attempt to identify potential decisions and evaluate the feasibility, economic implications, and research evidence for or against each alternative.

Historical Problems: The Effects of Day Care

Maternal-Child Attachment

The earliest problem faced historically in infant intervention research was posed primarily by clinicians, well aware of findings of severe disturbance in hospitalized infants separated from mothers (Bowlby, 1952), findings of growth failures in institution-reared infants (Dennis & Najarian, 1957), and even findings of a marked lag in language development in infants reared in the countryside by paid peasant women (Brunet & Lezine, 1965). A major concern was that intervention programs which involved separation of mother and infant for lengthy daily periods would tend to weaken the mother-infant bond despite the best intentions of interventionists to prevent developmental deficits (such as the downward drift in IQ observed in longitudinal studies of low-income infants) by optimizing the developmental milieu of the infant. Fear of tampering with the development of mother-infant attachment was responsible for decisions of some center-based programs not to take infants younger than six

---

*An abbreviated version of this paper was presented as a workshop at the Merrill-Almer Institute Conference on Research and Teaching of Infant Development, Detroit, February, 1972.

months of age into a program. Addressing themselves to this concern particularly, Caldwell and her associates (Caldwell, Wright, Honig, & Tannenbaum, 1970) used in-depth maternal interviews to assess mother-infant attachment patterns of 21 two-and-a-half-year-old home-reared infants, and 18 infants who had spent at least one year in an infant care program. No dilution of the maternal-child attachment relation was found as a result of attendance in the intervention program. Keister (1970b), whose infant care program included infants as young as three months, and whose attention to the health and socio-emotional needs of infants was meticulous, likewise reports no difference in research results comparing infants in her program with home-reared controls. Erikson's thesis that the quality not the quantity of mothering is what counts seems to be borne out by such results. Additionally, as Stevenson & Fitzgerald (1971) have pointed out, the growth failures encountered in group care may well have resulted from inadequacies in the environmental settings in which the infants were reared.

Individual Differences among Infants

Bowlby, in a letter to Dr. Bettye Caldwell, has raised another interesting clinical problem with respect to infant intervention and attachment. He questioned whether intervention which involves early separation of infant and mother might in fact enhance dependency needs or anxieties in certain infants rather than dilute them. Growth of emotional independence from the mother might then be hindered. Such effects may not be visible when mean attachment scores are examined for a project. Mean scores may even mask attachment-dilution effects in some infants. Attention to the growth careers of individual infants in any intervention project thus seems of paramount importance. Only regard for the progress of each individual child in a program can alert us to those infants, or perhaps types of infants, for whom certain kinds of intervention—in a day-care setting for example—may not be suitable.

Long-Term Effects

The problem of long term effects of day care or intervention centers on emotional-social development is even more complex. The relative "infancy" of such intervention projects has until the present precluded the possibility of finding large samples of older children who have experienced intervention for one or more years in infancy and whose attachment patterns with parents can be assessed in relation to that experience. Another yet-to-be adequately assessed research area is the possibility raised by Kagan & Whitten (1970) that the long-term effects of extensive infant intervention may detract from the parent's basic responsiblity for child-rearing. One could in turn argue, however, that such responsibility may be tenuous or stressful for a parent initially. The services and support then offered by a family-oriented intervention program may serve rather to foster the growth of attachment and parental responsibility over time.

Intervention and Peer Relations

The long-term effects of early group care on peer relations is of historical and cross-cultural interest. Freud & Dann (1951) found that concentration camp orphans, institution-reared after the war, showed intense attachment and loyalty to each other. Recently, Lay & Meyer (1971) have found that infants reared together in one intervention program and then kept together in another program showed a marked preference for each other's company despite the addition of other pre-schoolers into the continuation program. Such strong peer preferences may be viewed both as a problem and a benefit of an infant program.

Planning Problems: Choice of an Intervention Model

Factors Which Influence Choice

In planning an infant care project, a program director may declare himself with respect to one intervention model or utilize attractive features of several models. His model may be based on philosophical or psychological convictions about what are the optimal conditions for infants and families to flourish. The model may meet the needs of working mothers in priority to other considerations. The model may be chosen with strong consideration of its exportability. That is, the director may be interested in developing a curriculum and designing environmental supports which are both replicable and disseminable to other communities and projects. From an economic point of view, models which provide one adult for every one-to-two babies may simply be unfeasible, unless large commitments are made by volunteers, and the logistics and training aspects of such commitments can be met. Legal constraints may be paramount.

Some states forbid group care of infants outside a home. For the home-care model, in which a neighborhood mother is trained to care for infants in her home, little research evidence of effect on child development is available. Such a setting may restrict an infant's access to a variety of environments such as play yards, or stores, since there is no other adult to share caregiving tasks.

Data from a variety of intervention models are currently available to assist in the decision-making process (Appalachian Regional Commission, 1970; Butler, 1970; Grotberg, 1971). Aside from differences in degree and kind of structuredness, programs differ also in the settings in which they occur and the persons involved in program delivery.

The Center Model

Rather extensive use has been made of outside-the-home centers for infant intervention by Caldwell & Richmond (1968), Dusewicz & Higgins (1971), Gallagher (1972) at the Frank Porter Graham Child Development Center, Heber (1971), Keister (1970a), and Sigel (1971). In general the rationale for choosing such a model involves the provision of important services such as baby-sitting, pediatric care, and the provision of nutritious meals. Choice of a center model may also involve the recognition that a "more intensive and cumulative contact with the social and non-social environment" can thus be provided (Sigel, 1971, p. 9). Infants in center-based programs, whether such programs are highly structured or follow child-choice of activities, often register considerable developmental gains during their enrollment (Caldwell & Richmond, 1968; Fowler, 1972a). They have also been reported to exhibit marked enjoyment of activities and social interactions (Keister, 1970b). Center-based programs can often provide a more "total" environment to shape and reinforce those multiple developmental processes and competencies which have been identified as "goals for education" (Biber, 1969, p. 11). Where infants are persistently at nutritional deficit within the home environment, the use of a center model may provide that consistent boost in nourishment which the infant requires to maintain good health and lessen proneness to respiratory infections and to hemoglobin deficiencies (Osofsky & Osofsky, 1970).

One drawback to the center-based model exclusively concerned with infants is that an aura of "we-know-best-for-baby" professionalism may alienate the parents and community from the intervention program and contribute to the isolation of already alienated poverty parents from involvement with one more educational institution. Another consideration is the costly nature of such centers. Unless a center intervention program is supported by research or community funds, individual parents may find it impossible to finance such services for their infants.

The Tutorial Model

A more economical model which has been tried is the tutorial model. Trained child development personnel attempt, usually within a home setting, to extend the range of experience and competence of an infant. Using special cubicles set up within a university setting, Palmer (1970) has investigated both a carefully sequenced concept training program and a concept discovery program with older infants. Both versions of the tutorial model proved successful in producing cognitive achievements superior to those of control infants. The tutorial model, which concentrates on encouraging infant developmental advances and which involves parents very weakly if at all, has proved effective in sustaining infant developmental scores, or improving them relative to controls, during the time the intervention is ongoing (Painter, 1968; Schaefer, 1970). Learning materials, games, songs, and ideas, developed by infant tutors for these models, testify to the concern and ingenuity manifested by the tutors. The tutorial model, involving two or fewer hours per session, has the advantage of meeting objections that day care intervention models which involve removing the infant from the home for many hours of the day may have deleterious emotional effects. However, tutoring which does not involve parents has been found to produce regression of scores several years after the experience (Schaefer, 1970). Such tutoring may have negative consequences for an infant because learning situations and family interactions occur separately for him. Additionally, this model may not suit the needs of many families for more extensive service for infants.

Home-Visit Model

Children who have participated in infant development programs sometimes fail in follow-up studies to sustain earlier gains. It has been assumed that lack of parental involvement and lack of follow-up or continuity in intervention may be responsible for such declines. Parent visitation models have been introduced to ensure continuity of the intervention process. Giesy (1970), Gordon (1969), Gray (1971), Lally (1971), and Weikart *et al*. (1969) have trained home visitors in their programs with low-income mothers to offer supportive suggestions and demonstrations in the areas of nutrition, child development, Piagetian games, toy creation, and language development. Levenstein's (1971) Toy Demonstrators during their home visits suggest alternative ways to use toys and books, which are offered as gifts to mothers, to encourage infant growth.

The recently announced Home Start program (Kapfer, 1972) will use the home visitation model exclusively to help parents enhance the total development of their children. Some of the thirty-three national Parent-Child Centers, which focus on infants under three years of age, provide home vistation. The function of this outreach component is either to reinforce center-based learning, to involve other siblings, or as a mechanism to deliver social services to parents.

The Parent-Group Model

A parent model which has been found successful in programs for older pre-schoolers by Karnes *et al*. (1968), and by Nimnicht (1970) is characterized by teaching of parents in groups. Parents then return home and are better able to apply intervention techniques and behaviors with their own children. Stern (1971) reports increased language performance scores for Head Start age children whose parents participated in meetings where group process techniques encouraged expression of feelings and needs. Models which involve parents to a marked degree in their infants' growth would seem to meet several basic clinical and sociological objections to intervention programs. Parent models strengthen rather than weaken parent-child responsibilities and bonds. They ensure a longer-term intervention than the few years most funded project personnel function. They offer the potential of 'vertical diffusion'' to other children in the family (Gray & Klaus, 1970). When they train the mother herself as a change-agent, they may decrease her sense of powerlessness— and not only in her mothering-and-educating role. If the mother's sense of self-competence and achievement with regard to child-rearing has been sustained, she may more successfully relate to problems of poverty or ethnic discrimination as they affect her and her family. Involving parents in infant intervention programs makes explicit the philosophical conviction that a program must support and supplement but not supplant parenting. Such involvement may increase the trust and cooperation of low-income families and serve to decrease drop-outs in research programs where high subject attrition makes longitudinal data difficult to interpret.

A program which includes parents can help make clear that difference is not automatically equated with deficit (Cole & Bruner, 1971). Cultural differences, reflected in food patterns and holiday activities, for example, should be respected and incorporated into programs wherever feasible and with the parents' help. Parent participation can ensure that the match between an operating model and the population served is a good one. Participation may be of varied sorts. The parent may do volunteer work in a center program, be in a teacher-aide training program for parents of enrolled infants, or represent participative management as when parents and teachers together select and purchase toys for a program. In some Parent-Child Centers, parents on the Policy Advisory Committee aid in the selection of staff, project administration, program planning, and recruiting client population. Unfortunately there is very little data available on the impact of decision-making parents, who certainly vary in their degree of participation, on the programs operated.

Staff Selection

If a center-based program is planned, certain logistical problems must be solved: ordering equipment, leasing buses, arranging diaper service, and securing pediatric and food preparation services. Whatever the setting of the program, however, staff selection and training are of critical importance. Recent failures to discover which of a set of parametric variations on intervention models is more effective for promoting child development may be due to this staff variable. Many methods—sequential learning, discovery, polar concepts, verbal bombardment, Piagetian task, or open classroom—may succeed in fostering a young child's development when the personnel involved are committed to children, enjoy children's growth, and are sensitive to ways to facilitate that growth. Thus, the director with a genius for selecting, training, and keeping personnel may in the end find sustained infant developmental gains in his program no matter what his curriculum or model may be nor how fancy his toys nor how sequential his learning lessons.

Babies and children come to understandings and competencies through many routes. Given a varied environment and a baby normal at birth and adequately fed, the adult who varies, patterns, and regulates the input an infant receives, and who also nourishes the infant's self-initiated attempts to cope, to comprehend, and to communicate in his world is the indispensible catalyst for infant growth. Even in a center environment where other infants are available for interactions and as sources of stimulation, research indicates that the adult remains during the first two years of life the prepotent dispenser of social and cognitive transactions (Honig, Caldwell, & Tannenbaum, 1970; Maudry & Nekula, 1931).

Automated Teachers Versus Human Ones

The importance of the adult for early infant development cannot be over-emphasized. Recent studies which program babies' cribs show us that, indeed, babies' behaviors can be controlled by external programmed object-stimuli (Friedlander, 1970; Watson, 1971). However, the extensive use of toys and automated equipment is no substitute for people. Do we want babies to exhibit smiles primarily to three-dimensional cut-outs or tape-recorder playbacks? Or do we want babies to relate to people initially, to trust people as the sources of comfort, of interesting events, and of rewards? Automated equipment should be considered an adjunct to, not a substitute for, human teachers in infant intervention programs.

The Ideal Caregiver

Who is the ideal candidate for intervention program staff— whether working directly with parents or infants? He or she should have: love for babies, cheerfulness, patience, willingness to learn (from parents and babies as well as psychologists and supervisors), comfortableness with quirks and customs of people, a knack for seeing the learning potential in ordinary situations such as a dropped mitten or a new food at mealtime, and the ability to recognize and take joy in small successes. If this prescription seems to be too good to be true, then at least let us keep it as a firmly held ideal while addressing ourselves constantly to the problems that arise in trying to find or create such caregivers.

Sometimes bilingual skills will make the difference in staff effectiveness with families. Sometimes strong hips for carrying a baby will make the difference in easing a disconsolate infant's crying during his first days at a center intervention program.

Staff Diversity

Hiring some women, some men, some professional, and some

paraprofessional staff will enable an intervention program to ensure a diversity of life styles, and of life experience in the personnel serving parents and children. It is wise in hiring infant teachers to include some trained as nurses, who offer important skills in health care and can be taught special-curricular games and social skills with babies. When paraprofessionals are selected for an intervention staff, special training techniques such as role-playing and small-group workshops have been found to be particularly effective (Lally, Honig, & Caldwell, 1973). Careful staff selection procedures enhance a program's chances of training a cadre of knowledgeable and effective caregivers. Such care may also minimize chances of interpersonal frictions, with their attendant effects on staff morale, and minimize chances that personal moods of caregivers will interfere with the quality of responsive care for infants.

Staff Training

Theoretical Problems

Consideration of theoretical issues in conceptualizing the role of the caregiver may be of relevance in the process of staff selection and training. Is the care giver to be considered primarily a source of emotional-tactual satisfactions *a la* Harlow or Spitz? Is he or she simply a source of reinforcements *a la* Gewirtz? Is the caregiver, as Lewis & Goldberg (1969) would have us believe, a source of contingent reinforcers which teach the infant that he is important and competent because his behaviors have consequences and thus motivate him to accomplish a wide range of behaviors? If the intervention program director is more interested in infant development than in proving that one theory of caregiving function is more effective than another he will probably answer "yes" to all questions. In so doing he may increase the probability that his intervention procedures will succeed, because he is not artificially fragmenting caregiver functions facilitative of infant development. Awareness of the value system underlying the intervention research is important to those responsible for training staff (Starr, 1971).

The Role of the Home Visitor. Some problems which concern the director responsible for staff orientation and training are tied to his conceptualization of the multifaceted role of the home visitor, who is often a woman selected from the same social milieu as the parent. Weikart *et al.* (1969) suggest that the home visitor perceive herself as a guest having a positon of low power in the home. She may also be a casual friend and information-giver (with respect to learning games and alternate ways of discipline), or offer toys and books (Levenstein, 1971). She may give suggestions for and then participate in family activities and outings (Giesy, 1970). In Lally's (1971) program she may also occasionally serve as a counselor, as a guide to social agencies and community supports, and as a workshop teacher of, for example, tie-dyeing or clothes-making activities requested by a group of mothers. Strong emphasis may be placed on the home-visitor's ability to increase a mother's pleasurable social interactions and teaching behaviors with her infant. Which component of this complex role may be most effective in helping a given mother to enjoy and facilitate her infant's growth is possibly an unanswerable research question. Again, the director's concern with infant development may support a decision to sensitize home visitors to the potential effectiveness of any or all of these roles so that they can be used when warranted by the home situation and by material as well as infant needs.

The Role of the Teacher. The role of the classroom teacher in fulfilling program goals has been conceptualized in several ways. Shall he or she create a learning environment which permits the learner to explore freely and is self-pacing? A Piagetian viewpoint may dictate that this is the only way "learning-that-sticks" ever gets done. Shall the teacher, instead, structure and pattern the infant's activities so that the infant-learner can make a series of interconnected discoveries about his physical or social-cultural world? Bereiter & Engelman suggest (1968, p. 512) that the teacher is someone who by direct, highly controlled instruction can nourish not only positive learning attitudes and abilities but also divergent thinking and creative spontaneity in tasks. Perhaps a categorical either-or position here is simply nonproductive for an infant intervention program. Recognition of the child's need to program his own time, to use his own investigative methods, and to move at a pace unique to his capacities has never meant that the adult totally abdicates a facilitative role in this process. As Bruner (1971, p. 105) succinctly phrases it, the caregiver must "provide the occasion for the child to move successfully toward a sense of competence."

Katz (1970), in an analysis of teacher role models in early childhood programs, has distinguished among three potential teacher role models in intervention settings: the nurturant maternal model, the therapeutic model, and the instructional model. Again, it is important, when surrogate rearing of infants is involved, to make sure a variety of role models, congruent with infant developmental needs and daily activities and routines, is available. The intervention program director who is determined to research the relative effectiveness of any of these models, and who insists that one role model exclusively be assumed by a given teacher, may short-change the infants in his program.

Practical Problems

How best or most effectively can staff training be accomplished? A preservice training program for infant caregivers may be implemented in several weeks or several months. A program director concerned with the quality of program for infants and with staff morale will build a continuous inservice training component into the program. Finding time to arrange for inservice workshops, discussions, and case conferences is often a vexing problem. Using infant nap hours, or recruiting volunteers to replace teachers for an hour, may provide the time slots needed for training. Another method is to assign a program supervisor to rotate among classrooms, model various skills, and offer helpful suggestions when teachers ask for them. In a home visit program, one day a week may be devoted entirely to inservice training and conferences.

The amount and time given to training will be constrained by available planning funds, federal guidelines, community wishes, and certainly by the skills and sensitively levels of the trainees themselves. Some recent publications offer technical assistance, specific guidelines, and suggestions for infant teacher training (Day Care Resources Project, 1971; Honig & Lally, 1972).

If it is feasible, a director may decide to suspend a program for a week or two annually in order to carry out intensive retraining workshops. This kind of intensive effort at reorienting and retraining staff offers positive motivational consequences for teachers. It also offers a director a chance to bring all program staff members—including bus drivers, teachers, home visitors, and cooks—together into a training program. Diaries turned in each day by participants can help trainers redirect their efforts daily toward greater clarification of certain topics and consideration of other topics trainees wish to have placed on the agenda.

Program Operation

Staff Assignments

If infants under 15 months are to spend a good part of their waking hours with caregivers other than their own parents, special needs for attachment must be met. Babies in the first year of life particularly need a "special person"—someone who is there to comfort, to play loving games, to bring forth laughter, and to reassure a tiny adventurer that he may touch or creep or explore beyond the former boundaries of his known world. Infants who attend intervention programs may be multiply-mothered or mothered by a person too overwhelmed with her problems to cope with a baby's demands for "specialness." In such cases it is even more important to make sure, despite the sharing of tasks which goes on in the ordinary nursery, that each infant grows to know whom he can count on, his very own, his "special person." Assigning three or four babies in the first year of life can nurture such a special relation. Directors and caregivers need to be flexible however. If a baby quiets or "lights up" for another caregiver more easily, perhaps a switch should be made. Not all babies and caregivers "take" to each other. Self-selection by an infant can be compatible with ensuring him a special person.

How Many Babies?

How many infants and staff shall be included in a given program? Available funds must of necessity be considered. As Keister (1970a, p. 12) has observed, "The actual monetary cost of a program that gives individual care to babies is inevitably going to run high." To be considered also are the peculiar changes in the quality of staff interactions with children and children's response to a program environment which can occur when too many people are clustered together. One of the teachers in an open classroom setting with 45 two-to-three-year-olds explained, "I can't keep the skill levels or special needs of so many children in my head." If the 45 toddlers are broken into groups of 15 with three teachers responsible for each group, then it becomes easier for a caregiver to focus on and be alert to each child's special needs or difficulties. However, such an arrangement may have shortcomings too, because each toddler now has access to less equipment, and to fewer peers from whom to choose his playmates. An alternative solution might be to keep the larger group of older infants intact but assign each teacher special responsibilities for a few children within the larger group.

Funding agencies may consider it more facilitative of infant development to encourage directors to plan smaller programs for infants. Yet cost analysis and the requirements of a research design may exert pressure to include large numbers of infants in a program. Directors may solve some of the research problems entailed by small samples by a decision to pool assessment measures with other infant centers rather than to try to provide for the needs of hundreds of infants in one necessarily bureaucratized organization.

The ratio of staff to infants in a program is an additional factor which affects the quality of intervention efforts. Fowler (1972b) has found that even with ratios as seemingly favorable as one teacher for two infants, the number of daily structured learning sessions which could be carried out with individual babies was far fewer then initially planned.

Time Decisions

Some day care decisions reflect the often complex relation between service needs and child development needs. How much time should an infant spend in an intervention center? What age should he enter? How long should a program plan to offer care, whether home-tutorial or center-based? Sometimes intervention centers try to meet parent needs and offer care from 7:30 a.m. to 6:00 p.m. Indeed, the French créche system has been offering just such care for decades. There is no research yet available in our culture to tell us whether a few hours' stay at a center differs in its impact on social-personal or cognitive attributes from a 10- to 12-hour stay.

Age at entry into a program has received some research notice. Caldwell & Richmond (1968) found no particular advantage accruing on Cattell IQ tests to infants entering their program earlier or later. Fowler (1972a) found a pattern of mean cognitive gains by advantaged infants which favored both earliness of entry into and length of time spent in his program. Gordon (1969) found that infants in his home visit program showed no gains at the end of two years of age if the intervention had occured during the first year but not during the second. Heber (1971) reports that infants entering from birth with their mothers into an intervention program with intensively enriched curriculum, and a one-to-one teacher-infant ratio, exhibit markedly high IQ scores (33 IQ point mean gains) compared to controls after several years in the program. Lally (1971), who has recently developed a program which brings nutrition information and child development skills to mothers from the sixth month of pregnancy onward, has reported for a small group of experimental infants that Cattell IQ scores average 10 points higher than controls at six months of age. In general, no intervention programs which emphasize the quality of infant care offered and the importance of the family to the infant have shown detrimental effects of center attendance on infant development.

Program Content

Program supervisors in search of materials will find that suggestions for infant tasks, toys, and games have become more available in the past few years (Caldwell, 1971; Forrester, et al., 1971; Gordon, 1971; Gordon & Lally, 1967; Painter, 1971; Segner & Patterson, 1969; Upchurch, 1971). Although program ideas should be offered in detail and frequently to teachers, programs should also encourage teachers to create their own materials, games, and variants thereof. Particular stress should be placed on the use of caregiving routines to set the times and locales where learning activities are encouraged. During inservice training the importance of activities, such as reading to babies or providing many opportunities for coordination of vision with prehension, can be emphasized through presentation of research findings such as those of White (1968) on the advantages accruing to institutionalized infants for whom crib stabiles were provided along with a visually enriched environment.

Difficulties may lie not in clarifying program goals and content to caregivers but in finding ways to teach caregivers to monitor their own behaviors and readjust them in line with program goals so that intended intervention behaviors are visible, measurable, and sustained. For example, in a recent study (Meyer & Lindstrom, 1969) of classrooms in Head Start, a program certainly dedicated to improving the self-image of disadvantaged youngsters, a great deal more caregiver blame than praise was found to be distributed to youngsters. Some teachers do not hear their own negative voice tones. They do not remember not to shout negative commands from a distance to infants but instead to go over to the infant who is, for example, happily pulling soiled diapers out of a pail. Some teachers who get compliance from some toddlers in a group do not remember to reinforce those toddlers with positive reinforcers. Instead, teachers may fret at or concentrate on those children who, for example, did not come right away for tooth-brushing time. Sharpening the observation skills of teachers and providing feedback to them on the nature of their interactions with infants can boost program quality.

Supports for Personnel

Options for handling personnel problems may be decided upon before difficulties arise. Prevention of interpersonal frictions among teachers, for example, may best be handled by (a) clear structuring of grievance mechanisms, and (b) by frequent small staff meetings to discuss any confusing program operations or policies which may contribute to friction. Role-playing with staff members is often useful in teaching effective ways to handle parental complaints or discipline problems with children.

Assessment Options

Although a host of IQ, personal-social, and achievement measures exist for older children and even for preschoolers, the paucity or unreliability of instrumentation in infancy has raised thorny issues for intervention programs. Research to determine effective teaching processes and infant curriculum components has likewise been sparse.

Infant Assessments

Developmental Tests. Developmental quotients in infancy have long been considered to be nonpredictive of later IQ scores (Bayley, 1965). Yet obtaining such infant test scores was often a necessity if one purported to look for developmental gains from an intervention program. Recently some programs have administered Piagetian sensori-motor scales to assess the effects of a specifically Piagetian program on infant development (Honig & Brill, 1970; Weikart et al., 1969).

Learning and Conditioning Measures. Conditioned responses such as vocalizations or head-turning have been considered as indices of early learning. In intervention programs designed for infants at risk, an infant's inability to respond to conditioning procedures may be used as an index of fuctional deficit prior to nutritional supplement or medical and other treatment. Lewis and Goldberg (1969) have suggested that response habituation measures may distinguish among infants reared in enriched or improverished environments.

Naturalistic Observations. Efforts to monitor development, particularly in socio-emotional areas, with ecological assessments are becoming more widespread for infants and older preschoolers. Honig, Caldwell, & Tannenbaum (1970), using an elaborate numerical coding system, APPROACH, designed to be applied in naturalistic settings, tallied the frequencies of such activities as conversing, demonstrating, information-giving, and dramatizing, directed to and from infants (and older preschoolers) and adults in classrooms. Lay & Meyer (1971) have recently reported 9000 one-minute time samples of naturally occurring behaviors, such as verbal and gestural interactions, in a group of 3- to 5-year-olds. Escalona (1972) suggests that we need to explore the variety and range of social contexts that occur day by day in infant lives and record all encounters between a baby and other persons. Ricciuti (1970) has developed an elaborate observational code to record infant postures, locations, and behaviors. Fowler (1972b) has devised an observational grid which yields a profile of infant socio-emotional and cognitive competencies. Quite recently, a group of Upstart project directors has begun a collaborative effort to develop social-emotional measures of trust and persistence in infants during the first two years of life. Such collaborative efforts will facilitate the sharing of infant developmental research data.

Language Development. Quite a few language measures, such as the ITPA and the Peabody, exist for older children and preschoolers. However, they are scarce for the infancy period. Additionally, the relation of early babbling to later verbalization has not been well clarified. Cameron, Livson, & Bayley (1967) suggest that clusters of early vocalizing and language items are better predictors of later Binet IQ scores than are standard tests. Some early tests of language exist, but many require gross judgements of infant competence. In assessment, single instances of competence may lead to assumptions of widespread language skills which are not in fact present. An Early Language Assessment Scale (ELAS) in use at the Syracuse University Children's Center measures infant vocal and verbal communications, as well as gestural and verbal decoding of the meanings of objects, sounds, words, facial expressions, and gestures (Honig & Caldwell, 1966). Slobin (1972) has proposed that we look at all the words a baby uses in different contexts such as bath time or messy play.

Product vs. Process Measures. In general, there is a downgrading nowadays of "product" compared to "process" measures of child development. Although this emphasis on qualitative variables is important, problems still remain. Just how does one assess "learning to learn," "joy and love of learning," "development of decision-making strategies," "social sensitivity," "variety and persistence in problem-solving attempts," "increasing ability to defer gratification or tolerate frustration" and other such qualitative characteristics of intervention success? The author believes one should opt for observational strategies, using behaviorally-defined categories of such qualities. These observations should be carried out not only in a center intervention program but in the home and later in the school and other life settings where the transfer of such successes must occur as the ultimate "pay-off" of any intervention program.

Tester Training. In many cases, a program director will find that infant testers need to be trained specially for his program. Few universities teach infant testing. Few teach the particular skills and styles—almost magician-like—which are often required either to interest a nonverbal baby in using strange, new materials, or deftly to recuperate toys clutched from a prior item administration. If possible, interdepartmental efforts should be made (among psychology, special education, and human development programs, for example) to set up a special course on infant assessment.

Where a particular linguistic or ethnic group is specially represented in the intervention program, the director may want to train personnel from these groups to carry out infant testing and family assessments rather than hire psychologists who have a background in child development and in testing.

Caregiver Assessment

Confirmation of teacher styles and skills in intervention programs has not kept pace with eloquent formulations of program objectives. A problem faced by any program, regardless of intervention strategy, is to ensure that caregiver behaviors in fact reflect program models in theory. Katz (1969) has made poignantly clear that a designation of "cognitively-enriched preschool program" compared to a traditional nursery program may in fact turn out to amount to more commands and restrictions placed on youngsters rather than the stated goal difference of specific increased curricular enrichment.

An observational rating scale "Adult Behaviors in Caregiving" (The ABC scale) recently developed by Honig (1972) at the Syracuse University Children's Center attempts to checklist the occurrence, during 2-minute periods, of teacher inputs to infants in six major areas: language facilitation, positive reinforcement, negative reinforcement, Piagetian tasks, physical exercises and games, and bodily and environmental caregiving. Differences in teacher inputs in each area are readily apparent from frequency tallies. Inservice training can be used to bolster areas where a given teacher's input has been judged insufficient. Such a scale also pinpoints imbalances in teacher sharing of, for example, clean-up jobs. Thus inequalities which could lead to staff friction can be adjusted by a director who uses such information judiciously, with sensitivity to teacher needs as well as program needs. A further advantage to observational systems lies in their adaptability to all daily caregiving routines, which are teaching situations par excellence with babies.

Maternal Measures

Since the ultimate goal in intervention is not only to prevent deficit but to ensure that the infants leaving projects will be sustained in sociable and cognitive ventures and adventures by family efforts, an important problem lies in the nature of the measures by which one can, with more or less confidence, assert that such sustenance will henceforth be offered.

Both Gordon (1969) and Lally (1971) have made use of home-visit observational checklists. However, such checklists can possibly be influenced by halo effects. The mother who has forced a home visitor to reschedule a weekly visit four times, because she neglected to be at home each time, may receive lower scores than the mother who is at home and accepts materials from the visitor, although the maternal interactions with infants may be quite similar.

Maternal Tempo and Style. More subtle problems of gauging the input of program on maternal care practices exist. These problems have nothing to do with the "what" of intervention tasks but rather with the "hows" and "whens." Hess and Shipman (1967) showed several years ago that maternal teaching styles differed markedly among black mothers from different social classes. In our zeal to teach mothers intervention techniques we may become too enamored of "what" to do with infants, such as: show the baby pictures and get him to label objects thereon, or help the baby complete a puzzle. The author has recently, with Dr. Robert Mercurio, coded videotapes of low-income mothers in teaching situations with their infants. What was often devastatingly evident was that some mothers had learned the ends but not the means of teaching interactions with infants. If the intervention program director were to assess what those mothers did, indeed they questioned, they informed, they conversed, they demonstrated. However, their tempo and pacing was often breathtakingly rapid for an uncomprehending toddler. The variety and number of inputs was changed so quickly that often the infant literally had no time to respond—either accurately or compliantly or ineptly!

A maternal style which offers (1) judicious patterning of a variety of appropriate inputs, (2) attention to saliency and tempo of adult offerings and responses and to figure-ground clarity, plus (3) a constant adult alertness to the infant's interests and capabilities as well as to the adults' intentions in teaching, is hard to teach and hard to measure. Also, to say that "caregiver loving and child learning" are inseparables for infants is a far different matter from translating such dicta into subtle and creative interaction patterns between mothers and infants, or, for that matter, as Lally (1969) has noted, between home visitors and infants.

Despite instrumentation difficulties, an over-all evaluation plan should include some assessment of the effect of intervention on the family. A true concern with the long-range continuing development of infants does not permit satisfaction only with five more Piagetian scale points or ten more IQ points gained by infants immediately prior to exit from the program. Child development experts are certainly not philosophically agreed that the prime goal of intervention is "acceleration" of infants. However, they are concerned that more positive contacts with adults become available to infants and young children to sustain whatever development an intervention program has nourished and encouraged. A positive measure, for example, can be as basic as finding out that a project mother, who continues to use physical punishment, is now able to offer reasons along with her swats.

Non-obtrusive Measures

Nonobtrusive measures of program effectiveness present almost as many problems as psychometric or observational assessment. For example, "days in attendance" at a center may not correlate highly with infant developmental score gains. Some nonworking mothers who learn special games from the home visitor may keep their infants at home once in a while and sometimes play these learning games. In such cases, attendance records will not reflect the amount or quality of program input to infants.

Using a nonobtrusive measure, percent of home visits successfully accomplished, Lally (1971, p. 35) has found a significant correlation with infant Cattell IQ scores.

Recycling Information Back into the Program

One important decision a program may need to face is how to get assessment information gathered by testers, observers, home-visitors, and even site visitors, back to the intervention personnel in a useful, understandable form. Feedback of this sort makes intervention personnel feel how important their efforts are. It keeps them in touch with other persons' assessments of where the infant is at in all his developmental endeavors. Feedback generates ideas for program improvement. Such ideas may range from new furniture-rug arrangements which entice a toddler to sit down with a picture book to new workshops which increase parental participation in a program.

"Sleeper" Effects of Program

Sometimes the social and cognitive facilitating effects of a program on family or infant functioning may not "show up" right away. Effects which can show up a few years later might be (a) an increase in organized behaviors in school and home, (b) decreased parent-child frictions in the family, (c) higher classroom achievements scores than controls, and (d) more socially cooperative behaviors with peers than may be usual in children from poor, overcrowded environments, where daily stresses often increase chances for negative interactions. Funding problems may arise in attempts to monitor not only "who benefits from what," but "under what circumstances is the effect sustained?" (Beller 1972, p. 36).

Evaluation

Evaluation Design

The pre-post intervention vs. control group model has some built-in hazards when dealing with low-income populations, due to geographical mobility and life crises which cause subjects to disappear from the community or not to appear for testings. Longitudinal controls are to be preferred, but are often impossible to maintain when populations are highly mobile. Cross-sectional controls are easier to obtain, but it may be difficult to establish that they come from a sample identical initially to the intervention group. Additionally, some differences between retested intervention infants and cross-sectional controls must be attributed to the former's familiarity with testing.

Motivational Factors. In some cases evaluation attempts are confounded by complex motivational factors which make comparisons of infant development within or outside of intervention programs more difficult. Such a factor is involved when one mother agrees to place her infant in an intervention research program at six months and another mother refuses (yet perhaps regrets her decision a half-year later when her baby is busy creeping into things!). As long as most infant programs are dependent on mothers voluntarily accepting daily, if brief, early separations from infants, then the motivational variable will have to be considered. Differences in maternal feelings and attitudes ultimately may affect subsequent infant development more than any specific care or teaching practices in the home or in intervention programming. It is often difficult to arrange conditions so that mothers consent both to having very young infants in a program and to having the babies randomly assigned to the program or to control groups.

Another problem in defining an adequate control group for intervention infants stems from the nature of the family disorganization which may be present in certain populations. Pavenstedt (1965) has vividly described the differences between lower-lower and upper-lower poverty cultures. Where a lower-lower class mother of a control group infant is unable or unwilling to make the effort to bring her infant in for developmental assessments, data may not be available for that infant. From a similar family, an intervention infant may be picked up daily, brought into the intervention center, and tested or observed at will within that setting regardless of the mother's cooperation or lack of it in arranging for testing. Such infants may have no adequate controls since assessment may require a degree of parental cooperation which may not be forthcoming from the "matched" control family.

Such a problem again raises the ethical issue of a project's responsibility to provide auxiliary services to families. Provence (1969), in her research intervention project, assumes that services to parents which support their development as adults will make services for children more effective. If pediatric, social work, medical, and other services are made available through a project to families, parents are more likely to trust the members of a research team. Thus more information about parents and children will be available to the project. Certainly the chance for parental involvement in project goals, for and with their children, becomes more likely.

Dissemination

Programs, whether they are designed to optimize infant growth directly or to nurture parental abilities, need to share their experiences with others in the field. Journals which limit acceptance purely to data-based papers or to published reports of completed programs pose a problem in communications for ongoing programs. A director may alleviate this problem by asking initially for adequate funds to disseminate his program findings to others engaged in such research. Hopefully, finding techniques and media for sharing problems and successes will be the least of the problems encountered in program efforts to serve infants and families with greater mutual trust, joy, and effectiveness.

References

Appalachian Regional Commission. *Programs for infants and young children.* Washington, D.C.: ARC, 1970.

Baley, N. Comparisons of mental and motor test scores for ages 1-15 months by sex. birth order, race, geographical location and education of parents. *Child Development,* 1965, *36,* 370-411.

Beller, E. K. Research on teaching: Organized programs in early education. In R. Travers (Ed.) *Handbook for research on teaching.* New York: Rand McNally, 1972, in press.

Bereiter, C., & Engelmann, S. Observations on the use of direct instruction with young disadvantaged children. In J. Frost (Ed.) *Early childhood education rediscovered.* New York: Holt, Rinehart & Winston, 1968.

Biber, B. *Challenges ahead for early childhood education.* Washington, D. C.: National Association for the Education of Young Children, 1969.

Bowlby, J. *Mental care and mental health.* Geneva, Switzerland: World Health Organization, 1952.

Bruner, J. Overview of development and day care. In E.H. Grotberg (Ed.) *Day care: Resources for decisions.* Washington, D.C.: Office of Economic Opportunity, 1971.

Brunet, O. & Lezine, I. *Le développement psychologique de la première enfance.* Paris, France: Presses Universitaires de France, 1965.

Butler, A. L. *Current research in early childhood education: A compilation and analysis for program planners.* Washington, D.C.: American Association of Elementary-Kindergarten-Nursery Educators, 1970.

Caldwell, B.M. Home teaching activities. Little Rock, Arkansas: Center for Early Development and Education, 1971.

Caldwell, B.M. & Richmond, J. The Children's Center in Syracuse, New York. In L. L. Dittman (Ed.), *Early child care: The new perspectives.* New York: Atherton Press, 1968.

Caldwell, B. M., Wright, C. M., Honig, A. S., & Tannenbaum, J. Infant day care and attachment. *American Journal of Orthopsychiatry.* 1970, *40,* 397-412.

Cameron, J., Livson, N., & Bayley, N. Infant vocalizations and their relationship to mature intelligence. *Science,* 1967, *157,* 331-333.

Cole, M., & Bruner, J. Cultural differences and inferences about psychological processes. *American Psychologist,* 1971, *26,* 867-876.

Day Care Resources Project. *Handbook on day care.* Vol. 1-8. Office of Child Development, U.S. Dept. of Health, Education, & Welfare, Washington, D.C.; Government Printing Office, 1971.

Dennis, W. & Najarian, P. Infant development under environmental handicap. *Psychological Monographs,* 1957, *71,* No. 7, 1-13.

Dusewitz, R. A., & Higgins, M. J. Toward an effective educational program for disadvantaged infants. Paper presented at the annual meeting of the American Educational Research Association, New York City, February 1971.

Escalona, S. K. Basic modes of social interactions: Their emergence during the first two years of life. Paper presented at the meeting of the Merrill, Palmer Institute Conference on Research & Teaching of Infant Development, Detroit, February 1972.

Forrester, B. J., Brooks, G. P., Hardge, B. M., & Outlaw, D. C. *Materials for infant development.* DARCEE, George Peabody College for Teachers, Nashville, Tennessee, 1971.

Fowler, W. A developmental learning approach to infant care in a group setting. *Merrill-Palmer Quarterly,* 1972, *18,* 145-176. (a)

Fowler, W. The development of a prototype infant, preschool and day care center in Metropolitan Toronto. Year I Progress Report: Program development. Toronto, Ontario: Woodbine Project, Ontario Institute for Studies in Education, 1972. (b)

Freud, A., & Dann, S. An experiment in group upbringing. *Psychoanalytical Study of the Child,* 1951, *6,* 127-168. Friedlander, B. Z. Receptive language development in infancy: Issues and problems. *Merrill-Palmer Quarterly,* 1970, *16,* 7-51.

Gallagher, J. J. Perspectives: A Progress Report on Child Care. Chapel Hill, North Carolina: Frank Porter Graham Child Development Center, University of North Carolina, 1972.

Geisy, R. *A guide for home visitors.* Nashville, Tennessee: DARCEE, George Peabody College for Teachers, 1970.

Gordon, I. J. *Baby learning through baby play.* New York: St. Martin's Press, 1971.

Gordon, I. J. Early child stimulation through parent education. Final report No. PHS-R-306, Washington, D.C. Children's Bureau, Department of Health, Education, and Welfare, 1969.

Gray, S. W., & Klaus, R. A. Educational intervention at home by mothers of disadvantaged infants. *Child Development,* 1970, *41,* 909-924.

Gray, S. W. Home visiting program for parents of young children. Nashville, Tennessee. *DARCEE Papers & Reports*. 1971, *5*, No. 4.

Grotberg, E. H. Day care: Resources for decisions. Washington, D. C.: Office of Economic Opportunity, 1971.

Heber, R. Rehabilitation of families at risk for mental retardation: A Progress Report. Madison, Wisconsin: University of Wisconsin Rehabilitation Research and Training Center in Mental Retardation, 1971.

Hess, R. D., & Shipman, V. C. Cognitive elements in maternal behavior. *Minnesota Symposia on Child Psychology*, Vol. 1. Minneapolis: University of Minnesota Press, 1967.

Honig, A. S. Adult behaviors in caregiving, (ABC scale). In Lally, J. R., Progress Report, 1971-72, Syracuse University Children's Center, No. PR-156 (C-6) Office of Child Development.

Honig, A. S., & Brill, S. A. comparative analysis of the Piagetian development of twelve-month-old disadvantaged infants in an enrichment center with others not in such a center. Paper presented at the annual meeting of the American Psychological Association, Miami, September 1970.

Honig, A. S., & Caldwell, B. M. The Early Language Assessment Scale. Unpublished manuscript, Children's Center, Syracuse University, 1966.

Honig, A. S., Caldwell, B. M., & Tannenbaum, J. Patterns of information processing used by and with young children in a nursery school setting. *Child Development*, 1970, *41*, 1045-1065.

Honig, A. S., & Lally, J. R. *Infant caregiving: A design for training*. New York: Media Projects, Inc., 1972.

Kagan, J., & Whitten, P. Day care can be dangerous. *Psychology Today*, 1970, *4*, 36-39.

Kapfer, S. Report of first National Home Start Conference. Washington, D. C.: Office of Child Development, 1972.

Karnes, M. B., Studley, W. M., Wright, W. R., & Hodgins, A. S. An approach for working with mothers of disadvantaged preschool children. *Merrill-Palmer Quarterly of Behavior and Development*, 1968, *14*, 174-184.

Katz, L. G. Children and teachers in two types of Head Start classes. *Young Children*, 1969, *25*, 342-349.

Katz, L. G. Teaching in preschools: Roles and goals. *Children*, 1970, *17*, 42-48.

Keister, M. E. Final Report. A demonstration project: Group care of infants and toddlers. University of North Carolina, Greensboro, North Carolina, 1970. (a)

Keister, M. E. *The good life for infants and toddlers: Group care of infants*. Washington, D.C.: National Association for the Education of Young Children, 1970. (b)

Lally, J. R. Selecting and training the parent educators. In I. J. Gordon, Final Report, No. PHS-R-306, Washington, D.C.: Children's Bureau, Department of Health, Education, & Welfare, 1969.

Lally, J. R. Development of a day care center for young children. Progress Report, 1970-71, Syracuse University Children's Center, No. PR-156 (C-6) Office of Child Development.

Lally, J. R., Honig, A. H., & Caldwell, B. M. Training paraprofessionals for work with infants and toddlers. *Young Children,* 1973, *28,* 173-82.

Lay, M. J., & Meyer, W. J. Effects of early day care experience on subsequent observed program behaviors. Final report, National Program on Early Childhood Education, Syracuse University, 1971.

Levenstein, P. Mothers as early cognitive trainers: Guiding low-income mothers to work with their toddlers. Paper presented at the biennial meeting of the Society for Research in Child Development, Minneapolis, April 1971.

Lewis, M., & Goldberg, S. Perceptual-cognitive development in infancy: A generalized expectancy model as a function of the mother-infant interaction. *Merrill-Palmer Quarterly of Behavior and Development,* 1969, *15,* 81-100.

Maundry, M., & Nekula, M. Social relations between children of the same age during the first two years of life. *Journal of Genetic Psychology,* 1931, *39,* 393-398.

Meyer, W. J., & Lindstrom, D. The distribution of teacher approval and disapproval of Head Start children. Final report. Office of Economic Opportunity, Contract Number OEO-4120, and the Evaluation & Research Center, Project Head Start, Syracuse University, 1969.

Nimnicht, G. P. Overview of a responsive program for young children. Unpublished manuscript, Far West Laboratory for Educational Research and Development, Berkeley, California, 1970.

Osofsky, H., & Osofsky, J. Adolescents as mothers. *American Journal of Orthopsychiatry,* 1970, *40,* 825-833.

Painter, G. *Infant education.* San Rafael, California: Dimensions Publishing Company, 1968.

Painter, G. *Teach your baby.* New York: Simon & Shuster, 1971.

Palmer, F. H. Socio-economic status and intellective performance among Negro preschool boys. *Developmental Psychology,* 1970, *3,* 1-9.

Pavenstedt, E. A comparison of the child-rearing environment of upper-lower and very low-lower-class families. *American Journal of Orthopsychiatry,* 1965, *35,* 89-98.

Provence, S. A three-pronged project. *Children,* 1969, *16,* 53-55.

Ricciuti, H. Categories employed in descriptive scanning of nursery environment. Unpublished manuscript, Cornell University Research Program in Early Development and Education, August, 1970.

Schaefer, E. S. Infant education research project. Paper presented at the Conceptualizations of Preschool Curricula Conference, Center for Advanced Study in Education, City University of New York, May 1970.

Segner, L., & Patterson, C. *Ways to help babies grow and learn: Activities for infant education.* Denver, Colorado: John F. Kennedy Child Development Center, University of Colorado Medical Center, 1969.

Sigel, I. An early intervention program for two-year-old children. Presidential address, Div. 7, meeting of the American Psychological Association, Washington, D.C., September 1971.

Slobin, D.I. Cognitive prerequisites to grammatical development in children. Paper presented at the meeting of the Merrill-Palmer Institute Conference on Research and Teaching of Infant Development, Detroit, February 1972.

Starr, R.H., Jr. Cognitive development in infancy: Assessment, acceleration, and actualization. *Merrill-Palmer Quarterly of Behavior and Development,* 1971, *17,* 153-186.

Stern, C., & Marshall, J. Increasing the effectivess of parents-as-teachers. Paper presented in Symposium "The Parent as Educational Agent" at the annual meeting of the American Educational Research Association, New York, 1971.

Stevenson, M. B., & Fitzgerald, H. E. Infant-toddler Day Care Unit: Standards for infant care in the United States and Canada. Report of Early Childhood Research Center, Michigan State University, Office of Economic Opportunity (OEO) Grant No. CG-9931, April, 1971.

Upchurch, B. *Easy-to-do toys and activities for infants and toddlers.* Greensboro, North Carolina: Institute for Child and Family Development, University of North Carolina, 1971.

Watson, J.S. Cognitive-perceptual development in infancy: Setting for the seventies. *Merrill-Palmer Quarterly of Behavior and Development,* 1971, *17,* 139-152.

Weikart, D. P., Lambie, D. Z., Wozniak, R., Miller, N., Hall, W., & Jeffs, M. Ypsilanti Carnegie Infant Education Project. Progress Report, Ypsilanti, Michigan, September 1969.

White, B. L. Informal education during the first months of life. In R. D. Hess & R. M. Bear (Eds.) *Early education.* Chicago: Aldine, 1968.

13. Programs of Child Care: The United States Need and What Should Be Done*

Dorothy S. Huntington

In 1967, Katherine Graham, the president of the *Washington Post*, used this title for an address she gave to a day care conference: "Does America Hate Children?" She went on to say that:

> "Americans are terribly accustomed to telling themselves that they love children. We love our children to a fault, we say. We have created a child-oriented society, we confess blushing at the thought of our own generosity and devotion. The American regard for motherhood, we tell ourselves, is legendary. But, if we look to the hard evidence, we discover something very different in this country's attitude toward its children. Beginning at the beginning, we discover that we have an infant mortality rate and a maternal mortality rate far higher than, for example, Japan's. The United States, as Professor Moynihan points out, is the only industrial nation in the world with no kind of family allowance whatever. In Congress the continuous debate over aid to the families of dependent children makes it clear that the American politician's regard for motherhood is entirely platonic—it discourages any thought of sex, and it tries to express its devotion with as little money as possible."

> "The maximum Federal contribution to the support of an old lady on relief is $75 a month. The maximum for a dependent child is $32—reflecting, apparently, the conviction that it is cheaper to feed a 12 year old boy than an old lady, and easier to find a big apartment than a small one. We can find similar examples of discrimination against children sowed throughout our national welfare system. But to me, the gravest of our sins against the nation's children are the sins of omission."**

*This article is a modification of a paper originally presented at the Community Pediatrics Section, annual meeting of the American Academy of Pediatrics, San Francisco, California, October 17, 1970. It is reprinted from the *Journal of Clinical Child Psychology*, 1972, I, 3, 12-15

**In the *Proceedings of the Conference of the Maryland Committee for the Day Care of Children*, October 27, 1967, "Day Care Is Your Business".

Let us now consider, in 1972, what those sins of omission are, for this country is rapidly approaching a crisis in its system of developmental child care.

The word crisis as represented in Chinese calligraphy is a composite of the two characters "danger" and "opportunity". The quality of the lives of millions of children is clearly endangered; we have the opportunity to change this, to change for the better the lives of our future generation, *if* we have the commitment. We *must* prevent the development of the personal and social dysfunctions associated with poverty, ill-health and disorganization, enhance the development of the handicapped and provide optimal care for all our children.

In the past, child care projects have referred almost exclusively to day care and many people know only about day care projects. It is an interesting exercise to ask yourself when day care services were first offered to children; you probably will answer in two different ways, depending on your age. If World War II is a hazy episode to you, you probably think day care originated in the early Sixties. If World War II is real to you, you probably remember the Lanham Act that provided money for day care services for the children of women war workers. Rosie the Riveter enjoyed child care services that few modern women can possibly afford.

Actually, day care was a Civil War phenomenon: the Nursery for Children of the Poor in New York City was established in 1854. "These early services, called day nurseries, were offered as philanthropic assistance: first, to children of Civil War widows; then, in the latter part of the 19th century, to children left alone during the day while their immigrant mothers worked in domestic service or in factories."[1] Paralleling this growth of day nurseries with their increasing emphasis on health care, nutrition and child development, was the growth of the kindergarten movement for the children of the privileged classes.

The daytime care of children received major impetus from the Civil War, World War I, the Depression and World War II. The Community Facilities Act—the Lanham Act—passed in 1941 made federal funds available to the states on a 50-50 matching basis. By July 1945, 1,600,000 children were in nurseries and day care centers financed largely by federal funds. When these funds were curtailed at the end of the war, almost all the centers closed. Only in the state of California and in New York City did the programs largely remain active, under other funding auspices.

Nonetheless, following World War II came a new emphasis on

experimentation, social action, child development research and education, maternal and child health, but no innovative programs to meet the needs in a rational way of a large segment of our population—our children. Only in the last five to ten years has any real change taken place, a change noted by the beginning awareness that child development programs might mean something of great importance to *all* families. Where is the new concept evolving?

New Concepts in Child Care

Day care for children of working mothers, to be sure! But add to this day care services both full and part time that have heavy emphasis on removing the deleterious conditions of life for disadvantaged children, day care programs with important educational and emotional-social emphases. Consider also "drop in" centers for mothers who need to shop for a few hours, or go to a clinic for care, or go to the welfare office, and who have no one with whom to leave the children and no money to take them along via public transportation; or care centers for children of students with classes to attend; day care services that include what is necessary for specific groups of children: educational components, health care, nutritional supplementation, and socialization in the broadest sense. Add to this new approach, educational programs such as nursery schools, Headstart, home intervention projects where both children and parents are offered supportive educational services; parent and child centers where parents work together to design and carry out their programs. We are talking about programs for children and parents, family *strengthening* programs that examine the real needs of children and parents in a coordinated sense and then try to meet those needs in a rational way.

What functions do such programs serve? For some children, the provision of the conditions that enhance their future potential: provision of physical protection; absence of physical abuse; food; medical and dental care; education; recreation; just plain growing in circumstances that provide the emotional, social and intellectual nourishment any child has a right to expect.

For the parent, these programs allow working without the constant worry about what is happening to the children; they allow adolescent parents to remain in school; they supply relief from overwhelming stress; they enhance the parents' self respect and strengthen the ties to their children. Training and economic opportunities via jobs in the child development programs are also made possible.

The Need for Developmental Child Care

Who are the children needing such child development services? About 4 out of 10 mothers with children under 18 years were in the labor force in 1970 as compared with 3 out of 10 in 1960 and less than 1 out of 10 in 1940. This trend is expected to continue. While employment of the mothers is the main reason for the need for services, these same services are desperately needed for children with mental or physical handicaps, emotional disturbances, poor family relationships and poverty living conditions.[2]

Many forces have converged to accelerate the need for child care. The report of the Child Development-Day Care Forum of the 1970 White House Conference on Children refers to employment of mothers outside the home; family mobility; urbanization; community mobilization to fight poverty; the rise in single parent families and the choice of alternative life styles by many young parents; pressures to reduce the number of parents on welfare; and the realization of the vast opportunities for early education in the broadest sense.

The social institutions traditionally responsible for child care have generally treated the new needs simply as more of the old. For decades, "day care" has been part of "child welfare" where it has been "tended by a devoted few, condescended to by many". It is still widely believed that only mothers on the verge of destitution seek employment and outside care for their children; that only disintegrated families where parents are unfit to give even minimal care seek outside support. The need for supplementary child care is often viewed as the result of other pathology in the family, its use justified only in forestalling greater disaster for the child.

The child welfare concept of day care—as a service for poor and problem families—has contributed to the resistance to enlarging services to cover broader segments of the population. There has been a lack of community understanding of and commitment to developmental child care, inadequate community coordination and information on available programs, and distress at the high cost of quality care. The needs and uses of child care services have changed more rapidly than our understanding of the situation and our ability to respond to it.

Developmental child care is no longer needed primarily to buttress disintegrating families. Changes in economics, divorce, education, cultural values and other areas have led to a variety of family situations. The working mother is no longer a "misfit", and the family is not the simple mother/father/child picture usually assumed. By the end of this decade, it is possible that most American children will have working mothers, and there is no reason to think that these mothers will be less concerned than other mothers about the care their children receive, or that their employment will, of itself, lead to destructive deviations from normal parent-child relationships.

Next to the growing number of employed women, the second force in the increasing demand for making available supplementary child care to all citizens grows out of recent discoveries of the importance of early experience for human growth and development. Psychologists, pediatricians, psychiatrists, educators, nutritionists, and other investigators continue to document the critical significance of the first years of life. The central finding is that during the years when a child's body, intellect and psyche are developing most rapidly, his conditions of life will profoundly influence his later health, motivations, intelligence, self esteem and relations with other people.

Every moment of a child's life involves learning: what he can and cannot do, what adults expect and think of him, what people need and like and hate, what his role in society will be. His best chances for a satisfying and constructive adult life grow from a satisfying and constructive infancy and childhood. Sound development cannot be promoted too early. It is becoming increasingly clear that supplementary child care holds an important potential for providing all children with the essentials of experience that support optimal development. What then is the challenge?

The Urgency of Action

There are two clear issues in developmental child care for American children: the comprehensiveness and quality of care which all children deserve; and the responsiveness and flexibility of social institutions to the changing needs and desires of American parents. Simply keeping the child in a center for a few or for many hours without applying our utmost expertise and common sense for his sound development is as cruel and absurd as feeding him only the minimal nutrition required to sustain life and expecting a vigorous and healthy body. We must respond as a nation to the changes that we as individuals are living, changes in our views of family roles and of the needs of our families with children. Our lives are changing more rapidly than our institutions. We must develop a network of voluntary supplementary child care, flexible enough to support family life, able to promote the full development of our children, and readily available to all families with children. We must commit our heads and our hearts as well as our pocketbooks to this task.

There is, above all else, an urgent need for political action. "Perhaps we cannot prevent this from being a world in which children are tortured, but we can reduce the number of tortured children. If we do not do this, who will do this?" Albert Camus' familiar statement has very direct bearing on the action that needs to be taken. As 535 members of Congress, a President, a vast Executive Branch, and hundreds of special interest lobbyists compete for power, it is hard to find anyone whose primary concern is to reduce the numbers of tortured, dependent children. Beyond this, it is almost impossible to find anyone who is concerned with the fullest development of *all* of America's children. After all, the children have no vote and therefore must be meaningless.

As psychologists dedicated to the well being of children, you ought to be shocked at the lack of national attention to the critical developmental needs of children in this country. Child care programs must be recognized as developmental services with tremendous potential for positively influencing and strengthening the lives of children and families.

Children need spokesmen. The establishment of the new Office of Child Advocacy is a first step, but there must be powerful advocates in every community and at every governmental level. Legislators must be informed about the basic needs of children, and they must know the consequences of neglect of these needs. Political action is a powerful tool. Money must be raised; programs must be coordinated for maximum impact; the public must be educated. As psychologists you could play new and exciting roles in *action* programs as advocates for the basic rights of children to be well born and well nurtured in the broadest sense.

How can we arrange for the optimal nurturance of today's children at a time of profound changes in the American family and its living conditions? Developmental child care should meet not only normal supervisory, physical, health and safety needs but should also provide for the intellectual, social, emotional and physical growth and development of the child, with opportunities for parental involvement and participation. The family and home remain the central focus of the child's life. Parents must retain the primary responsibility for rearing their children; but society, in turn, must recognize its role in the ultimate responsibility for the child's well-being and development. Developmental child care is a service for all children of all ages from infancy to school age. Regardless of the hours, the auspices, the funding source, the name of the service, or the child's age, the program should be judged by its success in helping each child develop tools for learning and growing, both in relation to his own life style and abilities and in the context of the larger culture surrounding him.

A good program must focus on the development of warm, trusting and mutually respectful social relationships with adults and other children. Such relationships form the basis not only for the personal and social development of the child but also for his future ability to learn from and about others. The program must help develop a positive identity so that each child sees himself and his background as worthy of respect and dignity. A child's positive image of himself as a member of an ethnic, cultural, linguistic or religious group is basic to a strong self concept. Cultural relevance, therefore, is not a separate political issue, but an integral part of human development. Those in charge of programs must be knowledgeable of and sensitive to the values and patterns of life in the children's homes. To help correct past inadequacies and injustices and move toward a truly human heritage for future generations, children must also learn about diverse cultures and their contributions to modern America. We are a multi-ethnic society, and children must learn the value of this from the very beginning. You as psychologists need to become much more knowledgeable about other ways of life, to expand your own horizons, in order to help others become richer people.

In terms of services currently available, any of you who work in hospital out-patient clinics will be poignantly aware of the care arrangements currently forced on women. Babies are cared for by 3 year old sibs; children are locked alone in apartments; neighbors care for five or six children who sit on the sofa all day watching TV. The "latch-key children" care for themselves. According to the latest estimate, day care in licensed homes and centers is available for only about 640,000 children. It is estimated that several million children need the service.

Any of you with patients having handicaps—physical or mental— know how difficult it is to find nurseries that will accept these children and give them the kind of social, emotional, educational and physical experiences they so need. "Lack of adequate child care facilities has been found to be a major deterrent to solution or even significant progress in providing greater educational opportunities for children, reducing the welfare burden, giving greater dignity and self respect to mothers on welfare, filling critical manpower needs in shortage occupations and providing real freedom of choice in lifestyle for women."[3] Our current systems force dependency on people as a way of life; we really make little effort to help people develop more adaptive and rewarding coping mechanisms.

Child Care Programming: An Ecological Approach

What is the need, then? A vast system of custodial day care services, in which children are housed away from their parents for a few or many hours a day? *No!* Programs in other countries show us why the answer must be an unqualified *NO*. What is needed is attention to the ecology of the child and family, attention to what goes on in the network. There must be an integration of thought and of services before any of this will make sense. An ecological approach would lead to an awareness of the interrelationships of significant developmental factors and the provision of care that would supply the personal, social, educational and health "nutriment" so needed. It would lead to an awareness of the conditions fostering despair, hopelessness, a sense of powerlessness and being trapped in poverty or depression. The programs to change these conditions must be geared to the myriad of interacting and synergistic conditions of economic and psychological disadvantage—not just to one or another at a time.

In terms of pratical programs, where does this complex view lead? We must have programs for *children* with special needs—the economically disadvantaged, the migrants, children essentially without families: the "neglected and dependent", for the physically and mentally handicapped, for the emotionally disturbed. We must have programs for *families* with special needs—the working mothers, the one parent families, the teenage mothers, the students, the psychologically pressured. We must have programs for *groups* with special needs—programs oriented toward re-establishing pride, enhancing self-esteem, providing jobs and a sense of community and the neighborliness that is so lacking.

Programs must have within them a variety of services so that the services meet the needs of the individual children and families. No *one* model answers everyone's problems. The services might include health care; homemaker emergency services; community action; employment; before and after school care; full and partial day care for all age children, including infants; a drop off service; educational, social and recreational opportunities; 24 hour care and week-end hours for shift workers; someone to go into a home and work with chilren and the parents; whatever is needed and may be creatively organized by the consumer of the services. There are many different kinds of families and children with many different kinds of needs requiring different solutions.

This leads to another consideration—that is, the focus of control of these services. In the past, the professionals decided what they thought was best. Sometimes they were right, sometimes very wrong. At best, the consumer could acquiesce and passively use the service. At worst, he could go away. The decision making process now is being re-shaped—it is now the community that wants to decide what is desirable and appropriate to their own individual needs, and it is through this process of decision making and responsibility that families and groups are experiencing—many for the first time—a sense of effectiveness and competence.

Where does this lead us? Essentially to a period of social change that is reinforcing the positive changes in the lives of the families involved. For example, a high level of parent participation in the Head Start program was associated with high involvement of the Head Start program in bringing about institutional change; the more stages of change in which the Head Start program participated, the greater the benefit, scope and duration of the change.[4] The parents themselves change as they become re-involved with other people and sense their own increasing ability to have an effect on the world. The knowledge that your behavior *does* make a difference, that you can effect changes on other people and institutions is basic to a positive sense of self esteem. Of vital importance is the reconstituting of the community network of services—fragmented children and fragmented families are not helped by fragmented services. The child cannot be redeemed without redeeming the community.

"Generations ago, as society became industrialized and urbanized, family roles and functions were fractionalized among a variety of community institutions—educational, vocational, recreational, child care and health. These institutions carried out their functions under the aegis of especially educated personnel, often supported by legal requirements and usually with sharply delineated boundaries separating home and institution. Today we are witnessing and experiencing a resurgence of parental role and responsibility in those areas. Hitherto restricted to family roles within the home, parents are following their children into these institutions to take part in policy making, decision-making, service-giving. The home has begun to encompass the institution in behalf of the children."[5]

The assumption that has been too clear in the past—that one could effect a lasting change in children without effective changes in the parents—has been proven false repeatedly in such a variety of programs from exquisitely expensive individual psychotherapy to educational intervention programs for the disadvantaged.

Many legislators decry the cost of programs for children and families, yet their knowledge of the costs of present alternatives is sadly deficient. Social cost accounting must be carried out in a long term framework; a hard dollars and cents look at the cost to society of non-productive citizens, the welfare structure, hospitals and courts, and long term residential institutions *vs.* the cost of preventive services to children and families. This society pays a very high price indeed for the dependency it forces on many of its citizens. Nowhere is there to be found now a rational assessment of the costs of preventable waste of human potential.

This is not simply a problem of poverty—all socio-economic groups have children with handicapping conditions: the Children's Bureau has estimated that there are 450,000 children under 21 with cerebral palsy, 2,600,000 mentally retarded children, 3,200,000 with speech impairments and 5,000,000 to 10,000,000 who are emotionally disturbed (one in every four families). Where are the comprehensive, coordinated services for these children? Where are the services that will permit them to fulfill their potential, that will optimize their own development, and preserve the strength of their families? A relatively small investment in preventive and supportive services—in daytime care programs, enrichment programs in homes and centers, special school programs, homemaker services, protective environments (like sheltered workshops for adolescents), recreation facilities, special health programs and clinics—all *family oriented* services—would save this country untold billions of dollars in wasted human beings.

The Psychologist as Child Lobbyist

Given all this, then, how may psychologists best help in developing appropriate services in their communities? In two vital ways: first—by becoming *change agents*—by working for coordinated and adequate services that will expand the options currently open to families, that will expand the options open for the future of children, services with high and enforced standards to insure that they help rather than hurt children. Use your knowledge of child development to ensure quality of programs and to emphasize the importance of family involvement. Second—you can be invaluable by lobbying for financial support for these programs.

Mr. Nixon has committed himself verbally to early childhood, but his actions have spoken otherwise. His veto of the Comprehensive

Child Care Act of 1971 was again a message implying "We don't care about our children". It indicated most poignantly, in addition, the President's lack of awareness of the family strengthening potential inherent in programs that enhance self respect through providing direct parental participation in the conduct and overall direction of prgrams for their children. The Mondale-Brademus bill (The Comprehensive Child Care Act) provided for such parent involvement, for training, for in-home services, for jobs, for policy councils, provisions that are family strengthening in the broadest sense. HR 1, Mr. Nixon's Welfare Reform Act, allows for no family involvement or control of the custodial day care services that will be provided the children of working mothers. There is no family centered approach here, and it will diminish both parental authority and parental involvement with their children. In addition, the money being provided for day care is so minimal, there will be no possibility for child development services within the framework of the day care program.

As psychologists, we must all use our power to make clear what our commitment to our nation's children *must* be—then we will truly be practicing the art and science of the human psyche.

References

1. Mayer, Anna and Alfred Kahn. *Day Care as a Social Instrument*. New York: Columbia University School of Social Work, January, 1965, page 21.
2. *Day Care Facts*. Washington, D.C.: U. S. Department of Labor, Women's Bureau. May, 1970. WB-70-213.
3. A Matter of Simple Justice. The report of the President's Task Force on Women's Rights and Responsibilities. Washington, D.C.: Government Printing Office. April, 1970, 0-383-452.
4. Datta, Lois-Ellin. "Head Start's influence on community change". *Children,* September-October 1970.
5. Adair and Eckstein. *Parents and the Day Care Center*. New York: Federation of Protestant Welfare Agencies. 1969.

14. Preschool Enrichment and Learning*

Jerome Kagan

America has been, for the most part, an optimistic community, convinced of the correctness of its direction, and childishly confident that any obstacles that deflected its linear progress could be swept aside through a combination of intelligence, diligence, and permissive funding. One of the psychological premises upon which this optimism rested was the belief that errors in an individual's development could be corrected, and those too refractory to remediation could be set straight in the *next* generation by making *right* what went awry the first time. The dour mood that pervades the country at the present time is due, in part, to our failure to meet the standards we set for ourselves. We are either dismayed, angry, or apathetic because no healing ideology capable of inviting national commitment and halting further social disorder seems to be forming. We realize that our good mood will not return until equal opportunity becomes a reality, but recognize, simultaneously, that such a goal can only be obtained if progress in school, which is a major avenue to power in society, correlates only with effort and talent, and not with income, dialect, or color. There is, therefore, a preoccupation with the nature of intellectual growth in the child, and the title of this paper is one reflection of this interest.

The popular interpretation of the unfortunate fact that poor children find school difficult is that early experiences in the family, rather than demons, floating wombs, or excessive secretion of body humors, are the villainous cause of unsatisfactory academic achievement. It is possible that we, like the Greek and medieval physicians, have an exaggerated faith in the validity of our diagnosis. For it is unlikely that interactions with parents are the sole determinant of the complete sweep of psychological development. However, it is probably safe to assume a kernel of truth to the idea that the child's experiences with adults during the first five or six

---

*Vanuxem Lecture presented at Princeton University. December 8, 1970.

years have a nontrivial influence on his future abilities and motivation. Since an increasing number of educated women want careers outside the home, and many poor women have elected to work in order to contribute to the economic stability of their families, our society has been nudged to create sources of supplementary care outside the home, and pushed to the tip of a major structural alteration in the form of child care. It is likely that we will soon have several million children under age six cared for outside the home by adults who, in most instances, are complete strangers to the parents. Since there is no firm body of data or theory that allows us to predict the consequences of this arrangement, we should worry a little about its possible sequellae. Hence, the question of what to do with young children is relevant whether the location of child care be the home, a neighbor's apartment, a trailer, or a freshly built day care center on a busy city street. How do we arrange the environment so that the child's growth is optimal?

Let me state a prejudice in the clearest form possible. One cannot prescribe the correct experiences for a child unless one specifies the environment to which he must adapt. The skills, strategies, beliefs, and motives that are useful in one environment may be irrelevant or, in some instances, debilitating in another. We allow our children to express their anger because we believe that suppression of this emotion will produce an overly inhibited and tense child, and that an excessively inhibited adolescent will not fare well in our competitive society. The Eskimo, by contrast, try to prevent expression of anger in older children because they believe it will destroy the close feelings of cooperation that must be amintained if one lives continually with six others in an area of 1000 square feet. Unfortunately, most citizens prefer to assume a more absolute posture than the one I am advocating; they believe in a fixed and special set of psychological attributes that permit an adult to be happy and successful and a parallel set of environmental experieces that allow such a psychological house to be built. This is much too simple a view. There are too many different profiles of successful psychological adjustment to ensure the truth of the first proposition, and too many local theories of child-rearing to bolster the second. The rural, poor mother in West Virginia believes that a slap on the bottom will teach her child to inhibit childish crying or teasing of a younger sibling. The middle-class Princeton mother is sure that deprivation of a privilege will accomplish the same goals. The Utku mother living northwest of Hedson Bay knows that there is nothing she can do until the child is old enough to understand that whining and teasing are wrong—until the child acquires what the Utku call "ihuma," which is best translated as "reason." And we should not be surprised that most seven-year-olds in all three cultural settings have stopped both of these undesirable behaviors. There are many ways to socialize a child, and a relativistic attitude toward psychological growth is the only rational attitude to promote. There is no wrinkled guru who possesses the universal "how-to-do-it" secrets of human development. Despite the intellectual attractiveness of this conclusion, our hearts boldly resist it and persuade us that some experiences must be more beneficial to growth than others, and we continue to search for a statement that summarizes them. Although there is no neat recipe for growth, it is true, nevertheless, that there are some *principles* of psychological development and it is these principles that I shall consider. Let us first distinguish among the three great psychological systems; namely behavior, cognition, and motivation.

The domain of overt public behavior is most easily specified. The child's repertoire of public actions is best described by its functions. Some responses are used to gratify biological needs. Others are used for defense—physical as well as psychological. Still others are employed to gratify learned desires and further psychological growth. Some behavioral systems, like the motor coordination necessary for walking or playing tennis, are acquired through the processes of *conditioning*. Other response systems—like language—are potentiated through mere exposure to the proper set of environmental events. The child's speech emerges naturally, though mysteriously, as a result of listening to a talking environment. Apparently structures in the temporal lobe have been specially prepared by nature for the reception and organization of language. Given the raw material of hearing people talk, these brain structures manufacture language products in their host. Still other behavioral systems are acquired through observation of others, followed by imitated practice. Learning how to open a window is an example of this last category. Thus, if one prefers to use the word *learning* to cover all these types of *change*, then it is appropriate to speak of different modes of learning.

Cognition—or more simply thought—is our second system, where cognition refers to a set of mental units and a coordinated set of processes that manipulates these units in the intricate ballet of thought. The primary functions of cognition are (1) to allow the child to recognize the past, (2) to understand new experience, and (3) to manipulate his symbols, concepts, and rules in order to solve a problem. The basic units of cognition include schemata, images, symbols, concepts, and rules. The basic processes include perception, memory, inference, evaluation, and deduction; they are organized by special executive processes that are responsible for the permanent registration of experience, as well as its transformation and activation when problems have to be solved. Although we shall return to a discussion of the five units and five processes later, it is worthwhile to discuss now the idea of the executive, since it has only recently attracted the attention of psychologists.

All children learn a language which enables them to label discrete aspects of their experience. These linguistic structures are placed in long-term memory and retrieved, as if by a special mental rake, by an executive process that organizes knowledge as it retrieves it, much as a construction foreman directs the depositing of bricks, boards, and pipes around the building site and, at the proper time, retrieves them from the correct location, and organizes them into the proper architectural form. There are important differences among children in the efficiency with which this executive operates.

Consider the following empirical finding. Four-year-old children are shown a row of six familiar objects: a pin, button, cup, fork, doll, and scissors. The examiner assures himself that the child can name each of the six objects correctly. Now the examiner touches four of the six objects once in a random order, perhaps button, fork, doll, and scissors, and then asks the child to touch the objects in the same order. The four-year-old performs poorly, the eight-year-old does very well. We know that the younger child's failure is not due to absence of a language label for each of these simple objects. We also know that a four-year-old is capable of remembering much more information than is required in this problem. For if he is asked to examine 60 pictures from magazines, for about two seconds each, and is then shown 120 pictures, 60 of which are new and 60 of which he looked at earlier, and asked simply to say which ones he saw, he is correct 90-100% of the time. Some children make no mistakes when tested two days later. The four-year-old can remember 48 hours later that he saw 60 pictures, if all he has to say is "yes" or "no,' "old" or "new." But he cannot reconstruct a temporal pattern of only four events. Our explanation of this apparent paradox is that the young child did not activate the language label that he had in his repertoire while the adult was touching the objects. He did not use his knowledge to help him remember the temporal pattern he watched. Proof of this conclusion comes from a study in which five-year-olds, eight-year-olds, and adults looked through the 60 pictures under two different conditions. One group was given no special instruction, as in the experiment cited above. The second group was told to label the picture in some way. Then all the subjects were shown 120 pictures—60 old and 60 new—and asked to say which ones they saw earlier. For adults, who naturally activate a conceptual set of labels for experience, it did not make much difference which group they were in. They performed well under both instructions. However, for the children, especially the five-year-olds, those who were instructed to label benefited enormously and their performance was much better than those five-year-olds who examined the pictures under no special instruction, and who apparently did not activate any label for the pictures.

A second example comes from the Kpelle of Liberia, who do not have a written language. A list of 16 words was read to the Kpelle adult, eight of which belonged to one conceptual category, like weapons, and eight to another conceptual category, say edible foods. The subject was asked to remember these words and to recall them when the complete list had been read. The subject remembered about as many words as an American adult on the very first reading. But with succeeding readings of the list, Americans improved dramatically, while the Kpelle did not. It appears that the Kpelle did not have the mental set or disposition to organize the eight "weapon" words into one conceptual category and the eight food words into another, even though they have the individual words for the category. However, the more education a Kpelle had, the more his preference resembled an American. Education teaches the use of categories. The executive strategy of organizing experience into conceptual categories is one of the functions strengthened by formal education. We must make a sharp differentiation, therefore, between possessed knowledge and the active use and organized retrieval of that knowledge to solve a problem.

Consider a final example of the executive process from the infant. A ten-month-old infant was allowed to play with a simple toy—say a toy animal—for a few minutes. Then six minutes later he was given a pair of toys, a new one and the one he had played with earlier. Some children went directly to the new toy. Others first visually scanned each of the two toys two to three times, and only then crawled to the new one. We do not believe that it is a coincidence that the infants who stopped to scan both toys had mothers who were more interactive and playful with them. This one-to-one interactive activity between caretaker and infant may facilitate the development of the executive process that compares the past and present and retrieves relevant knowledge in time of conceptual conflict. The child who scans both toys, we believe, was activating his memory of the earlier experience with the old toy. He was thinking before acting.

The third major system—after behavior and cognition—refers to motives in the broadest sense and includes the varied goals the child desires to attain, his expectancy of obtaining them, and the affect that occasionally accompanies motivation.

If these are the three systems that form the bedrock of psychological development, we can ask about their relation to the title of this paper. The phrase "preschool enrichment" usually means providing experiences that will make poor children from ethnic minority groups similar to middle class white children in behavior, cognition, and motivation. A more relativistic definition of enrichment would be concerned with how one arranges the environment so that the largest number of children eventually come to possess the behaviors, cognitive structures, and motives that will be most adaptive for their particular cultural setting. To illustrate, Black English frequently omits syntactic forms of the verb to be. Thus, "I goes home" means the same as "I am going home." The former sentence is different from standard middle-class English, but it is not necessarily a cognitively deficient sentence. Hence the primary issue surrounding "what should be enriched" is as much an ethical as it is a scientific issue. Our society must decide on the profile of psychological qualities to be promoted. During the first six years of life we usually leave these decisions to parents. But since our culture is creating institutional care for preschool children, this issue cannot be ignored. We must make a value choice.

Each social community has an implicit catechism of ideal traits for its children. I suggest that most Americans would support the following statement of developmental goals—a sort of psychological platform for children. Each child should believe he is valued by the adults who care for him so that he will develop an autonomous identity, be self-reliant, and come to believe he can determine his own actions and values. We should note that these simple premises are not shared by all societies. The Japanese, for example, reject our stress on individual identity and self-reliance and are convinced that an adolescent should not be completely self-determining. He should be ready and willing to rely on others for help and affective support. Americans, by contrast, regard such behavior in a late adolescent as immature and excessively childish. Each of us is a unique bundle of talents and temperaments with a best fit in some particular context. My profile happens to be in harmony with the community in which I live, and thus there are occasional moments of serenity.

But I can imagine a half-dozen environments in which I would be miserable.

Each parent, parent surrogate, and educator must toss a prophetic fishline forward in time and estimate the talents, motives, and beliefs that will be most useful for 1990. Fortunately the set of traits to celebrate cannot be totally unrelated to those we promote now for there are sociological constraints on the amount of social change that will occur, as well as biological limits on man's psychological elasticity and imaginative capacity to invent a totally novel set of goals. It is reasonable to expect, therefore, that as far as cognitive processes are concerned, we shall continue to value the child who has a rich store of concepts and rules and effective strategies for registration of experience and retrieval of knowledge. The more specific talents that fill out that abstract formula will probably include reading competence (despite McLuhan, since reading is so much more efficient than listening), quantitative skills, the ability to write coherently, and the capacity to discriminate effective from ineffective arguments. The required motivational processes will include, at a minimum, the wish to be intellectually competent, an expectancy of obtaining that goal, and a firm personal identity.

As promised earlier, we shall now consider in more detail the cognitive and motivational processes that make development appear progressive. First, we shall consider the cognitive structures that should be enhanced at home and in preschool educational centers. The basic units in cognition are schemata, images, symbols, concepts, and rules.

Schemata. The schema, which is the infant's first acquired cognitive unit, is a representation of the salient aspects of an event. Although the schema is neither an image nor a photographic copy of the event, it does preserve the arrangement of the significant elements that define the event. Your schema of Atlantic City is likely to contain water as a critical element. The critical elements of a schema give it distinctiveness and, like the cartoonist's caricature, exaggerate the most salient attributes of the event.

During infancy the salient elements can include the sensory feedback from the infant's actions toward an object. Thus, a baby can represent, or come to know, his favorite rattle in terms of its visual appearance as well as through his actions toward it. Piaget believes that sensorimotor interactions with objects during the first year of life are necessary for cognitive growth, and he talks of the acquisition of sensorimotor schemes.

Most enrichment programs for infants—as well as toy departments—emphasize play with attractive toys. The single most common element in all day care programs for infants in the United States is the presence of toys that permit the infant to shake, rattle, push, and pull them and receive feedback from this manipulation. It is assumed that these experiences help to teach the child about the object and, as a dividend, persuade him that he can have an instrumental effect on the world. Although this notion seems intuitively reasonable, it is not so obvious to all parents and professionals. Some Dutch physicians in the eastern part of Holland instruct the mother to minimize the amount of stimulation and play that the infant experiences during the first 10 months of life, and they lie alone in cribs, with no toys, for the first 40 weeks. Moreover, these children are intellectually adequate at age five, although they are a little retarded on American tests of intelligence at one year. Furthermore, limbless infants born to mothers who had taken thalidomide have no opportunity to manipulate toys. Yet their cognitive development seems perfectly adequate. Thus, despite the intuitive reasonables of the idea that play with toys should be necessary for mental development, the empirical data force us to question the strong form of that proposition.

Images. A schema is not synonymous with a visual image, for the child can have schemata for voices, odors, and textures. The image is a mental picture and is a special and more elaborate structure which is related to the schema and more easily manipulated. However, like the schema, it preserves the unique pattern of physical qualities in the event. Perhaps the best way to regard the relation between schema and image is to view the former as the basic skeleton from which the more detailed holistic image is built. A schema is used in the construction of the image when cognitive processes perform work on it.

Symbols. Symbols are qualitatively different from both schemata and images, for unlike the latter two, a symbol is an *arbitrary representation* of an event. The best example is the name for a letter, a number, or an animal. A child who can name the arbitrary collection of lines we designate as the letter "M" and can point to an "M" when asked, possesses the symbol for that alphabetic letter. In most children, symbolic function begins around 15-18 months, but can begin as early as one year. Most enrichment programs encourage the development of symbols, especially linguistic symbols, by encouraging the caretaker to begin to name objects in the child's environment as soon as the teacher feels the child can understand them.

Concepts. All concepts are symbols but they are much more than that. A concept stands for a set of common characteristics among a group of schemata, images, or symbols, and is not a specific object. A concept is a representation of a feature or features common to a variety of experiences. Consider the drawing of a cross. The 8-month-old infant possibly represents the cross as a schema. The 3-year-old, who may call it a cross, presents it as a symbol. The adolescent who regards it as the cross of Christianity and imposes on it a relation to religion and church possesses the concept.

One of the serious difficulties preschool children have is that they regard many concepts as absolute rather than relative. When the 4-year-old first learns the concept dark, he regards it as descriptive of an absolute class of color—black and related dark hues. The phrase "dark yellow" makes no sense to him, for dark signifies dark colors, not relative darkness.

It is important to help the child appreciate both the absolute and relative qualities of many concepts and to persuade him that the same concept can have several different meanings in different contexts. The set to appreciate the relativity of conceptual dimensions can be promoted by a number of game-like problems in which the child has to name the multiple attributes of objects. A banana is yellow and brown and long and soft and smooth and sweet and sticky. A rock is good for breaking glass but bad for bouncing. A glass is good for drinking, fair for making musical melodies, and absolutely useless for drawing. The child himself is many things, he is a boy, the son of his father; he is the smallest child in the family, but the largest child in his classroom. It is possible to help the young child appreciate the multidimensional quality of concepts, and this victory seems to facilitate other intellectual conquests.

Rules. There are two kinds of rules. One states a relation between two concepts. The rule "water is wet" states that the concepts water and wet are related, for one of the dimensions of water is the quality wetness. A second type of rule is a mental operation of routine imposed on two or more concepts to produce a new one. Multiplication is a rule imposed on two numbers to produce a third. We call these rules transformations. Jean Piaget claims that there are discrete stages in the acquisition of rules. The appearance of stages in the child's thought sometimes results from the fact that rules that are learned initially stubbornly resist retirement, for they have been so effective in the past. A child's rule, like a scientific theory, is never replaced through criticism alone, but only by a better rule.

Having considered the basic units of schema, image, symbol, concept, and rule, we turn now to the cognitive processes that manipulate these units in thought. Cognitive processes include two general types, undirected and directed. Undirected thinking refers to the free flow of thoughts that occur continually as the child walks home or stares out the window. Directed thinking, by sharp contrast, refers to the processes that occur when the child tries to solve a problem. He knows there is a solution and he knows when he has arrived at it. This problem-solving process typically involves the following sequence: comprehension of the problem, memory, generation of possible solutions, evaluation, and implementation.

Comprehension of the Problem

Understanding the problem, which must be the first event in problem solving, requires selective attention to the salient aspects of an event and organized interpretation of information. Most problems are presented in the verbal mode and, therefore, the richer the child's vocabulary—that is, his language concepts—the more successful his understandings. This is one reason why the majority of preschool programs emphasize the teaching of words. However, all concepts are not linguistic, and if the child becomes overly accustomed to using only language to understand a problem, he may fail to develop other strategies. Hence, problems and information must be presented in nonverbal modes, including pictures, sounds, and action.

The preschool child has difficulty focusing attention on more than one event at a time. If he tries to listen or watch many things at once he often becomes confused. Hence, the teacher should guarantee that she has the child's attention when talking to him. The best way to accomplish this goal is to have an adult working 1:1 or with only a small group of children. Since it is impossible to have a half-dozen licensed teachers in every preschool center, paraprofessionals must be used. Mothers, older children, and college and high school students are an excellent reservoir of needed talent and help.

Memory

Memory refers to the storage of experience. There are two major kinds of memory, short-term and long-term memory. This differentation is based, in part, on special structures in the central nervous system which seem necessary for long-term memory. Information in short-term memory is typically available for 15 to 30 seconds. The easy forgetting of a new telephone number after it has been dialed is a good example. Unless one makes a special effort to transfer the perceived information to long-term memory, some or all of it will be lost. Young children display poor memory because (a) they have a less adequate set of cognitive units to encode information for placement in long-term memory, (b) they have not learned the trick of rehearsal and do not spontaneously repeat events to themselves in order to aid transfer to long-term memory, and (c) they are not efficient at retrieving what they know. Enrichment programs should include exercises in which the child is taught memory tricks, ways of grouping words, numbers, or pictures, and strategies of free associating that will aid later recall. Moreover, anxiety is memory's major enemy; it interferes with focused attention and with the ability to recall the past. Curricula should help the child develop strategies for placing new knowledge in memory, and for efficient retrieval, while keeping distraction and anxiety tamed.

Generation of Ideas

The comprehension of a problem and remembering it are typically the first two processes in any problem-solving sequence. The third process is the generation of possible solutions, the thinking up of alternative ways to solve the problem. The child is motivated to seek solutions whenever he comes across a problem he does not understand, one for which he does not have an immediate answer. The child sees his mother weeping or watches a bird unable to fly. These events create a state of uncertainty because he cannot explain the event. He wants to resolve this uncertainty, to understand the experience, and so he dips into his reservoir of knowledge and searches for ideas that will allow him to explain what he has seen. One of the major obstacles to the generation of good ideas is the possession of beliefs that conflict with good solutions. A set of firmly held ideas that are inconsistent with the required solution is one cause of rejection of the correct idea, should it occur. Anxiety over possible criticism for suggesting unusual ideas also can be inhibiting, for fear typically blocks creative solutions. The easiest and most common reaction to fear of error is to withdraw from the task or, if the fear is mild, to inhibit offering answers. Every preschool teacher recognizes this syndrome, for each group has a few children who are intelligent but overly inhibited. They know more than they are saying and censor good ideas because they would rather avoid making a mistake than risk the joy of success. The teacher must reduce these fears by encouraging guessing and convincing the child that honest approximations are better than no response, that any attempt is better than none.

Evaluation

Evaluation refers to the degree to which the child pauses to evaluate the quality of his thinking and the accuracy of his conclusions. This process influences the entire spectrum of thought, including the accuracy of perception, memory, and reasoning. Some children accept and report the first hypothesis they produce and act upon it with only the barest consideration for its quality. If correct, they are called ebullient; if not, unruly. These children are best called impulsive. Others devote a long period of time to considering their ideas and censor many hypotheses. These children are reflective. If correct, they are called wise; if incorrect, dull. This difference among children can be seen as early as two years of age and seems to be moderately stable over time. Fortunately, the child's disposition to be reflective or impulsive can be modified by training, and teachers should consider this factor in working with young children.

Implementation of Ideas: The Deductive Phase

Deduction or implementation is the application of a transformational rule to solve a problem, once the solution hypothesis has been generated. There are basic changes in the child's understanding and use of rules during the first 12 to 15 years. Some psychologists assume the child merely learns more good rules each day, storing them for future use, and there is no rule that is necessarily too difficult for a child to comprehend and apply. The alternative view, which I find a little more congenial, is that some rules are inherently too complex for young children to understand. Hence, there must be maturational stages in the development of thought.

Let us summarize this section on cognition by noting the general changes that occur during the period from one through six years of age. The richness of the child's supply of symbols, concepts, and rules increases each year and these units undergo continual reorganization as a function of experience, especially experience that causes him to question what he knows.

The original function of thought is to help the child make sense of his experiences. If he witnesses an unusual event he does not instantly understand, he reaches back into his mind to pull out an explanation that will put him at ease again. The child becomes increasingly concerned with the amount of agreement betweeen his concepts and those of others, and he becomes more apprehensive about making mistakes. Hence his conception of problems and the rules he activates to solve them begin to approach that of the adult community. The second function of cognition is to communicate thoughts and wishes to others. Finally, thought permits the pleasure that comes from having a good idea, which is one of the basic sources of joy nature has permitted us. You will note that I have refrained from using the word "intelligence" or IQ. This was a purposeful act for I believe we should think of mental phenomena as a set of coordinated but separate processes—not as a global capacity. Let me defend this prejudice.

The Concept of Intelligence

Human beings like to rank order people and things into categories of good, better, best. We are not satisfied with noting that the rose is a deep red but feel pressed to add that it is the loveliest flower in the garden. We automatically give a goodness-badness score to most of our experiences. We also perform this evaluation on ourselves, for homeliness is bad and attractiveness good; weakness bad and strength good. Of the many attributes of mankind, three typically receive special attention in all cultures. We usually evaluate physical qualities, inner feelings, and skills. There are very few cultures that do not have special words to describe how a person looks, how he feels, and how competent he is—and these words imply that certain appearances, feelings and skills are good, while others are bad.

But each culture's decision is somewhat arbitrary and may not be valid for another group or for its own membership at another time in history. In 17th century Europe, women whom we would regard as hopelessly overweight and unattractive were viewed as beautiful, and a comparison of a Rubens' nude with that of a Gauguin reveals the changing standard of attractiveness.

The skills that are tagged good or bad also vary with time and social group, although every society sets up certain talents as most desirable. Bushmen must be skilled at hunting and tracking and those who possess this talent are given a designation that has a connotation similar to our word intelligent. "Intelligent" is the word society applies to those people who possess the mental talents the society regards as important. But those talents change with time. In the late nineteenth century, Francis Galton suggested that those with extremely sensitive vision and hearing were intelligent because the dominant brain theory of the day emphasized the importance of transmission of outside sensory information to the central nervous system. Today we emphasize the salience of language and reasoning because our theories of the brain have changed. But, like Galton, we still use the word intelligent to designate those who have more of those skills we happen to believe are "better."

From a scientific point of view we should exorcise words like intelligent because they are primarily evaluative and explain very little. But this will not happen because most members of our society —scientists as well as nonscientists—believe that this word has an explanatory power that derives from differences in our brains. So let us consider possible meanings of this word.

There are at least four different meanings of the concept of intelligence that deserve mention. The first is not very psychological; the remaining three are, but are different in conception.

Intelligence as Adaptation to the Environment. The ability to adapt to the specific environmental niche in which an organism lives and grows is, for the biologist, the most important attribute of an animal species. Successful adaptation requires resisting predators, maintaining a capacity to reproduce the next generation, and the capacity to cope with new environmental pressures by learning new habits and by alteration of anatomy and physiology. Evolutionary history tells us that some species, like the opossum, have survived for many thousands of generations; others, like the graceful heron, are about to become extinct. If intelligence is defined as the ability to adapt to an ecological niche, then the opossum must be more intelligent than the heron. Since this conclusion contradicts our intuitions, this view of intelligence has never become popular. But that attitude is a matter of taste, not logic.

Piaget's View of Intelligence. Piaget believes that intelligence is the coordination of mental operations that facilitate adaptation to the environment. Hence, in one sense, Piaget promotes the biological prejudice described above. The growth of intelligence is the resolution of the tension between using old ideas for new problems and changing old ideas to solve new problems. Intellectual growth is adaptation to the new through alteration of old strategies, and the intelligent child is the one who has the operations that allow him to solve new problems.

Ease of Learning New Structures and Skills. The most popular laymen's view of the concept of intelligence assumes that the more intelligent the child the faster he will be able to learn a new idea or skill. This belief rests on the notion that there is a generalized receptivity to acquiring new competence, regardless of their specific nature. This faith is opposed by the belief that there are important differences depending on what specific skill is being learned. The man who learns a foreign language quickly may not have such an easy time learning to sail. This tension between a generalized intelligence and a set of specific intelligences is the subject of much controversy among psychologists and is reflected in our ambivalent attitude toward experts. We announce preference for the doctrine of specific intelligence by surrounding the President of the United States with counsellors of different expertise—economists, social scientists, physicists—assuming that insight into inflation is most likely to come from the person who has gained knowledge in economics. As citizens we tend to seek advice from varied people according to the problem. We ask for help with our investments from a broker and advice on building a house from an architect. However, there are still lingering beliefs in a generalized intelligence, for the society is still willing to listen to the advice of a Nobel laureate in physics on how to solve the racial crisis in our schools, as if brilliance of insight into atomic structure indicated profound understanding of social-psychological problems. It is this issue that characterizes the intense controversy surrounding the current use of intelligence and the value of the IQ score. Parents and teachers who believe that intelligence reflects the capacity to learn new skills with ease are often impressed with the intelligence test because a 10-year-old's IQ score does predict, to some degree, grades in high school and college. Is this possible because there is a general ability to learn that is stable over time and domain? Or is it because the skills that are taught in most high schools and colleges are intimately related to the skills measured on the intelligence test? The ability of the IQ obtained at age 10 to predict high school English grades may merely reflect a specific intelligence. In this case, it is the capacity to master English concepts and vocabulary. One reason why this last conclusion is attractive is that there is no question on the standard IQ test that requires the child to learn any new concept, idea, or skill.

The IQ Test. The notion that the IQ score defines intelligence is much different from the three conceptions considered above. Unfortunately, it has gained wide acceptance by Americans. Typical American parents are anxious about their child's IQ and attribute more value and mystique to it than to most characteristics their child possesses. Many believe that a person's IQ score is inherited, does not change very much over the course of life, and can be measured in early infancy. These beliefs are gross exaggerations of the truth. Although most people regard intelligence as the ability to learn a new skill as a result of experience, the majority of questions on intelligence tests do not require any new learning, but ask the child whether he knows a particular segment of knowledge. Hence, the IQ test does not measure the central attribute that most people believe defines intelligence.

However, the intelligence test is an excellent measure of how much the child has learned about the dominant concepts in his culture. That is why the IQ score is a good predictor of school grades.

Since middle-class chilren are more consistently encouraged than lower-class children to learn to read, spell, add, and write, rather than to keep away from police or defend oneself from peers, the child's IQ, social class, and school grades are all positively related. The IQ is an efficient way to summarize the degree to which a child has learned the vocabulary, beliefs, and rules of middle-class American society. The IQ is extremely useful because it can predict how easily a child of 8 years will master the elements of calculus or history when he enters college. However, the specific questions asked on intelligence tests have been chosen deliberately to make this prediction possible. The child is asked to define the word "shilling" rather than the word "rap"; he is asked to state the similarity between a "fly" and a "tree," rather than the similarity between "fuzz" and "Uncle Tom"; he is asked "what he should do if he lost one of his friend's toys" rather than what he should do if he were attacked by three bullies. IQ tests are not to be discarded merely because they are biased toward measuring knowledge that middle-class white Americans value and promote. But both parent and teacher should appreciate the arbitrary content of the test. It is not unreasonable that if the printed word becomes subordinate to tape recorders and television as ways to present knowledge, one hundred years from now our culture—like the early Greek orators— might place higher value on the ability to imagine a visual scene than on richness of vocabulary. We may have a different test of intelligence a century hence because the skills necessary to adapt successfully will have changed. Perhaps the groups we call intelligent then will be different from those who have that label today.

It will always be true that some people will be better adapted to the society in which they live than others, and man is likely to attribute their more successful adaptation to the possession of a set of superior talents. The society will then make a test to measure these talents, and label the score as an index of "intelligence." This process is bound to continue as long as man continues to evaluate himself and others. What will change is the list of talents he selects to celebrate.

Motivation. Let us now briefly examine the two problems surrounding the relation between motivation and the issue of enrichment. The pivotal assumption can be stated plainly. Too many poor children in our country enter school with minimal motivation to master school tasks and no expectancy of succeeding. Since the school directs its tutoring procedures toward the average child, the second grader who has not learned to read or write is hopelessly behind four years later. Perhaps five to seven percent of these children, but probably no more, have subtle nervous system pathology that is undiagnosed, and normal curricular procedures may be inappropriate for such children. But the vast majority of children who fail to show satisfactory progress in school do so because they enter that embattled house with frail motivation for mastering the arbitrary requirements of the primary grades, and a high expectancy of failure. But these children are motivated for some goals, and the teacher must graft a desire to read onto the wishes that happen to be dominant. Motives, in the most general sense, are desired goals the child is uncertain of attaining. Many of the desirable things we seek are experiences we are not sure we can attain. During each successive stage in development, the profile of these uncertain delights changes, and so do the salient motives. The typical 5-year-old is uncertain about his sex role identity and whether he will be accepted and respected by extrafamilial adults. Hence, he is motivated to acquire traits and skills that help define his masculinity (or femininity and help him gain signs of acceptance from others. The teacher, and I use this term in its most general sense, and should capitalize on these motives. The best structure for a young child in a learning situation is a one-to-one relationship with an adult. Such an arrangement is most likely to convince the child that the adult is aware of his existence and cares about his victories, joys, doubts, and fears. A one-to-one arrangement is most likely to persuade the 5-year-old that intellectual skills are appropriate to his burgeoning identity and most likely to guarantee that his smallest victory will be praised. These experiences can thwart the temptation to withdraw, which continually shadows potential failure.

Since we do not have enough certified teachers to meet the one-to-one requirement for every child, we must use high school and college students, parents, and interested adults in the neighborhood as part of a nationwide plan. This suggestion is practical, economical, and a reasonable derivative from theory. It is difficult to understand why we did not think of it earlier. The goal of the tutor, be he student, parent, or neither, is to persuade the child to involve himself in a cognitive activity so that he can produce evidence of the competence hidden within him.

If there is anything new to these ideas, it is the simple plea that we stop thinking of the disadvantaged child as having a deficit in words or numbers that has to be "made-up," a mental cavity that has to be filled as we feed a child deprived of protein or carbohydrate. A more appropriate image is the tempting of a shy deer out from behind a tree in order to try our menu, in the hope that he will come to prefer it to his usual diet. Persuasion, not enrichment, should be the essence of educational procedures. We must convince a great many young children that the attainment of the intellectual talents that our society happens to promote holds a potential for joy, since mastery of the competences valued by a culture can be one route to the self-actualization that everyone requires.

If we are successful, we will be able to use Remy de Gourmont's criteria for documenting our victory, for he suggests that "to judge how high a child's talent will reach do not attend so much to his greater and smaller facility for assimilating technical notions, but watch to see whether his eyes are occasionally clouded with tears of enthusiasm for the work."

15. Psychological Services in Project Head Start[1]

Paul Wohlford

Traditional direct services for the emotionally disturbed child have generally failed to reach low-income families. Two recent sociopolitical developments have offered some promise to correct this problem. First, many anti-poverty programs with mental health-related components are directed to children, such as Head Start and comprehensive health care. Second, community psychology or community mental health programs both directly treat current emotional problems and attempt to prevent future emotional problems. Psychological services for *all* children are, or should be, a large component of any community psychology program. However, children from low-income families require special attention which they have not yet received.

Direct services for current problems of children at the present time are provided by outpatient child guidance clinics, which for the most part are suited to serve a middle-class rather than a lower-class clientele (Adams & McDonald, 1968). In providing preventive programs, community psychology offers the promise of a breakthrough in the attempt to reach children from low-income families. Disappointingly, the promise has not yet been fulfilled for several reasons.

First our society has not devoted the resources necessary to make headway on the immense task. Federal, state, and local governments have generally not allocated sufficient money to test the new

[1]This article is a revision of "Providing Direct Service and Preventive Programs for Children in Poverty," which was presented as part of the Section I, Division 12 symposium, "New Direction for Clinical Child Psychology," at the meeting of the American Psychological Association, Miami Beach, September 1970. This article was written by Dr. Wohlford in his private capacity prior to his present position. No official support or endorsement by the Office of Child Development or the Department of Health, Education and Welfare is intended or should be inferred. The article is reprinted with permission from *Professional Psychology*, 1972, 1, 2, 120-128.

community psychology concepts. To do this, the nation must shift its priorities, replacing the Indo-China war and the limitless drain of the nation's resources for military technocracies, with ecological, educational, community psychology, and other programs of pro-human and pro-survival value. Budgets of domestic programs, like the National Institute of Mental Health, suffer wicked cuts while military expenditures sail merrily through congressional committees, often escalating en route. Individuals and professional organizations must speak out against the lunacy of military plunder and have the courage, like the American Orthopsychiatric Association (1969) did, to come to grips with the fundamental issue of reordering national priorities. Can the American Psychological Association be far behind? I hope not.

A second reason why community psychology programs have not provided necessary services for low-income children may be that there has not been a sufficiently long period, say 15 to 20 years, to develop these services and demonstrate the potentials of the program, let alone to provide research evidence about these methods. On the other hand, is such evidence—at least a generation away—really necessary? I think not.[2] In Project Head Start, the government mounted a massive new educational program for poor children based on a substantial, though not overwhelming research foundation. Indeed, Head Start's justification from research evidence is still not free from controversey (*Harvard Educational Review,* 1970). At the present time in community psychology, there is an available body of demonstration projects and firm research evidence, piecemeal and limited though these may be, that is comparable to that available to Head Start at its onset.

Project Head Start itself is a promising delivery system for community psychology in which psychologists may have been already involved. The purpose of the remainder of this paper is to appraise Head Start psychological services over the past five years and to discuss some promising new models. Although limiting the scope of this article to Head Start, I wish to note there are many parallels between the creative and effective role of the Head Start psycholo-

---

[2]Others would agree. For example, "We cannot wait until all the answers are in, for the development of children does not wait . . . On the other hand, we cannot afford to base large programs or for that matter small ones—on dubious premises. One safeguard, of course, is to recognize the need for eternal vigilance against premature acceptance of instant revelations without demanding full credentials. Such vigilance is especially necessary in those concerned with treating children (Herzog & Lewis, 1970, p.376)."

gist and the role of a community psychologist in other programs serving low-income families.

There are several reasons for concentrating attention on Head Start. As a new program, Head Start is not as limited to old patterns as established institutions were and, thus, has a good potential for innovation. Second, Head Start reaches children at a period of stressful transition in their lives, as they cross the threshold from life in the family to life in society, the public school, during which time many emotional crises can be anticipated. Third, Head Start is no mere demonstration program, since it currently reaches hundreds of thousands of preschool children. Fourth, Head Start has an officially defined role for the psychologists (Office of Economic Opportunity, 1967; Project Head Start, 1970) which is clearly compatible with the role of the community psychologist. Last, in spite of much literature related to Head Start, there are few public reports of psychological services in Head Start, either written or presented. This is the area that I shall now discuss.

Psychological Services in Head Start

In what follows I shall draw primarily on observations from my experience with 10 Head Start programs in six states in the period from 1965 to 1969. The regularity of certain patterns has made me fairly confident of these generalizations, preliminary and limited though they may be. Perhaps a more important qualification is that in 1969 Head Start was moved from the Office of Economic Opportunity to the Department of Health, Education and Welfare in the new Office of Child Development under the directorship of Professor Edward Zigler.

The *Head Start Manual*, which appeared in September 1967, defined a very innovative role for the psychologist in the official Head Start guidelines and requirements for a psychological services program:

"Every Head Start program must have a psychological services program that facilitates effective interaction among staff, parents, children, and volunteers. The psychologist has important contributions to make in all phases of a Head Start program. His major role should be that of enabling staff, parents, children, and volunteers to relate to one another effectively to maximize benefits of the program. In order to do this, his functions should include (1) consultation with staff concerning needs for diagnostic evaluation of individual children, (2) arrangement of a follow-up on evaluation, (3) consultation with teachers and aides concerning diagnosed needs of individual children, (4) consultation with parents concerning needs for specific referral to special agencies, (5) liaison with local and regional mental health facilities and resources, (6) consultation with staff in planning, evaluating, and improving program operation, including curriculum development and services to children and families (Office of Economic Opportunity, 1967, p.39)."

To assure compliance with the guidelines, the Head Start application form has a checklist to specify each psychological service to be performed and who is to do it. Finally, the *Head Start Manual* specifies the minimum and maximum level of staffing psychologists according to the size of the program, ranging from at least one part-time Director of Psychological Services for small programs to a maximum of a program with one psychologist per 200 children.

With such a level of staffing, and with a prohibition against blanket IQ and achievement testing, the psychologists consultative role is reasonably safeguarded and, indeed, even demanded. The Head Start psychologist's functions require that he be responsive to the organization as a whole and not just to a part of the Head Start program. Effective functioning of a particular Head Start organization requires that all the interrelated elements are performing well *both* as individual units (e.g., educational program, social services) *and* as members of the team (e.g., teachers reporting their home visits to the social workers). If the psychologist is to help a Head Start organization function effectively as a whole, he must be tactful but effective in staff management matters, such as correcting overly rigid or authoritarian role prescriptions, replacing low quality staff, initiating staff training, and drawing Head Start parents into meaningful participation with their children. In short, the official structure set down by Head Start in 1967 seems to encourage psychologists to function at a high level of progressive, effective, and innovative community psychology.[3]

Too frequently, this has not happened. Indeed, in many cases, there isn't even a psychologist in the program, even on a part-time basis. Where there are psychologists in programs, they are usually not familiar with the guidelines or seem unable to follow them and consequently slide back into the old role of diagnostician-IQ-tester rather than consultant.

[3]The Head Start "Rainbow Series" on psychology (Project Head Start, 1970) may make it possible to implement the guidelines much more effectively than has been done. This official publication, staying within the guidelines of the 1967 *Head Start Manual,* essentially expands the content and gives practical tips on how to implement a psychological services program.

What accounts for the disparity between the promise and the reality? Quite simply, it has been permissible to ignore the Head Start requirements for psychological services and get away with it. The over-all program has explicit and implicit organizational rules, construed differently from area to area, city to city, but with a total pattern of what is permissible and what is not. As a psychologist who was called upon to assist Head Start, I encountered four distinct patterns of problems, each of which constitutes a syndrome, if we use the metaphor of viewing each Head Start organization as an organism.

Types of Problems Encountered

Naive, Overburdened Syndrome. Often, but not always, the Naive Overburdened Head Start program is found in rural areas where there is a scarcity of any professional consultation, including educational and medical as well as psychological. In such a program, the Head Start director may spend all his time attempting to secure minimally adequate buildings, food for lunches, and teaching personnel. Thus, he is too overwhelmed with the "necessities" to concern himself with the "luxuries" for the program. Identifying characteristics of the Naive Overburdened Syndrome include (*a*) lack of familiarity with the *Head Start Manual,* (*b*) desperate shortage of adequately trained and experienced key personnel including (besides psychologists) social workers, doctors, dentists, volunteer and parent activities coordinators, and supervising teachers, (*c*) poor understanding of basic dimensions of the preschool child's development among the staff, (*d*) chaotic administrative organization, (*e*) nonexistent communication among the staff on various levels, demoralized staff attitudes, and (*f*) no contact with other agencies.

Valid as his concern for the welfare of the children may be, a Head Start director of such a program may literally never have given psychological services a serious thought, not to mention planning psychological services or seeking local or out-of-town consultants to provide the services.

If psychological services are officially in Head Start, why have such programs been permitted to ignore them? The offices from which Head Start programs are directly authorized are themselves similarly overburdened with an abundance of work and a shortage of staff. They, too, give highest priority to those "necessities" like buildings, food, and teachers and lowest priority to "luxuries" like psychological services. Theoretically, the authorizing office has the power to compensate for weaknesses in programs by evaluating programs and supplying technical assistance where necessary. However, the authorizing office's inefficiency may compound the problems of a struggling Head Start program[4] and reinforce the program's denigration of psychological services.

For instance, if a Head Start program realizes that it needs psychological services, asks for them, and even receives visits by a consultant or two, typically there is no completion of the task and not even a report to which to refer. After months and years of languishing, the program staff feels further alienated and is thus less likely even to ask for assistance. If such assistance is again provided, it will be viewed with suspicion. If I may indulge in developmental speculation, such a program is likely to evolve from the Naive Overburdened to the next syndrome.

Disorganized, Indifferent Syndrome. If programs which once had vitality of interest and enthusiasm among the staff have problems which go unsolved due to administrative ineptness or whatever, the immediate result is a series of flare-ups. Over a period of months or years, the flare-ups may die down, as those people concerned either leave the program or become demoralized. The remaining staff become detached and indifferent. These attitudes have great survival value for the individual in this situation, but they contribute to and perpetuate the disorganization of the program. A key etiological factor in this syndrome is often a governing board of directors who themselves suffer from the same syndrome of disorganization and indifference.[5]

While in the Naive, Overburdened Syndrome there are no psychological services whatsoever, there may or may not be services in

---

*For example, outside consultants had visited a Naive, Overburdened Head Start program for a year and a half, but no reports had been sent to the center with suggestions for improvement. On my second visit to assist this program, the program had not yet received my first report. I repeatedly called the authorizing office to which I submitted my report, and finally reached the official responsible for this particular program. Yes, he had received my report, but "it must have slipped through the cracks in the floor somewhere" because he could no longer find a copy of it.

'The clash of the interests of the poor in the community with the interests of the community's dominant power structure may lead to both a stalemate in the conflict and an impotent board that can't make important decisions. In one such case, a white director of the parent agency resigned. His logical replacement, the black assistant director, was not acceptable to the Board because in this town, no black had ever received a salary of $15,000 per year. Although the Board was unable to make this and other important decisions for the welfare of the agency, its individual Board members exerted much influence over the hiring of Head Start personnel, running completely over the wishes of the Head Start director as well as others along the way.

the Disorganized, Indifferent Syndrome. If there are, they are typically provided by a volunteer or paid consulting psychologist who is called upon to evaluate a handful of children who usually exhibit behavioral problems. Some reports are filed away in the psychologist's office or Head Start director's office. The child's teacher is left in the dark. The psychologist, if he works at a public child guidance clininc, may have recommended that the child and his family come to the clinic for treatment. When several families don't show up, the psychologist labels Head Start as hopeless.

In the following example of a Disorganized Indifferent Head Start program, there was a Psychological Services director. There was, however, almost a complete lack of communication within the Head Start organization, specifically between central staff and several delegate agencies, which were actually conducting the Head Start program. There was no mechanism for implementing basic education programs and related components, such as psychology for inservice training, promotions on a performance basis, over-all screening and advisement of daily operations, staff selection and retention, staff performance, and priority selection in terms of assigning the budget. Thus, the Head Start director reassigned the titular Psychological Services director to other duties so that he had no time to perform his psychological services. The Psychological Services director had neither adequate training nor experience, and none of the volunteer psychology consultants was familiar with the functions stated in the *Head Start Manual*. Available community resources had not been used, and social services to support and complement an adequate psychological services program were nonexistent. The teachers' home visits and observations of children's behavior, also supportive of a psychological services program, occurred only rarely and not systematically as specified by the *Head Start Manual*, and there were no records of the children's progress or of parent contacts.

University Exploiter. Since universities are frequently (and sometimes unfairly) criticized for exploiting problems or programs in the ghetto, I am reluctant to give more ammunition to the critics. However, I have seen classic cases of exploitation by some universities and by some psychologists in them under the guise of training, research, and service. For instance, one university-based psychological consultant provided "I.Q." scores derived from the Bender-Gestalt Test for all Head Start children which the Head Start director posted (with names) on his office walls.

In another case, Dr. "X," a white university-based "psychological consultant,'' had no training or backgrond in psychology but rather in a specialty of education. He was quite frank in stating that he was interested in the local Head Start program, which was black, in order to control the curriculum. Dr. "X" and his assistant, who also had no background in psychology, hoped to unseat the Head Start director. When pinned down as to how he would function as a psychologist, he said, "I'd like to do a lot of coordination . . . speech and hearing and that kind of thing." He was not acquainted with the functions of psychology listed in the *Head Start Manual*. Finally, when Dr. "X" hurriedly resigned as psychological consultant, he recommended in his place a clinical psychology student who lost his fellowship because of poor grades. By recommending an inferior person to Head Start, Dr. "X" also revealed a disregard for the program, its goals, and a subtle, though distinct, racist attitude.

Sophisticated Slicker and Bureaucratic Zombie. The last syndrome is often seen as one composite syndrome, though each of its subsyndromes may be observed separately. For instance, in one example the Bureaucratic Zombie existed in a pure form, without pretense or psychopathic cover-up, exposing its dynamics, which were a classic vicious circle: bureaucracy led to poor morale among the staff, the poor morale led to a poor program, and the poor program led to more bureaucracy. In this case, teachers were required to complete 10 different forms each week or month. The forms, including a 15-page children's observation record, reduced staff morale, time, and effectiveness. The forms, once completed, were never used.

Psychological services in such a setting are often prostituted. Referrals for evaluation are made to psychologists or agencies whose perfunctory reports are often deficient. Usually these reports are used to remove the children from the Head Start program, rather than to improve their adjustment to the classroom situation. In summary, identifying characteristics of the Bureaucratic Zombie include the following: (*a*) Compliance with official program requirements if present on paper, not in actuality. (*b*) Highest priorities are always given to the administrative procedures, and thus child development concepts are often lost in the shuffle. Some very powerful administrative organizations and suborganizations resemble military organizations. The resemblance is often not coincidental. (*c*) In rigidly authoritarian hierarchies, communication proceeds in one direction only, from the top down. No complaints or suggestions for improvement are allowed to filter up to the Head Start director. (*d*) The staff at the level of teachers and teachers' aides are thoroughly demoralized and/or indifferent. (*e*) Since such great investment is made in *their* organization, contact with any outside agencies, individuals, or volunteers who may be able to help further the Head Start program is viewed with suspicion or hostility. Therefore, there is no meaningful collaboration with potential community resources.

Finally, the Sophisticated Slicker Syndrome, usually found in larger cities, is frequently a part of the Bureaucratic Zombie Syndrome. That is, the Sophisticated Slicker says, "Everything is fine with us. See, we've complied with all regulations, and we're doing a *great* job." Like every well-integrated psychopath, the Sophisticated Slicker has indeed complied with official procedures, at least superficially, or has a ready alibi prepared. As a kind of psychopathic overlay to conceal program deficits, the Sophisticated Slicker usually also combines with the University Exploiter, and less frequently with the Disorganized, Indifferent Syndrome. When psychopathic features are present, differential diagnoses among Head Start or organizational pathologies may be difficult to establish, as in the psychology of individuals.

As a last comparison between organizational and individual disorders, a good understanding of the nature of the disorder and its underlying etiology should facilitate treatment or remediation. That is, there are significant differences in the intervention strategy to correct deficits in Head Start psychological services, depending on whether it is a Naive, Overburdened program, a Sophisticated Slicker, or something else.

Problems Common to All Programs

There are certain weaknesses or deficits in the central or regional Head Start structure that are common to all the programs I have seen which affect the availability and nature of psychological services. First, programs have been annually handicapped by the unfortunate funding procedures of OEO or HEW and, ultimately, Congress. As a result, funds for psychological services may not be available until a given year has passed. Second, the selection of priorities appears questionable, raising the issue about how priorities are selected, a problem tied to the whole realm of the community's "maximum feasible participation." Third, the Head Start staff's efforts are diminished through a combination of the lack of delegation of authority and the lack of organization across services. There seems to be a lack of true *working* relationships at practically all levels. Fourth, the efforts of consultants have been diminished by a basic lack of communication and coordination between Head Start regional offices and local programs. OEO definitely lacked, and HEW probably lacks, an effective mechanism to enforce compliance with its policies and directives. The only mechanism available, cutting off funds or threatening to, has been ineffective because it was so drastic it was rarely used.

Certain basic changes are obviously needed to make Head Start more hospitable for delivering psychological services. Besides correcting the instability of the Congressional funding pattern, I recommend first that the Head Start structure, especially from the regional office to the local Head Start program, be tightened up drastically, in order to put muscle into the recommendations that are made. This would include more effective coordination and implementation at the regional level with new lines of greater, but flexible authority articulated to make the Head Start guidelines. Second, the members of the local community governing boards should be better informed of the extent and limitations of their duties and responsibilities to promote the functioning of the Head Start program.

Psychological Services in Head Start: Some Promising Models

Small-group psychological consultation. The small-group model of psychological consultation is recommended to correct problems that are often encountered in delivering psychological services and to facilitate director-level and center-level communication enhancing the delivery of medical, social, and psychological services, as well as education. Such a regular series of small-group meetings or conferences is needed to permit effective psychological consultation in particular, but it would also be an important addition to all aspects of the program. The regular Center (or Area) Work Conferences may be arranged as follows.

Natural geographical units should be determined for maximum cooperation and communication either at the Area or the Center level. All Center directors and all teaching and social services staff should participate in groups from a minimum of 10 or so to a maximum of 15 or 20 participants. The Work Conferences must be held regularly, every two weeks, or every week, depending on circumstances and objectives. Every Work Conference should have a decidedly professional orientation with at least a representative from the Head Start central staff in education or social services and preferably from both. A representative of one of these professions should chair each conference, except when it is more appropriate to have it chaired by the psychological consultant, who should attend at least one or two meetings per month.

The main objective of the Work Conference would be to focus on an individual child's development, with contributions being made by all staff who have any contact with the child or his family. Children in need of individual diagnostic evaluations would be referred to the psychologist who would discuss the need for referral, arrange the evaluation, including the family, and follow up on the evaluation's recommendations. Formal diagnostic testing is seldom needed. A Work Conference would describe the child and his family as fully as possible, describe what strategies the staff has already tried in dealing with the situation, evaluate the results of these strategies, and determine whether to continue the same course or plan a new course of action for bringing out the child's fullest potentials. During the intervening period between the Work Conferences, the teacher and others will have an opportunity to implement the new approach to working with the child. At subsequent conferences, there would be reports of progress or lack of progress with the new approach. Also, the Work Conference is a good vehicle for continued in-service training, but on a limited basis to allow time for continuing follow-up of children and families previously discussed.

Head Start parent meetings using participant groups methods. To cope with the almost universal failure to engage Head Start parents meaningfully in programs, new methods must be tried. The participant small-group method has proved successful in an initial pilot effort and on a larger scale (Wohlford, 1971). The purpose of this method is to intervene in the poverty cycle by changing attitudes and behavior among parents of preschool children. These changes in parental attitudes and behavior are intended to promote beneficial social interactions within families by improving the parents' own emotional and cognitive functioning and helping the parents to assist their children's emotional and cognitive development.

The participant small-group method, a modification of the sensitivity training laboratory method, was used with 120 Head Start parents in eight different series of groups, varying the membership, duration, and content of the group. The parents met intensively in groups of 10 to 15 for a two-month period and had skilled group trainers to help them, providing materials for their children's language development. Although the evaluation of this method is not finished, the good attendance and enthusiastic participation indicated that the method was quite successful (Wohlford, 1971).

Summary

In summary, when the psychologist serves Head Start, he must be more than a clinical child psychologist attending to individual children with specific problems, and more than a child psychologist attending to the developmental situations of groups of children. He must be a consultant to the Head Start program in the manner that Glidewell (1966) described. This means the psychologist must attend to the whole Head Start organization from top to bottom, director to children, and horizontally from potentially supportive agenices in the community to the Head Start staff, to the children and their parents. In the process of serving as a community psychologist, he will be called upon to perform traditional clinical services as well, as Sperber (1969) described.

Not all psychologists will like these splits in roles and in responsibilities to different agencies and individuals who are often themselves in conflict. Yet if we do not now have enough psychologists who are willing to accept these new roles and responsibilities, we must train psychologists who are. As I see it, that is the greatest challenge of this new direction in clinical child psychology and also a splendid opportunity for community psychology.

References

Adams, P. L., & McDonald, N. F. Clinical cooling out of poor people. *American Journal of Orthopsychiatry*, 1968, 3, 457-463.

American Orthopsychiatric Association. Communication from American Othropsychiatric Association to Joint Commission on Mental Health of Children. *American Journal of Orthopsychiatry*, 1969, 39, 383-388.

Glidewell, J. C. Persepctives in community health. *Community Psychology*. Boston: Boston University Press, 1966.

Harvard Educational Review, 1970, 40, No. 1.

Herzog, E., & Lewis H. Children in poor families: Myths and realities. *American Journal of Orthopsychiatry*, 1970, 3, 375-387.

Office of Economic Opportunity. *Head Start child development programs: A manual of policies and instructions*. Washington, D.C.; Community Action Program, Office of Economic Opportunity, 1967.

Project Head Start. *Psychologist for a child development center*. Washington, D.C.: Office of Child Development, U.S. Department of HEW, 1970.

Sperber, Z. Changing children's psychopathology: Is a social action—clinical process dichotomy possible? Paper presented at the meeting of the American Psychological Association, Washington, D.C., Sept. 1971.

Wohlford, P. Head Start parents in small groups: The Miami Parent Project.

Paper presented at the meeting of the American Psychological Association, Washington, D.C., September 1971.

Wohlford, P. The use of participant group methods with low income families. In R. M. Dunham (Ed.), *The family as a unit of study in social problems, Vol. II*. Washington, D.C.; U.S. Department of Health, Education and Welfare, Office of Education, Bureau of Research, 1970.

Part Four

ADVANCES IN EDUCATION

Schools are a place where clinical child psychologists should have enormous influence, yet in crucial areas—individualizing instruction, curriculum development, and, above all, personality enhancement—our input has been practically nil. There are exciting contributions for us to make to children in the schools, as the authors featured in this section demonstrate. What does the clinical child psychologist need to implement these innovative ideas?*

*power

16. Family Style Education:
A New Concept for Pre-School Classrooms Combining Multi-Age Grouping with Freedom of Movement among Classrooms.*

J. Ronald Lally and Lucille Smith

The program described below has been established as an alternate to teacher-centered and task-centered day care programs. It was thought that a sound day care model would be one which allowed the children to have similar movements and interactions to those they had at home. It was also thought that it was easier to solve Hunt's "problem of the match" by providing for children many experiences from which they could choose, rather than to have a teacher choose for the child. Most importantly, it was thought that many day care programs today stress cognitive skills with little regard for social skills. We felt that emphasis should be placed on giving very young children experiences and choices that would help to develop a concern for their needs and rights in relation to the needs and rights of others. We wanted to accomplish this socialization in a way that did not curtail cognitive growth, but would actually enrich it. Finally, we hoped to provide a structure in which the child could feel good about himself and his actions, and most importantly, one in which he could enjoy himself.

Daily contacts with children of varying ages and freedom of movement between rooms were thought to be necessary if the program was to be similar to the movements and interactions found in the home. It was thought that these daily contacts and freedoms would increase the number and kind of socializing experiences a child would have each day. By allowing him the choice of whom and what he would play with, we thought that situations would be

*Paper presented at annual meeting of American Psychological Association, Miami, September 1970. This investigation was supported by Grant No. PR-156, C.W.R.D., Health, Education and Welfare, for the Development of a Day Care Center for Young Children Project, J. Ronald Lally, Principal Investigator.

created in which the children could learn to consider and respect the needs, rights, and responsibilities of others in relation to their own needs, rights, and responsibilities. These choices would also limit the number of power confrontations between teachers and children, thus making it easier for the child to feel good about and enjoy himself. The over-all structure and rules for governance of the program are based on the idea that children are human and have rights as individuals.

A major goal of the program is to provide a richness of learning experiences from which children can choose, in a setting which is constructed to reward self-initiated activities. The teachers work toward this goal by viewing themselves as one of the many experiences available to the children. One of the teacher's tasks is to critically observe the children and then accurately assess their needs. The teacher uses this information so that she can organize and present an array of activities which match the child's developmental age. The teacher's most important task, however, is to be a model which the children imitate and identify with. Our teachers realize that the most crucial problem facing our world today are caused by the inability of people to interact peacefully with one another. We feel that it is essential that children should witness the teacher considering the needs and rights of other adults; not only the needs and rights of children.

The Program

The following pages describe the family-style program. It should be remembered that a great deal of the program focuses on the various social interactions that children have with each other and with teachers. These are not reported in detail. The physical environment of the present family-style program is comprised of four rooms and a hallway (see Figure 1), a gymnasium, a playground, and a cafeteria. These areas serve twenty-seven children ranging in age from eighteen to forty-eight months and are staffed by seven teachers. Each room contains materials relevant to a particular group of activities. The rooms are: A. Creative Expression Room; B. Sense-Perception Room; C. Small-Muscle Room; D. Large-Muscle Room.

The program structure and accompanying limits are defined mainly by the space set aside for particular activities. One rule used by the teachers in establishing limits was that use of materials and appropriate action should be defined for the different rooms. Con-

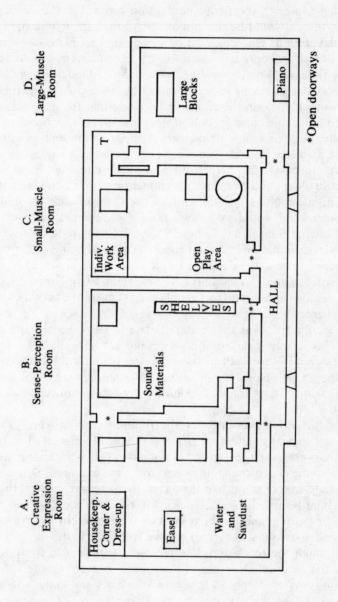

A.
Creative
Expression
Room

B.
Sense-Perception
Room

C.
Small-Muscle
Room

D.
Large-Muscle
Room

Housekeep.
Corner &
Dress-up

Easel

Water
and
Sawdust

Sound
Materials

S H E L V E S

Indiv.
Work
Area

Large
Blocks

Open
Play
Area

T

Piano

HALL

*Open doorways

cepts transcend rooms and concept links should be made from one type of activity to another. Teachers would not, for example, initiate running games in the Sense-Perception room; but the concept of faster-slower would be used in all the rooms, the gymnasium, and the playground. One constant limit was that all materials were to stay in the appropriate room. At first the teachers had to repeat many times, "Where does the book belong, Dougie?" or "Does that play dough belong in here, Angie?" but the children learned the limits quickly. Soon the children, knowing that the materials were not to leave the room, would drop the materials in the doorway. Finally, more and more items were returned to the shelves or tables where they were found. The older children had a great influence on the younger ones and helped them to understand the limits. Sometimes an older child would help a younger one take a toy back to the appropriate room, or would do it for the younger child. More often the older child would say, "No, no, Billy, take the car back," or "Look what Sharon has in here." The defined space also sets the behavioral limitations of each room. If a child wanted to run and happened to be in the Creative Expression room, he would be given the choice of going to the Large-Muscle room to run, or of staying in the Creative Expression room and doing some of the activities available there.

A second rule was that materials had to be respected and cared for. This simply meant that books could not be walked on, puzzle pieces could not be put in the water play, and dolls could not be hammered on. This did not mean that materials were not used in novel ways. It meant that children were not allowed to destroy them.

The activities presented in the different rooms were grouped together logically, and appear to be practically placed. The list of activities presented in Figure 1 is not all-inclusive because materials and activities keep changing as new ideas are explored. Some of the materials are constant, like the easel, the language master, the balance boards, and the small blocks. Puzzles, science displays, materials for pasting, and feel boxes (a box with different objects in it to feel and guess what they are) change from day to day.

Although the teachers relate concepts from one activity to the next, the different structure of the rooms seems to create different learning environments. These environments not only affect the behavior of the children, but seem to shape the role of the teacher. A brief description follows of the four separate environments and the style of the activities that go on in them.

The first room, the Creative Expression room, seems to dictate that the teachers move quickly from child to child or group to group. Teachers spend a great deal of their time making materials available and replenishing them. After the teachers help children get started on an activity, they move on quickly. They participate in the make-believe games and encourage and reinforce the spontaneous labeling that often happens at water play and pretend cooking. Many children come to the teachers talking about what they have made, and a great deal of creative description is encouraged. Teachers hang up finished products for the rest of the children to see, and help to prepare the children for the next activity. Teacher planning and preparation consists, for example, of creating open-ended activities that can be completed by young and old children alike, but with varying degrees of sophistication, and of collecting new and different kinds of materials for collage work, housekeeping, etc.

Wonderful things have happened to the children in this room. Make-believe play in the housekeeping and dress-up area is rich and fun-filled. Older children bring younger ones into make-believe "families" and encourage the young children to play various roles with them. Labeling games also include the younger and older children and significant events, to the older children, are pointed out, i.e., "Look at the bubbles when I blow on the pipe." The most encouraging finding was that the teachers did not see one child critical of the product of another, and a great deal of peer praise for jobs well done has been reported.

The Sense-Perception room seems to be more dependent upon the teachers' participation. Teachers are constantly approached by children who are confused or excited over peculiar occurrences. The teachers display materials, and indicate problem situations which move the children into experiences that foster the understanding of basic concepts, such as heavy—light, rough—smooth, high—low, etc. A great deal of individual work is encouraged, and a private space is made available for reading and language-master work. The teachers organize cooperative games, language lotto, felt board activities, etc., and initiate story telling and songs. The children seem fascinated with the Sense-Perception room and search each day for new things to stretch, to feel, or to observe in a mirror or under a magnifying glass.

The most difficult room for the teachers to keep in order is the Small-Muscle room. In this room are housed the materials for sorting, puzzles, Montessori materials, etc. The goal is to have scores of materials available on open shelves, and for children to come into the room and use particular materials, then replace them on the shelves and leave. At the present time the children do not have a sense of internal control which would maximize this room's utility, so teachers must make available a different group of activities each day.

The children seem to have particular partners with whom they like to work on puzzles, and these partners are not necessarily children they play with in the other rooms. The older boys seem to take pride in working by themselves, particularly with the hammer and nail sets, and peg board.

In the Large-Muscle room many of the concepts taught are the same, (high, higher, highest, round, left, and right), but the children use their bodies in game and dance to understand them better. The children use this room as a break from the activities presented in the other rooms and their "letting-go" is evident to the observer. Teachers use throwing and running to teach far and fast, but most of the activities in this room are free-flowing and boisterous. Loud talking, singing, and yelling are permissible and body contact is encouraged.

Individual work between teacher and child is scheduled by invitation. This work can be completed in any of the various rooms or in a private place like a table in the cafeteria. Usually a teacher will work individually with the children each day in the classroom. If a child is having a particular problem, his situation is discussed at a weekly meeting and a program is developed to help him in a particular area.

Table 1 contains an example of such a program.

In addition to the activities available in the four rooms mentioned above, two daily invitational routines have been established. Instead of a traditional snack time in which each child must participate, we have established a morning and afternoon snack period of 40 to 45 minutes in the dining room. A teacher, or a helping child, announces snack in each of the four rooms. The children come whenever they choose during the allotted time, select their snack items and serve themselves. A teacher is there for assistance. Children can stay for the entire snack time, or decide not to come at all. About five minutes before closing time the teacher again announces snack by reminding the children that this is the last call for snacks. At first we had children not getting snacks because they forgot to come to the dining room during the open times, but now if a

1. Use the Language Master and work toward the goal of independent use of the instrument by H.G.

2. Use a tape recorder: make up fun sentences, questions, and silly rhymes. Have H.G. listen and repeat the material where appropriate. Let him record his own phrases. Play them back and let him decode them aloud for you after listening to them.

3. Articulation lessons: H.G. needs work with the letter "r" in initial and second position in words such as "rain" or "drop." Tape a series of such words and leave a pause after each so that H.G. can practice repeating the word after hearing it on the tape. Demonstrate the labial position of "r" yourself to him and let him watch you and himself produce "r" sounds in a mirror. In the gymnasium, follow through by deliberate and frequent use of words like "run," "train," "throw." Get H.G. to repeat these words to ask as clearly as possible for toys such as "tricycle."

4. Grammar lessons: H.G. needs to learn the place marker sounds that signify actions or doers. Use pictures to elicit such distinctions as "sings-singer, plays-player, teaches-teacher."

5. Use physical activities, games, and sequences to promote auditory decoding and memory. For example, give two, three, or (later on) four directions sequentially. At first, these should be simple and involve minimal spatial dislocation (e.g., "Touch your nose, then your hair, then your shoes"). Later, these sequences may involve more complex geographic displacements (e.g., "Crawl under the table, go touch the door knob, then come back and sit in the rocking chair").

6. Use mislabeling of A) actions role-played physically by the teachers, or B) action pictures, in order to encourage both alertness in decoding pictorial symbols and attention to verbal symbols. For example, point to a picture of a dog lying down and say, "The dog is going home for his dinner." Encourage H.G. to correct you. Ask him how he can tell you were wrong and get him to explain what actually is happening.

7. To increase attention span for verbal materials: make up simple, amusing stories less than six sentences in length. Ask H.G. several questions after telling the story to check his comprehension and memory.

8. Analogy games: H.G. needs work with analogy concepts. Make-up a series of simple games using well-known words, body parts, foods, clothing items, etc.

Analogy games: "Gloves on on your hands
Shoes go on your____

"You see with your eyes
Your hear with your____

"You clap with your hands
You walk with your____

child misses snacks it is because he chose to. As in the other rooms, the items belonging in the dining room (food in this case) must remain there.

Gym or playground is the other invitational routine. The gym and playground are in different parts of the Center. For a period each morning and afternoon an announcement is made that the gym or playground is open and is available to the family-style children. The teachers work with the children both in groups and individually in the gym. Many of the children play with each other.

There are large jungle gyms, tricycles, balls, and room to play simple and complex games, from walking on masking tape squares and circles, to playing hide-and-seek. Three teachers supervise gym activities, freeing the other teachers to invite children out for one-to-one cognitive lessons. If the weather is pleasant, the playground is made available at this time instead of the gym. Similar games are played, but swings, a large slide, and a sand box are available for the outdoor play.

Lunch and naptime are the two remaining activities in the day of the family-style child. The tone of lunch is similar to the rest of the program. It is a learning and fun time. Even the very youngest child can serve himself at least one or two food items. If the children put too much on their plates, this can be a fascinating learning experience. The teachers converse with the children about the difference between taking only one spoonful of peas instead of two, or a small spoonful instead of a big one. The children experiment with new foods and pass things to one another. We have found that the young children learn a great deal from the older ones at lunch time, and both young and old children imitate the actions of the adults.

Nap time follows lunch. All but one of the rooms are closed and cots are placed in them. The children are allowed to get up and come into the open room if they cannot go to sleep.

Preliminary Findings

Although the family-style program has not been in operation long enough for us to get a full estimate of its strengths and weaknesses, some preliminary evaluation has been conducted. Of the twenty-seven children in the program, varying numbers received entry testing and mid-point testing on different developmental schedules. Seventeen children were assessed at both times on the Stanford-Binet, thirteen children on the Peabody Picture Vocabulary Test (PPVT), and fifteen children on the Pre-school Attainment Record (PAR).

No differences were found between the scores on the entry and mid-point tests or any of the measures. Table 2 contains the scores obtained at both test periods on the three measures used, and the amount of time children spent in the program between testing. Observation of the similarity of entry and mid-point test score means and the size of the standard deviations negated the need for tests of significance.

TABLE 2

Mean Scores and Time in Program for Family-Style Children

Measure	Entry Test $\overline{X}$	SD	Mid-Point Test $\overline{X}$	SD	$\overline{X}$ Time Between Tests	$\overline{X}$ Age at Post-test
Binet N-17	112.6	13.0	115.5	10.7	5.6 months	40.2
PPVT N-13	95.1	16.2	98.1	14.4	5.5 months	41.8
PAR N-15	120.5	21.5	123.0	18.3	8 months	38.4

Discussion

It appears that the Family-Style Program has not contributed to a decline in cognitive ability as measured by the developmental schedules reported above. This assumption is possibly a bit premature for the children tested have only participated in the program for part of a year. The data reported above, however, can be interpreted to support the switch in program style from a more restrictive age-grouped program to a freer Family-Style Program for at least this small period of time.

The most important contribution of the Family-Style Program is that children are helped to grow in areas that are not measured by the traditional tests of development. At this point, since we have little data on which to base our feelings, it is conjecture to say that children are gaining in ego strength, or are developing internal motivation toward learning, or are getting along better with each other. Teacher reports, however, indicate that something different is happening with the children since they moved to this program.*

The children are reported to be reacting to the mixing of ages nat-

*Author's Note: After this was written additional information was available. Emmerich's Observer Rating of Children was used for intensive observation of classroom behavior of 20 program children and a separate group of 20 low-income controls attending city preschools. Center children were found to be more involved, expressive, relaxed, active, energetic, stable, social, assertive, independent, constructive, purposeful, affectionate to others, socially secure, and flexible. They were also more rebellious.

urally and comfortably. The older children seem to be more observant and verbalize more about what it is like to be little. For example, two children were overheard talking about how different it is to be little and just learning to go up and down steps, from being big and knowing how to hop. There are questions about growth, "Was I little like Angie?" and interest in observing and helping in diapering and toilet training. The little children seem to have perfect models to imitate. When first moved into this setting, several of the children under two years of age increased their expressive language markedly and began to show immediate interest in toilet training. Behavior of the older children at lunch and snack times is mirrored in the behavior of the little ones. The older children have been helpful to and protective of the younger ones from the beginning of the program, and, because of praise from the teachers and the warm responses from the younger children for this help and protection, feel very good about themselves, and feel important. Older children have also started teaching the younger ones. It is common to see an older child labeling an object that he and a younger child are playing with and repeating, for example, "Car, car, car" and trying to elicit vocal imitation.

Because of the wide age range, the children and the teachers do not expect similar responses to materials and activities. This seems to foster cooperation, coupled with a better understanding of developmental differences. The structure of the program also allows for a freer selection of friends and work partners. It has been observed that some children seek out specific friends to play cards with, and others to work with in the Creative Expression room. It has also been observed that two of the children have become fast friends and move to all activities together.

The program has significantly affected teacher functioning. The teachers feel that the structure of the program has freed them to spend more time initiating activities, working with small groups or individuals, and planning special activities for particular children. They see that this structure has forced their role to change. One teacher stated, "I can still teach big and little, but not like I did before. Instead of making it a structured lesson, I must take advantage of the child's interests and activities." For example, if a child is building with blocks, this is a good time to help him learn about big and little. The teacher might have "structured" the experience by placing blocks of only two sizes on one of the work tables, but the children seem more receptive to the newer type of learning, and the teachers feel that it is more meaningful to them. The teachers are beginning to change their priorities and now seem to be more concerned about helping children make choices than with guiding them through particular activities. What the teachers used to judge as being too easy or too difficult might be just what the child wants and needs.

The wide variety of activities and materials used in this program have many levels of difficulty to meet the needs of all the children. This permits the child to play with pieces of equipment that one might not have programmed for a child of his age. He is free to go to a puzzle or game he may have mastered a year ago, and possibly get a good feeling on redoing the task. He may also try a task that is beyond his capabilities, and his need for assistance will propel him to seek the help of an older child.

Finally, the most striking thing about the program is that the children always seem happy. There is less crying and more inter-child laughter and verbalization. It is not that they were unhappy before, but now it seems that the combination of freedom with many opportunities to enter into a variety of experiences with other children of various ages, a teacher, or by himself, has really set an enjoyable individually-paced atmosphere that the children love.

17.   The Three-Pipe Problem: Promotion of Competent Human Beings through a Pre-School Kindergarten Program and Sundry Other Elementary Matters*

Eli M. Bower

*It is quite a three-pipe problem and I beg that
you won't speak to me for fifty minutes.*
—*Holmes to Watson in* The Red-Headed League

Pipe I: Individual and Social Competence and their Promotion

When one crosses the equator, it is expected that the event will be ritualistically celebrated by a dunking ceremony led by King Neptune and his henchmen. Similarly, one of the dunkings one must go through when entering the verbal land of juvenile delinquency is to define who or what juvenile delinquency is. At this point, many social and behavioral scientists do one of two things. Some go back to less arduous tasks. Others plunge in and are soon overwhelmed by the complex psychological and social currents which swirl around such a definition.

I will take neither alternative; instead I propose, first, that habitual rule- or law-violators who get caught are persons who have never acquired competencies in the use of symbols. Second, I propose that such competencies enable the individual to consensually validate himself and his environment when appropriate; they also enable him to move freely in space and time as he learns to use symbols creatively. The third part of the competency pie is the ability to integrate the validation component with the creative. To quote Sanford (1965; p.27) "By making the cultural world available to him

---

*This article is based on a paper presented to the Delinquency Prevention Strategy Conference at Santa Barbara, California in February, 1970.

and teaching him symbols and how to use them, we enable him to perform symbolically all kinds of psychological functions that would be impossible if he were restricted to transactions with 'real' things. One might say that this is the only way in which civilized adults can gratify the infantile needs which are still very much with them and which demand to be satisfied in some way."

The juvenile competency problem. I would like to more specifically identify the target group at which the strategy and plan presented in Pipe II will be aimed. The habitual rule-breaker and the ineffective or noncoping youth are part of the same ecological balloon. There are as many so-called sick persons in Federal penitentiaries, State prisons, and county jails as there are law-violaters in mental hospitals. It seems singularly unproductive to argue about the merits of two different types of garbage cans when neither is able, to any great extent, to do much about reducing its contents.

There are many ways in which children and adolescents fail to become competent adults. For example, a thirty-year follow-up of 524 child guidance clinic patients (Robins, 1966, p. 293) and a group of 100 nonpatients of the same age, sex, race, IQ, and neighborhood revealed that clinic children had more psychiatric illnesses and showed more rule-breaking behavior than their controls. Only four percent of the control subjects had five or more adult antisocial symptoms compared to 45 percent for the group seen in the child guidance clinic; 20 percent of the adult group seen in the clinic thirty years before were deemed to be free of psychiatric disease as compared to 52 percent of the control group. But to illustrate my point about garbage cans, the maladjustments of Robins' patients ran the gamut from alcoholism to zoocrasty, including occupational incompetence, burglary, high divorce rates, physical illnesses, hospitalization for mental illnesses, extensive dependency on community agencies, especially welfare, and a host of other maladaptive behaviors in-between.

Two other salvos of data from Robins' study need to be brought out. The more severe the antisocial behavior as a child (as measured by symptoms, episodes, and arrestability), the more disturbed was the adult adjustment. This is interestingly confirmed by a separate study (Glidewell, Mensh, & Gilden, 1957) in the same locality in which the investigators found a high positive correlation between the severity of complaints by parents of their children's behavior and the degree of maladjustment. Based on a symptom inventory using the mother as reporter, the investigators determined that there was 67 percent accuracy in predicting both presence and absence of emotional disturbance; 86 percent accuracy in predicting presence of disturbance; and 91 percent accuracy in predicting absence of disturbance.

The other salvo of data reported by Robins, which seemingly surprised her, was "that what we have found is not so much a pathological patient group as an extraordinarily well-adjusted group (p. 69)." The investigators had selected as a control or comparison group 100 elementary-school children from the same neighborhood as the patient group. These were children who had not been seen at the psychiatric clinic, had not repeated a grade, and had an IQ of 80 or more. "One would infer," notes Robins, "that a high proportion of those who as adults have psychiatric problems and social maladjustment must show very gross signs of difficulty while still in elementary school. While having repeated grades in elementary school certainly does not efficiently predict serious adult problems, having *not* had serious school difficulties may be a rather efficient predictor of the *absence* of gross maladjustment as adults (p. 70)."

There is, then, no clear connection between type of behavioral difficulty in childhood and type of difficulty in adulthood. It also seems clear we can do a better job of predicting the "good guys" than the "bad guys." O.K., then let's get "good guy"-oriented.

TABLE 1

Competence	*Incompetence*
1. Behavior varied and relaxed; anxiety utilized enhancingly.	1. Behavior driven; energy disproportionate or inappropriate to situation; anxiety utilized destructively.
2. Behavior has $xn+$ degrees of freedom.	2. Behavior stereotyped and repetitive; has $x-$ degrees of freedom.
3. Behavior encourages new sensory and conceptual inputs, i.e., can profit by experience.	3. Behavior discourages or filters inputs, i.e., does not profit by experience.
4. Behavior differentially open to others—considers feedback on self and usually accepts it.	4. Behavior in relation to others tends to extremes, either a pushover or Rock of Gibraltar.
5. Behavior integrated—primary and secondary processes of thinking connected.	5. Behavior fragmented—primary and secondary processes of thinking compartmentalized and separated.

Individual and social competence in children. The research cited by Robins (1966) and Glidewell *et al.* (1957) emphasizes the need to develop a conceptual and operational model of children which would help differentiate those having a chance of coping with themselves and their environment from those who do not. The beginning of such a model was developed by Bower (1969). I started at the behavioral level, differentiating social and individual competence from social and individual incompetence. The criteria for such a differentiation are presented in table 1.

The conceptual guidelines presented in Table 1 are, of course, at a pretty high level of abstraction. How does one pin them down operationally? Moreover, if one could differentiate those children veering towards social and individual incompetence from others, what, if anything, can be done to change their direction? To complicate things still further, if one could differentiate the positively-oriented children from the negatively-oriented ones and change the direction of the negatively-oriented children, could this process be institutionalized in such a way that a significant preventive effort might be programmed and administered for the population at large?

School: The point of concentration. Children and school go together like fish and chips. To a child with a learning or behavior problem the school is a micro-society from which he cannot escape. From society's point of view the education of children is one of the most prodigious and critical undertakings of the nation, the state, and the community. In the year 1970 there were more than 58 million children and youth in school, spending roughly five hours a day for about 180 days a year in an instructional relationship. Multiplying these apples, onions, and radishes, one comes out with more than 5 billion hours of planned professional interpersonnel interactions per year. How can we make these planned interactions go on more positively for more children?

The school seems to be, at present, the only social institution which has a ghost of an epidemiological chance of touching all children and all families. Some behavioral scientists and educators feel that by age 5 or 6 it may already be too late to do much about the direction in which a child's life is going. But then it may also be too late for some children when they are resting *in utero*. Whatever else may be said about the school (and in some large cities much can be said), it is a potential *linking* point between the two primary or KISS (Key Integrative Social System) institutions intended to civilize children (Bower, 1969, pp. 73-79). There is also a great deal of research to support the effectiveness of teacher ratings of the mental health status of children. Teachers have daily contacts with children in a normal group setting over a period of at least one year. The natural backdrop of age-appropriate behavior and experiences with different children each year give teachers a professional sense of when a child needs individual attention. This is not to say that teachers are clinicians or do not go off the deep end here and there. In some ways the teaching profession has never lived down the early Wickman study (1928). Since those days, much has happened.

Teachers as suspecticians. About 12 years ago, the State of California risked a sizable amount of funds and professional time (Bower, Tashnovian, & Larson, 1958) to find out if "emotionally handicapped" children could be identified early in their school life and if so, whether something could be done to head off or redirect this kind of development. Our research indicated that it was relatively easy to identify children with beginning learning and behavior problems within the school system using teacher-, peer-, and self-perceptions. At this point some of our mental health colleagues began to shake their heads. "Remember," they cautioned, "the old Wickman study (1928) in which considerable doubt was raised about the ability of teachers and schools to recognize the serious, much less the beginnings of, emotional or social disturbances in children and youth. How do we know," they asked, "that the children the teachers 'have identified are *really* and *truly* the mental health and juvenile delinquent problems of our society? In other words, how reliable and valid are teachers in this hazardous kind of prediction?"

Let me resurrect Wickman's (1928) study for those of you too young to have been exposed or too old to remember. I do so not to honor the past but to assist ths future. What Wickman did was to compare the ratings of 511 teachers and 30 mental hygienists on the seriousness of 50 behavior traits of children. What set the fulminating cap sizzling was his finding that the ratings of the teachers and the mental hygienists had zero correlation. Wickman, himself, was not at all dismayed by this result and was most emphatic and forceful in pointing out that the directions to each group had been significantly different. The teachers had been asked to rate the behavior of students as problems they faced in the classroom, in the here and now. The mental health people were directed to rate the traits on the basis of their eventual effect on the future life of the child. When the smoke cleared, teachers had rated as teachers, mental hygienists as mental hygienists, and the twain did not meet. Each group was looking at the children pretty much from its own professional biases and job-related firing line, as indeed it should.

So what happened? Two educators (Schrupp & Gjerde, 1953) examined 12 texts in psychology and educational psychology and found that only two books gave a clear and accurate statement of the study and its findings. Most of the presentations indicated that the disparity between the mental health judges and the teachers showed that teachers were way off beam. The basic assumption in all cases was that the mental health experts were right and that the teachers were wrong. Nobody called it the other way, and only rarely did an investigator say something about the problem of comparing papaya to pinocle.

In the study (Bower, *et al.*, 1958) mentioned earlier, we paid clinicians to do individual studies of children selected out as "emotionally handicapped" and found pretty good agreement between teachers and the clinicians. Where there was some disagreement, the weight of evidence often lay on the side of the teacher. The perceptual differences between teachers and other behvioral specialists is a myth which has surrounded possible action programs like the magic fire around Brunnhilde. The myth is that someone, somewhere, somehow can assess behavior and/or mental health as a characteristic or state of being independent of the social context and social institutions in which the individual is living and functioning. A study by Cohen (1963) compared the predictive skill of a teacher, a clinical psychologist, and a child psychiatrist in assessing and predicting the achievement level of 56 kindergarten children when they got into the first grade. Each professional person related to the children as he would in his normal professional practice. The teacher did what kindergarten teachers do, the clinical psychologist tested and observed, and the child psychiatrist employed a standard play observation situation. All three did a good job of predicting how each of the kindergarteners would do in the first grade, but the teacher did the best. The psychiatrist predicted more underachievement than actually occurred. In assessing his misfires, he found that some of the clinical anxiety which he picked up in some of the children and which he expected to lead to underachievement actually led to high achievement.

This is of course the nub of the problem—the evaluation of intrapsychic states separated from their social and individual implementation tells you nothing. The teacher, of all the professionals, may not know much about levels of anxiety but she cannot help but notice which children are hyperactive and how they manage it. Each child mediates his own feelings, cognitive abilities, personality traits, and physical self in his own way. The nature of this mediation is what teachers are constantly observing. What it comes to is that teachers' judgments provide the most economical and efficient perceptual platform for intercepting children moving in the wrong direction.

Competence and incompetence in relation to what? If the point of concentration for delinquency prevention is to be the school (or the home, the playground, or the well-baby clinic) one needs to focus on behaviors relevant to the school. The teacher tends to judge a child on the basis of his ability to perform the role of a student. Occasionally, quiet children who look like they might be learning something get through the teacher's net. This is expecially true of girls, who are more often seen as good students compared to boys. In fact, *they are* in the early grades. In the study of emotionally-handicapped children mentioned earlier (Bower, *et al.*, 1958, p. 57), teachers were asked to rate each child in their class on dimensions of aggression and withdrawal. The results, depicted in Table 2, were surprising. More students were scored as being overly withdrawn or timid than overly aggressive or defiant. However, if you were to ask teachers which children they wanted help with, they would give the aggressive ones priority for a rather simple reason. One aggressive kid can disrupt an entire class; a quiet child distrubs no one but himself. Note also in Table 2 that more than 10 percent of the students are overly aggressive or withdrawn most of the time; that boys are about twice as overly aggressive most of the time as girls; and girls are about twice as overly withdrawn or timid most of the time as boys.

Table 2

Is this child overly aggressive or defiant?

	Male		Female		Total	
Seldom or never	1579	54.0	1945	73.0	3524	63.0
Not very often	709	24.2	404	15.1	1113	19.9
Quite often	469	16.0	239	9.0	708	12.7
Most of the time	169	5.8	78	2.9	247	4.4
Total	2926	52.3	2666	47.7	5592	100.0

Is this child overly withdrawn or timid?

	Male		Female		Total	
Seldom or never	1700	58.1	1367	51.2	3067	54.8
Not very often	732	25.0	699	26.2	1431	25.6
Quite often	351	12.0	406	15.2	757	13.6
Most of the time	144	4.9	197	7.4	341	6.1
Total	2927	52.3	2669	47.7	5596	100.0

The percentage of students who do not seem able to play the student role seems to come out much the same in a variety of studies. In a Mental Health Survey of Los Angeles County done by the Department of Mental Hygiene in 1960 (p. 309), the teachers were asked to rate children in all grade levels on: 1) Is this child disturbed enough to be referred for psychiatric help? and 2) Is this child disturbed, perhaps not seriously enough to require psychiatric help but a problem enough to require more than his "share" of the teacher's time and attention? In kindergarten categories nominees for 1 and 2 add up to 6.1 percent. In first grade this jumps to 9.3 percent, rises to 10.1 percent in the second grade, hits a peak at 11.0 percent in the fourth and fifth grades and begins to drop in junior and senior high schools as many of the problem kids drop out. By the twelfth grade, teachers report only 1.9 percent of students in Category 1 and 3.3 in Category 2. The rest of the kids are out in the community raising hell.

The difficulties boys and girls have in school vary with the structure, the demands, and the professional perception of the teachers. A high school teacher sees the students more nearly as "subject matter" depositories; the elementary school teacher, especially the early elementary teacher, sees children as members of an extended family. For example, many kindergarten and first grade teachers object to formal rating or judging of their students in much the same manner as a mother avoids choosing favorites or black sheep among her children. The elementary teacher has a different frame of reference than the high school teacher, yet both are sensitive to the child who needs help (Bower, 1960). A teacher's major concern when a child is overly aggressive or is unable to learn because of his apathy is that she cannot teach him and therefore is unable to carry out her professional responsibility. This disturbs her and therefore makes the child a disturbing student. Similarly, when a child in a play group or nursery school cannot adhere to rules of games, or cannot take turns, the teachers and the group will find him a problem *in that setting* and, if it continues, will tend to isolate or evict him. A child who gives little or no emotional response to a mother (as in childhood autism or related disorders) will become even a greater problem in a family setting since emotional responsiveness is what makes a mother, and even at times a father, act like a warm, loving parent. The child "makes" the parent as the parent "makes" the child; the student "makes" the teacher as the teacher "makes" the student. It seems necessary to reemphasize that competent or incompetent behavior can only be evaluated or judged in relation to the primary or KISS institutions in which the behavior takes place. A play group requires rule-awareness behavior; a school requires one to pay attention; in a family one needs to be able to accept anger and demonstrate love. Life, for children, is lived within these primary institutions, each of which requires specific functioning skills and behavior appropriate to its goals. One can therefore define the effectively-growing child as one who has learned the competencies to make it through the KISS institutions—family, play, neighborhood groups, and school. As mentioned earlier, the competency most significant to people is their ability to conceptualize—to rehearse actions and their consequences in one's mind and to create actions therein — in short, to be able to symbolize.

Symbols and behavior. Many animals can think things. Human beings are probably the only animals that can think *about* things. Needing to live as social animals in social groups, they found it impossible to function in societies of other human beings unless some actions were regulated and controlled. To do this, they had to find a way to act without acting, to go beyond the present in anticipating the future. As Dewey (1930) pointed out many years ago, we can perform marvelous experiments by means of symbols wherein the results are also symbolized. "If a man starts a fire or insults a rival, effects follow . . . But if he rehearses the act symbolically in private, he can anticipate and appreciate its result. Then he can act or not act overtly on the basis of what is interpreted (p.151)."

However man came to invent symbols, it is by far the greatest single event in his history. Perhaps Helen Keller (1954) expressed it best by her dramatic recapitulation of how she learned that the object "water" could be transformed into the idea of water. "As the cool stream gushed over one hand she (Annie Sullivan) spelled into the other the word water, first slowly then rapidly. I stood still, my whole attention fixed upon the motions of her fingers. Suddenly I felt a misty consciousness as if something forgotten — a thrill of a returning thought; and somehow the mystery of language was revealed to me . . . That living word awakened my soul, gave it light, hope, joy, set it free." Earlier Helen had written, "The few signs I used became less and less adequate . . . I felt as if invisible hands were holding me and I made frantic efforts to free myself."

Helen Keller was handicapped by lack of sight and hearing. Others are handicapped by early experiences. Malcom X (1965) wrote: "I have often reflected upon the new vistas that reading opened to me. I knew right there in prison that reading had changed forever the course of my life. As I see it today, the ability to read awoke inside me some long dormant craving to be mentally alive. I certainly wasn't seeking any degree, the way a college confers a status symbol upon its students. My homemade education gave me, with every additional book that I read, a little bit more sensitivity to the deafness, dumbness and blindness that was afflicting the black race in America. Not long ago an English writer telephoned me from London asking questions. One was, 'What's your alma mater?' I told him, 'Books'."

Claude Brown (1965) writes of a similar experience during one of his "stays" at Warwick. There he meets the kindly wife of the Superintendent, Mrs. Cohen, who keeps telling Claude that he could be somebody. She tries to interest him in going to school but Claude sees little chance that he will. One day she gives him a book to read—*The Autobiography of Mary McLeod Bethune*. Claude reads it because he likes Mrs. Cohen and figures she'll ask him about it if he doesn't. This is followed with books about Jackie Robinson, Sugar Ray Robinson, Einstein, and Schweitzer. He is especially impressed by the latter two. Einstein was a cat who really seemed to know how to live. He reminds Claude of Papanek, a therapist he'd met at Wiltwyck, because both seemed to be able to control their lives and what they wanted or did not want to do. "I kept reading and I kept enjoying it. Most of the time, I used to just sit around in the cottage reading. I didn't bother with people and nobody bothered me. *This was a way to be in Warwick and not to be there at the same time*."

Similar episodes can be cited in James T. Farrell's (1935) earlier history of a group of delinquents on Chicago's South Side, Richard Wright's autobiographical *Black Boy* (1945) and *Native Son* (1957), Sylvia Ashton-Warner's *Spinster (1959)*, and in the *Life and Times of Frederick Douglas* (1881). Douglas, a slave, recalls his interest in the mystery of reading after hearing the Bible read aloud. He asks his mistress to teach him, which she does. She feels her husband would be proud of her accomplishment. He definitely is not and forbids her to continue "Very well, thought I, knowledge unfits a child to be a slave . . . and from that moment I understood the direct pathway from slavery to freedom in learning to read' (p. 67)."

Symbols and meditation. The basic symbol systems of a society are its: a) language for communicating and expressing primary processes of thinking, secondary processes of thinking, and their integration (words, syntax, and emotionalized expressions); b) language for communicating and expressing secondary processes only (mathematics); c) expressive sound (music); and d) expressive sight (painting, sketches, pictorial work, design, etc.). All are important in developing competence; however, creative and consensual use of language is primary.

A child learns language by listening. It is not formally taught but informally taught. It requires a mediating person to bridge symbol and object, event or feeling. Such a bridge is most often a person the child has learned to trust. He or she must also be one who can provide the conceptual and denotative glue which binds ideas and meaning to sentences, phrases, and words. The three major mediations which need almost immediate bindings for survival are space bindings (two objects like an automobile and a person cannot occupy the same space at the same time); time bindings; and human relationship bindings. As the child comes into contact with objects, events, and feelings in the presence of a mediating person, no different perhaps than Annie Sullivan, Mrs. Cohen, or Sylvia Ashton-Warner, there is an opportunity to create and transmit symbols by which the object, event, or feeling can be differentiated from other objects, events, or feelings. The process thereby enables the child to experience the world and bind it within his mind. Parents are potentially the best mediating persons for young children. But many parents feel they lose their effectiveness when their children are adolescents.

Mediating persons. Parents, however, are not the only potential mediators—teachers, peers, and other adults can also function in this capacity. In some cases extreme experiences can make a person his own mediator. For example (Esslin, 1961), comparison of the reaction of prisoners who have served time and that of a regular San Francisco theatre audience to *Waiting For Godot* indicated that the San Quentin group could differentiate and identify Becket's symbolism while the non prisoners could not. Similarly Hess (1968) and others have pointed out that middle-class mothers make better conceptualizers and mediators than lower-class mothers. Middle-class mothers tend to use more subordinate clauses which in time leads middle-class children to think of things happening *because* . . . The lower-class child is more often ordered and commanded and learns to mediate a world with less conceptual glue. One of the major outcomes of differences in mediating modes is that the middle-class child experiences a system of bound symbols which contain the possibility of controlling what happens to him and his environment; the lower-class child feels he is absolutely helpless in a world he never made.

Given a mediating person or persons, the young child picks up the necessary symbols to begin to separate himself out of his environment and differentiate himself from others in a clear and discrete manner. At the same time he is learning to attach symbols and meaning to a wide variety of his own experiences with objects, events, and feelings. Or, in some cases, there is little help in symbolizing and the few signs the child has available become less and less adequate.

If things go well, the child begins to create a clearly differentiated self and an effective internal map of the environment which helps him cope and grow. At this stage of development (ages 2-5) children learn to validate their symbols and at the same time "play" with them. They are not as yet so hemmed in by reality or the demands of adult learning that they cannot create their own idiosyncratic symbols or their own unique fairy tales. It is this ability to create meaning which begins to bridge the gap between the printed word and the mind in the process of reading. Reading is a kind of excitement between reader and printed page which is difficult to develop in a nonexciting reading experience. All one needs to get "hooked on books" is a couple of exciting reading experiences or some exciting experiences related to books.

The theoretical elements, then, which will go into Pipe II, Strategy and Plan for Action, are based on a) an early identification and intervention model with children and their families; b) competence with symbols as a goal; and c) the utilization of mediating persons in helping schools, families, and their children respond positively to family and school roles.

Pipe II: Strategy and Plan for Action

The basic strategy of this approach is to develop a pre school spring screening program for all families whose children are entering kindergarten. This will be integrated with a one-year and in some cases two-year kindergarten program in which screening will continue and during which specific interventions will be planned for those who need it.

Klein and Lindemann (1964) have outlined some of the elements of such a program and Bower and Lambert (1962) have put together a process for screening emotionally handicapped children. The *Sumter South Carolina Child Study Project* (Newton and Brown, 1967) has developed and used since 1967 a pre school checkup team for children entering the first grade.

This screening approach will differ in some ways from traditionally oriented screening. First, it will be geared in theory, practice, and in all communications toward helping *all children* to be more *effective* in school. Full-time personnel with case work or school psychologist backgrounds will be "given" positive titles and positive orientations. The titles might be something like child development consultant, school-home liaison worker, or supervising teacher. The initial screening and staffing with all families prior to the entrance of their children into kindergarten will include the prospective kindergarten teacher. The purpose of the initial contact is to get some rough and ready data on each child and his family, but more importantly, to set the school screening personnel and the family into a positive relationship. Indeed, one of the goals of this initial get-together is to search for strengths in the child and his family, the neighborhood, and the school ecology which can be identified, communicated, and discussed with the parents. In time, this data will be used by the teacher in curriculum building for the child when he comes to school in the fall.

If it seems apparent that some type of additional experience might be helpful to the child, such possibilities would be presented and discussed with the parents. In the Sumter program it was found that specific children needed some growth help prior to school entrance. One such group of kids needed school-related enrichment, adaptive skills, and peer-group experiences. These were enrolled in a six-week preparatory summer program. In this summer program, it was discovered that such children respond better to gradually introduced enrichment in a less stimulating room than the usual "give 'em all you've got" approach. Another group with apparent speech difficulties were intercepted via a parent education and speech skills program planned and administered by the Health Department. Another group of children of families who could not afford private kindergartens or nursery schools, or children with working parents or with parents with transportation problems were guided into a new program developed by the City Recreation Department with the help of the Project staff. These and other "intercept" programs were developed as needed. As these developed, it soon became apparent that the Screening Project was changing the nature and function of several family-serving, child-helping agencies. The Screening Project provided the impetus for many of these agencies to swing into action in a preventive enhancing manner with children and parents. Such changes in practice and agency goals were not temporary but became an integral part of the agencies' new concept of themselves. Nothing was asked of any of these community programs that was inconsistent with their goals or their budgets.

The Sumter program had the task of providing transitional preventive programs between home and first grade. Most California communities provide first-rate kindergarten programs as part of public education. This greatly expands the possibilities of gathering more accurate and valid screening data and provides a greater variety of preventive approaches the results of which can be monitored during the kindergarten year. In some cases it is possible and desirable to develop a two-year kindergarten program so that entrance into first grade will be a salutory rather than an automatic action. Laura Weinstein (1968) at George Peabody College in Nashville researched the thesis that there is an optimal absolute age at which children should be admitted to first grade. In her investigation she found that it is the age of the child relative to his classmates that seems to make the difference! Almost all researchers on this problem have found that younger children who entered first grade did significantly poorer in school work and academic achievement and that this state of affairs held up throughout the 12 public school years. Weinstein also takes note of the fact that this consistent and significant finding has been blurred by studies in which specially screened children who are admitted to first grade do well. Even here the evidence is far from convincing.

Children who start the first grade below the mean age of the classmates are *more likely* to be seen as emotionally disturbed by school personnel and more likely to be referred to a residential treatment center. This is probably more true for boys than girls and more true for children coming to bat with one or two strikes already against them because of environmental or emotional problems.

The results of breaking the lock step of entrance into the first grade are documented in one study by two investigators (Muller and Norris, 1967) who found that the differences between younger children and their classmates disappeared by the end of the second grade. Why? In this school system, new students were grouped by maturity and ability levels and did not enter a traditionally organized program until they reached the fourth grade. This, of course, loosened up the system so that children could be placed with comparable groups and reduced the pressure for grade level achievement.

Why then is this knowledge not plowed into programming? In part, there is the inertia of social institutions and all sorts of legislative and pseudo-legislative (I'm sorry, Mrs. Einstein, but since your son Albert was born at 11 P.M. on December 31 he will have to start school this September, not next September) fol-de-rol which schools use to maintain their own social sanity. Parents and schools face a mountain of legislative and administrative regulations if they attempt to change the processes of school entrance. Yet the mountain is easily conquered if one believes the view from the top is worth the effort.

Here and there a few school districts have rushed into developing full-scale individualized school entrance programs. Only rarely, however, have such programs managed to conceptualize their efforts as a home-school-community effort. Blain (in Bower, 1960) cites a school system in Pennsylvania where tests were used in predicting the probable success of preschool children. Where children had a low probability of success, parents were advised to wait before enrolling them. Some did; some didn't. The children whose parents waited as advised did significantly better. The children whose parents did not wait did singificantly worse. The lesson to be learned here is that school entrance is not a simple step from home to school one bright September morning. For many mothers, it is a giant step into freedom. For others, it marks the beginning of an achievement-oriented relationship between child and parents calculated to get the budding student into college. For all parents, this simple step is fraught with emotional tensions, worries, anticipation, doubts, and crises. After struggling for five years to play the most difficult, most potentially guilt-ridden role of our society, parents see their efforts go on public display for competitive judging. The first years of schooling not only represent a major crisis for the child but also for the parents. Parents begin to unconsciously ask such questions of themselves as: Have we given him what is necessary to make it? Should we have listened to Aunt Jane, Benjamin Spock, or our own intuition? Should we have given him more of our time and concern? With our genes and chromosomes, how come he's only doing a little better than average? What it comes down to for many parents is a test of themselves. Under such circumstances, anything the school might do to build positive mediational relationships should fall on eager ears.

Staff and goals. The staff would be made up of clinically-trained psychodynamically-oriented beavioral scientists (psychologists, a social worker, psychiatrist, experienced kindergarten teachers, and a secretary). Each screening group of three would be asked to see and monitor approximately 50 children and their families. Consultants may be used when necessary.

The screening procedure can utilize the model of the Sumter Child Study Project and modify as it goes along. Screening during kindergarten can proceed at a more leisurely pace except that liaison programs with parents will need to be developed almost immediately. All remedial and helping programs for children and parents need to be worked out and made operable within three months after the start of school.

The child's progress in kindergarten would be assessed by the teacher, staff, and parents. Children who may need an extra year in kindergarten would be indentified as early as possible so that counseling may be started with parents.

In large city schools, project staff may need to be drawn from students or specially trained personnel who would be enrolled in consultation and in service programs. Such a program was envisioned by Congressman Sam Gibbons (in H.R. 11322) who subsequently revised a bill to provide a program of Federal assistance to elementary schools and training institutions for the provision of child development specialists to work in preventive programs.

Pipe III: Evaluation of the Effectivness of the Action Plans

For the most part, children entering kindergarten would be treated as a cohort group on whom epidemiological indices would be kept. Such indices include height, weight, muscular coordination, social maturity, emotional development including ratings on conformity, spontaneity, capacity for enjoyment, and reaction to frustration. Level of speech and general coping ability would be assessed. These would be combined into a predictive index as the child continues through the grades. As the chart moves up, other rates to be kept include rates of illness, absence, reading achievement, arithmetic achievement, teacher ratings of conformity, spontaneity, capacity for enjoyment, and reaction to frustration. Such data would be analyzed via Markhov Chains or other multivariate analyses to determine degree of success of cohort in school-related tasks and to ascertain what kinds of remedial or preventive preschool, kindergarten, or early-grade programs had what kind of impact on what kinds of children. In time a pattern of successful intervening experiences would emerge which could be plowed back into the newer cohorts.

In the end, what is sought are cohorts which show more children becoming more effective in schools and schools becoming more effective with children.

References

Ashton-Warner, S. *Spinster*. New York: Simon and Schuster, 1959.

Bower, E. M. *Early identification of emotionally handicapped children in school*. Springfield, Ill.: Charles C. Thomas, 1969.

Bower, E. M., & Lambert, N. A process for in-school screening of children with emotional handicaps. Princeton, New Jersey: Educational Testing Service, 1962.

Bower, E. M., Shellhamner, T. A., & Daily, J. M. School characteristics of male adolescents who later became schizophrenic. *American Journal of Orthopsychiatry*, October, 1960, Vol. XXX, No. 4.

Bower, E. M., Tashnovian, P., & Larson, C. A process for early identification of emotionally disturbed children. Sacramento, California: State Department of Education, 1958.

Brown, C. *Manchild in the promised land*. New York: MacMillan, 1965.

Cohen, T. B. Prediction of underachievement in kindergarten children. *Archives of General Psychiatry*, 1963, Vo. 9.

Dewey, J. *The quest for certainty; a study of the relation of knowledge and action*. London: G. Allen & Unwin Ltd., 1930.

Douglas, F. *Life and times of Frederick Douglas*. Hartford, Conn.: Park Publishing Co., 1881.

Esslin, M. *Theatre of the absurd*. New York: Anchor Books, 1961.

Farrell, J. T. *Studs Lonigan*. New York: The Vanguard Press, 1935.

Glidewell, J.C., Mensh, I. M., & Gilden, M.C.L. Behavior symptoms in children and degree of sickness. *American Journal of Psychiatry*, July, 1957, *114*, No. 1, 47-53.

Hess, R., & Bear, R.M. (Eds.) *Early education; current theory, research and action*. Chicago: Aldine Publishing Co., 1968.

Keller, H. *Story of my life*. New York: Doubleday, 1954.

Klein, D.C., & Lindemann, E. Approaches to pre-school screening. *Journal of School Health*, October, 1964, 34, 8, 365-373.

Mental health survey of Los Angeles County. Sacramento: California State Department of Mental Hygiene, 1960.

Muller, W.D., & Norris, R.C. Entrance age and school success. *Journal of School Psychology*, 1967, 6, 47-60.

Newton, M.R., & Brown, R.D. A preventive approach to developmental problems in school children. In E.M. Bower and W.G. Hollister, *Behavioral science frontiers in education*. New York: John Wiley, 1967. Chapter 22.

Robins, L.M. *Deviant children grown up*. Baltimore: Williams & Wilkins Co., 1966.

Sanford, N. Ego process in learning. In *The protection and promotion of mental health in schools*. Washington, D.C.: USPHS D. HEW Mental Health, 1965, Mono. 5.

Schrupp, M.H., & Gjerde, C.M. Teacher growth in attitudes toward behavioral problems in children. *Journal of Educational Psychology*, April, 1953, *44*, 203-214.

Weinstein, L. School entrance age and adjustment. *Journal of School Psychology*, 1968-1969, Vol. 7, No. 3.

Wickman, E.K. *Children's behavior and teachers' attitudes*. New York: Commonwealth Fund, 1928.

Wright, R. *Black boy, a record of childhood and youth*. New York: The World Publishing Company, 1945.

Wright, R. *Native son*. New York: Harper, 1957.

X, Malcolm. *Autobiography of Malcolm X*. New York: Grove Press, 1965.

18. Emotional Education in the Classroom: The Living School*

Albert Ellis

Rational-emotive psychotherapy (RET) is a method of treating emotional disturbances that follows the educational model, instead of the commonly used medical, psycho-dynamic, or other models. Although it integratively employs emotive-evccative and behavioristic-activity methods, it somewhat uniquely *teaches* people, through many different kinds of educational modalities, that they basically cause their own emotional upsets and that by forcefully changing their thinking and actions, they can make themselves emote differently and thereby overcome their psychological hangups. Moreover, RET is used not only in one-to-one therapeutic relationships and in small therapy groups, but it emphasizes the educating of many different kinds of individuals (including children and adults in the so-called ''normal'' range of functioning) in rational-emotive philosophies and procedures, by using large group workshops, lectures, discussions, and forums, as well as tape recordings, TV presentations, films, and other audio-visual aids.

Cognitively, RET teaches clients and pupils the A-B-C's of personality formation and disturbance-creation. Thus, it shows people that their emotional Consequences (at point C) do *not* directly stem from the A ctivating events (at point A) in their lives, but from their Belief Systems (at point B) *about* these Activating events. Their Belief systems, when they feel disturbed, consist of, first, a set of empirically-based, rational Beliefs (rB's). For example, when they fail at a job or are rejected by a love partner (at point A) they rationally convince themselves, "How unfortunate it is for me to fail! I would much rather succeed or be accepted." If they stick rigorously to these rational Beliefs, they feel appropriately sorry, regretful, frustrated, or irritated (at point C); but they do *not* feel emotionally upset or destroyed. To make themselves feel inappro-

*Reprinted from the *Journal of Clinical Child Psychology*, 1972, I, #3, 19-22.

priately or neurotically, they add the nonempirically-based, irrational Beliefs (iB's): "How *awful* it is for me to fail! I *must* succeed. I am a thoroughly *worthless* person for failing or for being rejected!" *Then* they feel anxious, depressed, or worthless.

In RET, the therapist or teacher shows people how to vigorously challenge, question, and *D*ispute (at point D) their irrational Beliefs. Thus, they are shown how to ask themselves: "*Why* is it awful that I failed? Who says I *must* succeed? Where is the evidence that I am a *worthless person* if I fail or get rejected?" If people persistently and forcefully Dispute their insane ideas, they acquire a new cognitive *E*ffect (at point E), namely, the Beliefs that: (1) "It is not awful but only very inconvenient if I fail"; (2) "I don't *have* to succeed, though there are several good reasons why I'd *like* to"; (3) "I am never a *worthless person* for failing or being rejected. I am merely a person who has done poorly, for the present, in these areas, but who probably can do better later. And if I never succeed or get accepted, I can *still* enjoy myself in *some* ways and refrain from downing myself" (Ellis, 1962, 1971, 1972).

Children and RET

Quite logically, RET methods can be applied to children as well as adults, and sometimes more successfully. For children do not yet have deeply engrained the endlessly self-repeated, rigid irrational Beliefs that they may later hold as adults, they are often eager to learn new ways of thinking and behaving; and they are more available for reeducation. Consequently they can be taught, individually and in groups, principles and practices of rational living that adults may not allow themselves to hear or imbibe. To develop specific methods of applying RET to children's problems of living, the Institute for Advanced Study in Rational Psychotherapy started, in 1970, The Living School, a private school for normal children. The purpose of this school is to teach, in the course of regular classroom activities, the elements of both academic and emotional education.

In RET, we do not merely see the child as a product of his early environment; nor do we believe that he is naturally a fully healthy, self-actualizing, creative creature and that his parents and his society unduly restrict, constrict, and warp him so that he soon becomes alienated from himself and the world, hence moderately or severely disturbed. Instead, we think that his alienation, his ultra-conventionalism, and his emotional constriction or over-impulsiveness, result from his innate as well as his acquired tendencies to think crookedly, to be grandiosely demanding, and to refuse to accept hassle-filled reality (Ellis, Wolfe, and Moseley, 1972).

Children, in other words, *naturally* acquire several basic irrational ideas that they tend to perpetuate and to sabotage their lives with forever. They religiously, devoutly believe that they absolutely *need* and utterly *must have* others' approval; that they've *got to* achieve outstandingly and thereby, prove how worthwhile they are; that people who act unjustly or inconsiderately are bad, wicked, or villainous and should be severely condemned and punished for their villainy; that it is awful and catastrophic when things are not the way they would like them to be; that obnoxious situations and events *make* them feel anxious, depressed, or angry; that if they endlessly worry about something, they can control whether or not it happens; that it is easier for them to avoid than to face certain life difficulties and responsibilities; and that they absolutely *need* a well-ordered, certain universe. These are the same kinds of crazy ideas which most human adults more or less believe; but children often believe them more rigidly and profoundly (Ellis and Harper, 1972).

To combat this kind of irrational thinking, the Living School teachers use several methods of emotional education. While skills and arts are being taught, the teachers are constantly alert for unusual behaviors that indicate that a certain child may be helped by emotional guidance leading to personal insight and changed attitudes and actions. Thus, if a child displays an outburst of anger, frequent crying, physical mistreatment of other children, or rebellion against necessary rules and limitations of group activity, he or she may be singled out by the teacher for an immediate confrontation. The aim of this confrontation is not merely to point out to the child that his behavior is unusual or aberrant but, much more importantly, to show him or her how this behavior is self-created, how he or she has a choice between it and other actions, how ineffective emotionalizing and activity can be controlled, and how he or she can understand human behavior so that his or her overweening anxieties and hostilities may be controlled, and so that his or her potentialities for human enjoyment and more rewarding relationships with peers and adults may be fulfilled.

Each child is taught how to honestly acknowledge and identify his self-defeating (as well as his self-actualizing) emotional states. When, for example, he is needlessly upset, he is shown how to admit, "I am scared," "I am terribly angry," "I feel miserable." He is then asked such questions as: "Would you like to get rid of the feeling of being scared?" "Do you see the unpleasant things that happen to you when you are too scared?" "Do you realize that you made yourself scared?'' ''What do you think you were really telling yourself, or saying in your head, a few seconds before you began to feel scared?'' ''How could you change what you are telling yourself, to make yourself much less scared?''

If the child is temporarily unable—perhaps because he is too upset at the moment—to see that he did scare himself and that he could think and behave differently, the teacher may then take his problem to the other members of the class and ask them, ''What do you think Jimmie is doing to make himself scared? What do you guess he was telling himself a few seconds before he began to feel so scared?'' By getting them to speculate about Jimmie's problems, the teacher shows them that children do scare themselves, that they have alternative choices, that they can learn how not to scare themselves. She shows them how to empathize with Jimmie and how to learn from his needlessly making himself anxious. Then, when one of them has a problem and this is brought up in the classroom, they are more easily able to get at exactly what is bothering them and what they can do about it. What is more, Jimmie, who at that time is not so personally involved or upset, may be able to become better emotionally educated by listening to and partaking in the teacher-pupil discussions.

It is hoped that all the children in the class, by repetitions of this procedure, ultimately learn how to handle their own problems, to know that they have similar kinds of basic disturbance-creating procedures, to relate better to their peers, to accept life responsibilities more maturely, and to achieve a higher percentage of their potential for fuller and more creative living. The aim of this kind of emotional education is hardly to rid the pupils of all their emotional upsets or to turn them into little angels. But there is a persistent, long range effort to help them to help themselves and each other and thereby, to minimize their neurotic functioning.

In addition to the problems which are observed and highlighted in the course of regular classroom activities, the children at The Living School are given special periods where they can voluntarily bring out for open discussion any other troublesome issues, such as those that may arise in their family interactions, their social relations, and other aspects of their lives. During these group counseling periods they may spontaneously present their own difficulties; or they may raise issues about their classmates' behavior.

Thus, Mary's petulant, bitter refusal to walk alongside another child on a trip to the park or Eric's pulling a truck away from Joey can become topics for group focus soon after the incidents occur. A discussion of this nature may not only help Mary or Eric but may also lay the foundation for rules and procedures that contribute to the efficiency and safety of the class. Once a child's problem has been presented and a variety of opinions, values, and reasonings applied to it by the group and the teacher—and once a certain course of future action has been indicated and perhaps given as an emotionally educating "homework" assignment—future experiencing, catharsis, risk-taking, and problem-solving along similar lines are facilitated. Individual children become more able to deal with their problems and prophylactically to apply rational philosophies that will keep them out of trouble, and school rules gradually tend to become part of a democratically arrived at process.

In addition to the specific tackling of the children's difficulties in teacher-instituted and pupil-actuated sessions, principles of emotional education are presented to the children in various other formal and informal ways. Normal learning experiences—such as those incorporated in storytelling, drama, and play—are interlarded with principles of sane living; and these, in turn, sometimes lead to the discussion of specific psychological questions. If, in the course of formal or informal discussions, certain children are found to have more serious problems, special arrangements can be made for individual therapy, family consultations, and other forms of therapeutic intervention by the professional staff of the consultation center and training institute, the Institute for Advanced Study in Rational Psychotherapy, of which The Living School is a part. (Wolfe et al, 1971).

RET in the Classroom—Is It Effective?

Because RET is a mode of psychology that emphasizes the individual's *own* creation of his disturbed reactions to problems of life and his *own* ability to change his basic Belief System and to undo his emotional upsets, the children in The Living School are educated to understand and utilize their inner power or autonomy. They are *not* merely indoctrinated with, propagandized, suggestively taught, or "conditioned" with rational principles of behavior. Rather, they are continually shown how their own (and others') thinking processes work and are encouraged to deal with and think out difficult situations for themselves. Although various important modes of behavior modification, especially desensitizing homework assignments, are employed in RET, they are always used within an existential-humanistic framework and are not mechanically or mechanistically used to effect "good" behavior change (Lazarus, 1971).

Is RET effective? A good deal of experimental evidence now exists that tends to indicate that its basic theory as well as its clinical practice have been empirically confirmed. Much of this evidence is summarized in *Growth Through Reason* (Ellis, 1971) and will be discussed in more detail in "Rational-Emotive Therapy: Confirmation of Its Principles and Practice" (Ellis, 1973). Several papers have also been published showing that RET has been found valuable when used with children in regular classroom situations (Daly, 1971; Ellis, 1969a, 1971b, 1973b; Glicken, 1968; Lafferty, Dennerll, and Rettich, 1964; Wolfe et al, 1971).

RET's application to emotional education overlaps with and at the same time significantly differs from various other approaches to affective education that have been employed by other therapeutic schools. It is closest to the Adlerian approaches utilized by Dreikurs (1957) and Dinkmeyer and McKay (1973) and freely employs some of the behavior modification methods, such as those advocated by Homme et at (1970) and von Hilsheimer (1970). It utilizes but also significantly differs from the approaches of Glasser (1969), Leonard (1969), Maslow (1968), Neill (1964), and Rogers (1969). Instead of trying to create an atmosphere of schools without failure and with unusual warmth and support, as advocated by this last group of writers, the teachers in The Living School sometimes deliberately go to the other extreme and pretend that the children have failed at some task when they actually have succeeded. Their reactions to this "failure" are then elicited and analyzed, in an attempt to show them that although it is good (for practical purposes) to succeed and unfortunate to fail, they can always unconditionally accept themselves and strive for an enjoyable life *whether or not* they do well at academic or other pursuits. The Living School atmosphere, in other words, tries to help the children cope with, rather than avoid, competition and harsh reality and to equip themselves to meet adversities in their later lives.

Various means of encouraging the children to express themselves openly and authentically and to reveal their real feelings about themselves and others are employed. Through games, plays, role-playing, sports, art, writing, and other means they are stimulated to show what they truly think and feel. But just as rational-emotive group and encounter therapy does not merely *emphasize* authentic self-expression but also tries to show the group member that some of his feelings (such as assertiveness) are appropriate and healthy while other feelings (such as rage) are inappropriate and unhealthy, so do the teachers at The Living School try to help the children acknowledge and understand the feelings they express and consider the creation of alternative emotions when they are over- or under-reacting to stimuli.

Rational-emotive psychology makes concrete use of encounter methods with adults, particularly in the marathon weekends of rational encounter which the Institute for Advanced Study in Rational Psychotherapy gives in different parts of the United States and Canada every year (Ellis, 1969, 1972). These methods of affective encountering and release are also used with children. But it places them within a cognitive-behavioral framework and does not view them as sacrosanct or highly efficienct in their own right. For example, during classroom periods, children in The Living School are given exercises which may consist of telling each other off, deliberately doing something badly, or taking the role of other children (such as infants) who make mistakes. They are shown, in the course of these exercises, that everyone makes errors; that this is the human condition; that people learn by trial and error; that no catastrophe really occurs if they do poorly at some task; that others can easily be understood and forgiven for their errors; and so on (Knaus, 1972). Similarly, other active-emotive exercises are given and put in a cognitive-teaching context.

On the more behavioristic side, RET is one of the main psycho-therapies that has pioneered in the giving of explicit, activity-oriented homework assignments to clients. Teachers at The Living School use rational-emotive methods of working with children's problems in the classroom and of giving them concrete emotionally educating homework. Thus, if Robbie is shy and withdrawn in his relations with his neighborhood peers, he may be assigned the task of trying to make one new friend or acquaintance a week; and if Susan fights incessantly with her sister over which TV program they are going to watch, she may be assigned to giving in to her sister's choices for a few weeks, while convincing herself that it is not awful, horrible, and catastrophic that she is being deprived of the programs she most wants to see.

RET still has to be extensively tested when applied to children in classroom situations, and the Institute for Advanced Study in Rational Psychotherapy is arranging to begin controlled studies in these areas within the near future. One study by Albert (1972) showed that when used with fifth-grade students by a relatively untrained teacher, RET helped an experimental group achieve significantly lower anxiety scores on The Sarason Scale than were achieved by a control group. Many informal observations by teachers (both in The Living School and in other schools), by parents, supervisors and principals, and by others consistently seem to indicate that children are benefited when RET is employed in the classroom.

In many important ways, then, rational-emotive methodology can be applied to the emotional education of children. And what emerges at The Living School is a full-fledged meaning of this term. For RET is intrinsically didactic, pedagogic, instructional, and *educative*: more concretely and more fully, perhaps, than other widely used forms of psychotherapy. Not every therapeutic orientation is easily adaptable to teaching. Freud's psychoanalysis has largely failed in this respect, while Adler's individual psychology has succeeded much better. I think that it will eventually be shown that rational-emotive psychology is as beautifully designed for the educative process as this process is already largely designed for it. For schooling, essentially, is a concerted, long range attempt to help the child grow up in many ways and assume adult roles and responsibilities that will presumably be creative, productive, and enjoyable. And rational-emotive schooling is a concerted, long range attempt to help the child mature emotionally and become a reasonably independent-thinking, self-actualizing, minimally disturbed person.

And by person I mean *human* person. For RET is one of the most humanistic psychologies in contemporary use. It has no truck whatever with anything that smacks either of the superhuman or the subhuman. It believes that children are people and that they can fully accept themselves as enormously fallible, incredibly *human* beings, who have no magical powers, and who reside in an immense but still material and unmystical universe that doesn't really give a special damn about them and most probably never will.

RET holds that there are neither gods nor devils; that children (and adults) have no immortal souls or immutable essences; that immortality is a silly, grandiose myth; that there seems to be no absolute truth. RET holds that although reasoning and the logico-empircal method of validating reality have their distinct limits—because they, too, originate with and are employed by eminently fallible humans—they are the best means we have of understanding ourselves and the world, and we would do well to apply these methods rigorously in the understanding of children's (and adult's) life processes.

Rational-emotive education, teaches children to fully accept themselves as humans, to give up all pretensions of reaching heaven or finding the Holy Grail, to stop denigrating the value of themselves or any other person, to accept their mortality, and to become unabashed long range hedonists: that is, individuals who heartily strive to have a ball in the here-and-now *and* in their future lives without giving too much heed to what others dogmatically think that they *should*, *ought,* or *must* do. If clinical child psychologists will try this kind of psychotherapeutic education as they work or consult with schools, parents, and with children themselves, I think that they will encourage a humanistic way of life that will help us rear saner, happier, and more autonomous and creative individuals.

References

Albert, S., A Study to Determine the Effects of Emotional Education on Fifth Grade Children M. A. Thesis, Queens College, 1972.

Daly, S. Using reason with deprived preschool children. *Rational Living,* 1971, 5(2), 12-19.

Dinkmeyer, D., and McKay, G. *Raising a responsible child.* New York: Simon and Schuster, 1973.

Dreikurs, R. *Psychology in the classroom.* New York: Harper and Row, 1957.

Ellis, A. *Reason and emotion in psychotherapy.* New York: Lyle Stuart, Inc., 1962.

Ellis, A. Teaching emotional education in the classroom. *School Health Review,* November 1969a, 10-13.

Ellis, A. A weekend of rational encounter. In Burton, A. (Ed.), *Encounter.* San Francisco: Jossey-Bass, 1969b, 112-127.

Ellis, A. *Growth through reason.* Palo Alto: Science and Behavior Books, 1971a.

Ellis, A. An experiment in emotional education. *Educational Technology,* July, 1971b.

Ellis, A. *Executive leadership: a rational approach.* New York: Citadel Press, 1972a.

Ellis, A. *How to participate effectively in a rational encounter marathon.* New York: Institute for Advanced Study in *Rational Psychotherapy,* 1972b.

Ellis, A. Emotional education with groups of normal school children. In Ohlsen, M. M. (Ed.), *Counseling children in groups.* New York: Holt, Rinehart and Winston, 1972c.

Ellis, A. Rational-Emotive Therapy: Confirmation of Its Principles and Practice. *Counseling Psychologist.* 1973, in press.

Ellis, A., and Harper, R. A. *A guide to rational living.* Englewood Cliffs, N. J.: Prentice-Hall and Hollywood: Wilshire Books, 1972.

Ellis, A., Wolfe, J. L., and Moseley, S. *How to raise an emotionally healthy, happy child.* New York: Crown Publishers and Hollywood: Wilshire Books, 1972.

Glasser, W. *Schools without failure.* New York: Harper and Row, 1969.

Glicken, M. Rational counseling: a new approach to children. *Journal of Elementary Guidance and Counseling,* 1968, 2(4), 261-267.

Homme, L., with Csanyi, A. P., Gonzales, M. A. and Rechs, J. R. *How to use contingency contracting in the classroom.* Champaign, Illinois: Research Press, 1969.

Knaus, W. Five modules on emotional education. Mimeographed. New York: Author, 1972a.

Lafferty, J. C., Dennerll, D., and Rettich, P. A creative school mental health program. *National Elementary Principal*, April 1964, 43(5), 28-35.

Lazarus, A. A. *Behavior therapy and beyond.* New York: McGraw-Hill, 1972.

Leonard, G. *Education and Ecstasy.* New York: Macmillan, 1969.

Maslow, A. H. Some educational implications of the humanistic psychologies. *Harvard Educational Review*, Fall, 1968, 38(4), 685-696.

Neill, A. S. *Summerhill.* New York: Hart Publishing Company, 1964.

Rogers, C. R. *Freedom to learn.* Columbus: Merrill, 1969.

Von Hilsheimer, G. *How to live with your special child.* Washington: Acropolis Books, 1970.

Wolfe, J. L., et al. Emotional education in the classroom: The Living School. *Rational Living*, 1970, 4(2), 23-25.

19. Developing Understanding of Self and Others Is Central to the Educational Process

Don Dinkmeyer

The words of a recent popular song underscore a central problem in our society when they describe the "communication breakdown." While we may not be tuned in to the music of the day, we should not fail to grasp the message. Throughout our society there is a general lack of communication often described as a polarization between child and teacher, black and white, and even between peers. The problem is the product of the swift transition from an autocratic authoritarian type of society to a society which, for the first time, is attempting to cope with the problems of equality, democratic interaction, and the necessity for improved communication between all segments of the society.

Given this societal problem, it is important that educators look closely at their purposes and their products. While it is commonly accepted that the objectives of education are concerned with the development of the whole child—intellectually, socially, emotionally—it is equally apparent that there is a great disparity between what we say we value and our educational priorities.

Teachers talk about the development of the whole child and indicate their intellectual acceptance of this concept—as long as the whole child does not come to school! They accept the theory but they are not as willing or ready to deal with the child's social immaturity, feelings of inadequacy, anger, joy, and excitement. They would really, in many instances, prefer to deal with "an intellectual receptacle" in which they could place knowledge to be withdrawn and inspected at regular intervals. Anyone who observes classrooms closely and looks at the content of examinations and evaluation procedures will recognize instantly the dichotomy between the published objectives of education and the actual practices.

It is my contention that we can only facilitate the child's development as a person by becoming involved with his total being: his intellect, feelings, attitudes, values, purposes, and behavior. The continuation of a false dichotomy between cognition and affect (ideas and feelings), which has been promoted in the schools by an emphasis upon methodologies and evaluation, will fail to meet the need for educational experiences which are truly relevant.

It is time to consider the value of a student mastering the symbols of mathematics and language while remaining essentially ignorant in his understanding of self and others. What does it profit a man to master intellectual content which, due to lack of adequate understanding of self and others, he cannot utilize functionally? We must ask a fundamental question—Where in the school can the child examine critical questions related to: Who am I? Why do I behave as I do? What do I value? How can I relate more effectively with others? It is evident that there must be *planned* experiences for all children to help them to know, understand, and accept themselves. This humanization of the curricular process which focuses on learning as applied to self, sometimes referred to as personalized learning, enables a person to become more responsible for his choices and his human relationships. It certainly is basic to any intrinsic involvement with the curriculum.

It should be evident by now that while the educational curriculum has expanded at a rapid rate, we have tended to neglect opportunities to permit the child to explore, except by chance or on an informal basis, human behavior and human relationships. The assumption that we mature in self understanding and social-emotional growth without instruction and meaningful experiences must be challenged. Educators generally agree that a subject must be carefully planned, taught systematically, and evaluated. However, learning about self and human relationships has not been taught with the same attention that other subjects receive. An interesting hypothesis emerges from this apparent contradiction. Is it possible that a lack of attention to developing a more adequate understanding of self and others might account for many of the complex motivational problems, underachievement, the complaints about the irrelevance of the educational experience, and the increasing search for excitement in drugs, rebellion, and revolution?

When autocratic methods in education were relatively unchallenged, a stifling of emotions was possible. If the teacher was accepted as a disciplinarian and final authority, then the affective domain only existed to be controlled. Certainly this type of educational approach had a debilitating effect upon the development of the child, but it appeared to the onlooker that, on the surface at least, silence and learning were synonymous. It is now apparent that the increasing challenges from youth for equality and the insistence upon democratic participation in decision-making processes causes us to recognize that the autocrat can no longer survive in the classroom any more than he can on the political scene.

A book by Krathwohl, *et al.* (1964), *The Taxonomy of Educational Objectives: Affective Domain* provides a scholarly presentation of educational objectives in the affective area. However, despite interest and concern on the part of educators in regard to the relationship between affect and education, it is only in recent years that there has been much evidence that educators are truly involved in the development and implementation of educational programs which focus on feelings and human behavior. Richard Jones, in *Fantasy and Feelings in Education* (1968), reflected some of the concern that a number of educators had about the lack of educational experiences which involve a consideration of the feeling and attitudinal areas of life.

There have been a number of educational efforts in this area, such as *Self Enhancing Education* (Randolph and Howe, 1966). Ralph Ojemann's *A Teaching Program in Human Behavior and Mental Health* (n.d.) is another pioneer effort. Additional programs concerned with affective education include *Methods in Human Development* (Bessell and Palomares, 1969), *Dimensions of Personality* (Limbacher, 1970), *Values and Teaching* (Raths, Harmin, & Simon, 1966), and *Developing Understanding of Self and Others (DUSO)* (Dinkmeyer, 1970). The Association for Supervision and Curriculum Development has in recent years consistently expressed an interest in this type of instruction. However, at present we do not have any programs which appear to have been widely accepted by administrators, curriculum directors, and teachers as high-priority areas of instruction.

Thus, though we talk about commitments to the development of the whole child, actions speak louder than words. The lack of a required sequentially developed program in the area of self-understanding and human behavior testifies to this educational paradox. The expanded curriculum has enabled us to teach a child almost everything conceivable, except for one necessary ingredient—the capacity to understand and accept self and to function more effectively in human relationships. There appears to be a mythology that suggests that this type of understanding occurs through osmosis or magic. Learnings which are basic to the child's development have been assigned the status of concomitants rather than essentials.

Hence, we have not given our full commitment to this essential type of learning experience.

The failure to deal with feelings and attitudes in the classroom is commonplace. Teachers appear not to be trained to deal with the acceptance of emotional verbalization by their students. Flanders and Amidon (1967) found that acceptance of feelings accounted for only 5% of the verbal interaction in the classroom. Teachers appear to be more concerned with intellectual acquisition than the development of a positive self-image and the capacity to relate effectively with others.

Incidentally, it should not be implied that teachers are not interested in developing more effective relationships with children. Witmer and Cottingham (1970) have suggested that teachers are interested in increasing their guidance skills and providing for classroom experiences in guidance and affective education. They have really been victims of an educational gap in which they were told about the importance of the whole child but were not provided with methods or programs which would permit them to implement these concepts.

The responsibility for the lack of regularly programmed experiences in this area must be traced to teacher education institutions, educational theorists, psychologists, and publishing houses. Now there is common acceptance of the fact that we must close the gap between theory and practice. However, teacher education institutions have not traditionally taught skills which would assist teachers to facilitate productive group discussions of personal-social problems, lead role playing, initiate puppet activities, and in a number of ways become both skillful in classroom guidance procedures and acquainted with materials which have a guidance emphasis (Dinkmeyer and Caldwell, 1970).

This book is focused on new directions for clinical child psychology. It would seem that clinical child psychologists, who are concerned with development and prevention, would focus on helping the teacher understand human behavior, group dynamics, and communication procedures. They would make available specialized programs and would meet with teachers and groups to help them develop attitudes and skills which facilitate learning.

The 'C' group (Dinkmeyer, 1971, 1972) is a process which helps the teacher understand herself and her social relationships. This basic understanding and self-acceptance enables her to facilitate the child's growth. The 'C' group is a new tool for the pupil personnel specialist. It enables him to work with teachers in groups which are both didactic and experiential. The goal of these groups is to develop an understanding of the practical applications of the dynamics of human behavior while acquiring an understanding of self and human relationships. I shall conclude this paper with a description (Dinkmeyer, 1971) of the salient features of this new tool.

"The 'C' group is called a 'C' group because the factors that tend to make the group most effective begin with a 'c'

1. *Collaboration*. The group works together on mutual concerns as equals. There is no superior-inferior relationship. They are consultants to each other.

2. *Consultation*. The group consults by providing and receiving ideas about the specific application of new approaches to relationships with children.

3. *Clarification*. The group clarifies for each member what it is she really believes and how congruent or incongruent her behavior is with what she believes. Through the clarification of these beliefs, systems, and feelings it is possible to become aware of the congruency or incongruency between behavior, belief, and feelings. Participants come to learn how their beliefs and faulty assumptions keep them from functioning more effectively.

4. *Confrontation*. The group expects each individual to see herself, her purposes, and her attitudes and to be willing to confront other members of the group.

5. *Communication*. The group is a new channel insofar as it communicates in a holistic sense not only content but feelings. Teachers are now available to each other as 'whole persons.'

6. *Concern and Caring*. The group shows that it is involved both with its members and children.

7. *Confidential*. Discussions are not repeated outside the group.

8. *Commitment*. The group develops a commitment to change. Participants are concerned with recognizing they can really change only themselves. They are expected to develop a specific commitment which involves an action to change their approach to a problem, to be taken before the next 'C' group."

References

Bessell, Harold, and Uvaldo Palomares. *Methods in Human Development*, San Diego, Ca.: Human Development Training Institute Inc., 1969.

Dinkmeyer, Don. *Developing Understanding of Self and Others (DUSO)*. Circle Pines, Minn: American Guidance Service, 1970.

___ "The 'C' Group: Integrating Knowledge and Experience to Change Behavior." *The Counseling Psychologist,* vol. 3, no. 1, 1971.

____and G.M. Arciniega. Affecting the Learning Climate Through 'C' Groups with Teachers." *School Counselor,* vol. 19, March 1972.

____and Edson Caldwell. *Developmental Counseling and Guidance: A Comprehensive School Approach. New York: McGraw-Hill, 1970.*

Flanders, N.A., and E. J. Amidon. "The Role of the Teacher in the Classroom." Minneapolis Association for Productive Teaching, Inc. 1967.

Jones, Richard. *Fantasy and Feelings in Education.* New York: New York University Press, 1968.

Krathwohl, David R., Benjamin S. Bloom, and Bertram B. Masia. *Taxonomy of Educational Objectives, Handbook II: Affective Domain.* New York: David McKay Company, Inc. 1964.

Limbacher, Walter J. *Dimensions of Personality.* Dayton, Ohio: Geo. A. Pflaum, 1970.

Ojemann, Ralph. *A Teaching Program in Human Behavior and Mental Health.* Cleveland, Ohio: Educational Research Council of America, n.d.

Randolph, Norma, and William Howe. *A Program to Motivate Learners, Self Enhancing Education.* Palo Alto, Ca.: Sanford Press, 1966.

Raths, Louis E., Merrill Harmin, and Sidney B. Simon. *Values and Teaching.* Columbus, Ohio: Charles E. Merrill, 1966.

Witmer, J. Melvin, and Harold F. Cottingham. "The Teacher's Role and Guidance Functions as Reported by Elementary Teachers." *Elementary School Guidance and Counseling,* vol. 5, no. 1, October 1970.

20. *Learning Problems**

Howard S. Adelman

In recent years, a great number of children with learning and behavior problems have been grouped under one or more of three labels: *learning disabled (LD), emotionally disturbed (ED), educationally handicapped (EH)*. Despite all that has been written about these three groups, neither the nature nor the implications of the heterogeneity that exists in these populations has been widely discussed in the literature. In particular, little has been written about the likelihood that, in practice, the groups categorized as LD, ED, and EH include not only youngsters who actually have major disorders that interfere with their learning, but also youngsters whose learning and behavioral problems stem primarily from the deficiencies of the learning environment in which they are enrolled. The purpose of this article is (1) to discuss an interactional view of factors that determine school success and failure and (2) to relate this model to the heterogeneity that exists in the LD, ED, and EH populations.

Currently, at least as applied to youngsters in public school programs, the terms *specific learning disabilities, emotionally disturbed,* and *educationally handicapped* have been defined as follows:

The definition formulated by the National Advisory Committee on Handicapped Children identifies children with specific learning disabilities as "those who have a disorder in one or more of the basic psychological processes involved in understanding or in using language (spoken or written), which disorder may manifest itself in an imperfect ability to listen, think, read, write, spell, or do mathematical calculations. These disorders include such conditions as perceptual handicaps, brain injury, minimal brain dysfunction, dyslexia, and developmental aphasia." The number of youngsters who fit this definition has been conservatively estimated as ranging from 1 to 3

---

*Reprinted with permission from *Academic Therapy Vol. VI, 2,* Winter 1970-71.

percent of the school population, or roughly five-hundred thousand to one million five-hundred thousand students.

While seriously emotionally disturbed children have been defined in a variety of ways, all definitions tend to characterize such children as manifesting moderate to severe maladaptive behaviors with reference to the society in which they live. The components of such definitions usually include references to hyperactivity or withdrawn behavior, emotional lability, oversensitivity to stimuli, short attention span, difficulties in interpersonal relationships, such as tendencies toward fighting and other active or passive-aggressive actions, and underachievement. Such behaviors are seen, of course, as resulting from severe emotional, other than neurological, impairment. The number of youngsters in this category has been estimated, variously, from 0.5 percent to 10 percent of the school-age population.

As described in the California Administrative Code, Title 5, Section 3230, an EH minor " . . . has marked learning or behavior disorders, or both, associated with a neurological handicap or emotional disturbance. This disorder shall not be attributable to mental retardation. The learning or behavior disorders shall be manifest, in part, by specific learning disability. Such learning disabilities may include, but are not limited to, perceptual handicaps, minimal cerebral dysfunction, dyslexia, dyscalculia, dysgraphia, school phobia, hyperkinesis or impulsivity." In California, approximately forty-three thousand children, 8/10ths of 1 percent of the public-school population were enrolled in EH programs in 1969-1970.

At present, the majority of youngsters who come to be diagnosed as LD, ED, or EH have already experienced some degree of failure in their efforts to perform as requested in the classroom. It is well-documented that such failure produces effects that can confound efforts to diagnose, reliably and validly, the cause of the problem. In fact, it may be that such youngsters are so-labeled primarily on the basis of assessment data, which reflect little more than the effects of the school failure. Thus, it seems likely that many youngsters who are diagnosed as LD, ED, or EH are so-labeled on the basis of inferences derived from data that are of questionable "post-dictive" validity.

Despite the lack of reliable and valid etiological data, many professionals have tended to act as if all youngsters who are labeled LD, ED, or EH are handicapped by an internal disorder that has caused the learning or behavioral problem. Unfortunately, this emphasis on the "disordered child" has tended to restrict the range of efforts designed to enhance our knowledge regarding the etiology, diagnosis, remediation, and prevention of school learning and behavioral problems.

There is a viable alternative to this disordered-child model. This alternative view emphasizes the dynamic nature of the process by which school skills are acquired. Thus, the model stresses that a given youngster's success or failure in school is a function of the interaction between his strengths, weaknesses, limitations, and the specific, classroom-situational factors he encounters, including individual differences among teachers and differing approaches to instruction. Stated differently, with specific reference to children who manifest school-learning or behavioral problems, or both, this interactional model suggests that such problems result not only from the characteristics of the *youngster*, but also from the characteristics of the *classroom* situation to which he is assigned.

The Youngster and the Classroom

Throughout the following discussion, there is frequent reference to the characteristics of the youngster and the program in which he is required to perform. Therefore, there is a need to be more explicit as to just which characteristics are of major relevance.

The important characteristics of the youngster are conceptualized as his behaviors, skills, interests, and needs as they are manifested in the school situation. In addition, of course, it is recognized that all youngsters differ from each other in terms of (1) development—in sensory, perceptual, motoric, linguistic, cognitive, social, and emotional areas; (2) motivation—defined in this instance as the degree to which a youngster views a specific classroom activity or task as meaningful, interesting, worth the effort, and attainable through an appropriate amount of effort; and (3) performance—emphasizing rate, style, extent, and quality as the major variables.

The important characteristics of the classroom situation include the personnel, goals, procedures, and materials that are employed in the school's efforts to provide effective and efficient instruction. Of particular relevance for the following discussion, these situational variables are seen as combining differentially to produce classrooms that vary critically in terms of the degree to which the program (1) allows for the wide range of developmental, motivational, and performance differences that exist in every classroom; (2) is compatible (does not conflict) with the fostering of each youngster's desire to learn and perform; and (3) is designed to detect current and potential problem-students and is able to correct, compensate for, or tolerate such deviant youngsters. This dimension may be conceptualized as the degree to which the program is personalized.

Classrooms that are personalized usually have a wide variety of "centers," which are designed to foster and stimulate interest in learning; the teacher in such a classroom typically emphasizes individualized programs for each youngster, rather than a three-group, basal, text-oriented approach to instruction, and, in general, he attempts to minimize failure experiences, as well as tedious and boring activities.

It is recognized that many professionals do not feel that such personalized programs can be developed in regular-classroom programs that enroll thirty-five to forty students. Because of this factor, it should be noted that my colleagues and I have just completed a project that has successfully trained teachers of culturally disadvantaged youngsters to personalize classroom programs that contain large numbers of children.

Formal Hypotheses and Implications

The nature of the interaction of the child and program characteristics, then, is seen as the major determinant of school success or failure. The hyphothesized relationship between these two sets of characteristics and school success and failure can be stated formally as follows:

The greater the congruity between a youngster's characteristics and the characteristics of the program in which he is required to perform, the greater the likelihood of school success; conversely, the greater the discrepancy between the child's characteristics and the program characteristics, the greater the likelihood of poor school performance.

This hyphothesis suggests that there are children whose school difficulties are due primarily to the fact that their classroom programs are not effectively personalized to accommodate individual differences. Therefore, as a corollary, it is hypothesized that the greater the teacher's ability in personalizing instruction, the fewer will be the number of children in her classroom who exhibit learning or behavior problems, or both; conversely, the poorer the teacher's ability in personalizing instruction, the greater will be the number of children with such problems. It is unknown how many of these learning-problem youngsters are diagnosed as LD, ED, or EH at some point in their schooling. However, with the increasing interest in these areas, it seems probable that the number of youngsters assigned to one, or more, of these categories is increasing.

More specifically, it is hypothesized that there are at least three types of youngsters with problems within each category. In addition to (1) youngsters who do have major disorders that predispose them to school difficulties, there are (2) youngsters who do *not* have such internal disorders, but who simply do not function well in nonpersonalized instructional programs, and (3) youngsters who do have minor disorders, but who, under appropriate circumstances, are able to compensate for such disorders in performing and learning school tasks, for example, if the instructional process is approximately motivating. [1]For the purposes of this discussion, the nondisordered children are referred to as Type I learning problems; the children with minor disorders are referred to as Type II learning problems; and the youngsters with major disorders, namely, those with specific learning disabilities and serious emotional disturbances, are referred to as Type III learning problems.

In contrast to this view, the majority of states with public-school programs for the learning disabled and emotionally disturbed, having established two discrete categories, tend to assume implicitly that each group consists of a different and relatively homogeneous population, while a few states, such as California, encompass both LD and ED youngsters under the rubric *educationally handicapped* and tend not to differentiate among youngsters when they are assigned to this label. *Figure 1* summarizes three views of the LD, ED, and EH populations. The view being hypothesized here suggests that the majority of such youngsters are Type I and II learning problems and that only a small percentage actually come under the heading of *specific learning disability* or *seriously emotionally disturbed*. In this connection, it may be that a more fruitful use of the label *educationally handicapped* would be to employ this term for Type I and Type II problems and reserve the categories of *specific learning disability* and *seriously emotionally disturbed* for Type III problems.

The question of what the actual percentages are for these three types of learning problems is an intriguing one. From personal experience, the Type III group appears to be only about 10 to 15 percent of the total group currently labeled LD, ED, or EH; it is recognized, however, that without empirical data, such an estimate is easily challenged.

---

[1]The issue of compensatory mechanisms has not been well-studied, but there are many examples of highly motivated individuals who have overcome severe handicaps in their efforts to understand and to communicate with others.

Figure 1

Three Views of the Learning-Disabled, Emotionally Disturbed, and Educationally Handicapped Populations.

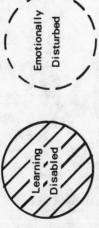

Majority view — Learning Disabled and Emotionally Disturbed students are categorized as separate populations.

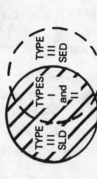

Minority view — Learning Disabled and Emotionally Disturbed students are grouped together and categorized as Educationally Handicapped.

Hypothesized view — The Learning Disabled and Emotionally Disturbed populations are seen as overlapping and as consisting of three major subgroups of youngsters with learning problems.

Type I   No disorder (problem results primarily from the deficiencies of the learning environment).
Type II Minor disorder (problem results from deficiencies in both the child and the learning environment).
Type III Major disorder (problem results from the child's deficits and/or disturbance, i.e., a Specific Learning Disability—SLD—or Serious Emotional Disturbance — SED.

In summary, what these hypotheses and inferences suggest is: (1) that the populations currently labeled LD, ED, and EH each consist of at least three major subgroups of youngsters with learning or behavioral problems, or both, ranging from those youngsters whose problem seems to stem primarily from the deficiencies of the learning environment to those who actually have major disorders that interfere with school learning or performance, or both; and (2) that there is a significant relationship between teachers' ability to personalize instruction and the type and relative proportion of the problem-youngsters who are likely to be found in these teachers' classrooms. Specifically, it is suggested that the more able the teacher, with reference to personalizing the classroom, the fewer Type I and II learning-problem youngsters will be found in his classroom. This hyphothesized relationship is shown in *Figure 2*.

At this point, then, it is emphasized that, in actual practice, the populations labeled *learning disabled, emotionally disturbed,* and *educationally handicapped* have been, and probably will continue to be for some time, heterogeneous with regard to both etiology and appropriate remedial strategies. This state of affairs, of course, is detrimental to efforts directed at developing a comprehensive and meaningful body of knowledge with regard to such youngsters.

Figure 2

The Hypothesized Relationship between Teachers' Ability to Personalize the Classroom Program and the Type and Relative Proportion of Learning-problem Children in the Classroom

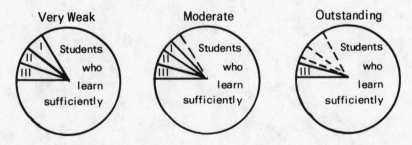

Type I — No disorder (problem results primarily from the deficiencies of the learning environment).

Type II — Minor disorder (problem results from deficiencies in both the child and the learning environment).

Type III — Major disorder (problem results primarily from the child's deficits).

Therefore, it seems reasonable to suggest that professionals who are concerned with developing such a body of knowledge need to devote ever-increasing effort to differentiating among the youngsters who are so-labeled.

21. Health and the Education of Socially Disadvantaged Children*

Herbert G. Birch

Introduction

Recent interest in the effect of social and cultural factors upon educational achievement could lead us to neglect certain biosocial factors which through a direct or indirect influence on the developing child affect his primary characteristics as a learner. Such a danger is exaggerated when health and education are administered separately. The educator and the sociologist may concentrate quite properly on features of curriculum, familial environment, motivation, cultural aspects of language organization, and the patterning of preschool experiences. Such concentration, while entirely fitting, becomes one-sided and potentially self-defeating when it takes place independently of, and without detailed consideration of, the child as a biological organism. To be concerned with the child's biology is not to ignore the cultural and environmental opportunities which may affect him. Clearly, to regard organic factors as a substitute for environmental opportunity (Hunt, 1966) is to ignore the intimate interrelation between the biology of the child and his environment in defining his functional capacities. However, it is equally dangerous to treat cultural influences as though they were acting upon an inert organism. Effective environment (Birch, 1954) is the product of the interaction of organic characteristics with the objective opportunities for experience. The child who is apathetic because of malnutrition, whose experiences may have been modified by acute or chronic illness, or whose learning abilities may have been affected by some 'insult' to the central nervous system cannot be expected to respond to opportunities for learning in the same way

---

*A working paper presented at the Conference on 'Bio-Social Factors in the Development and Learning of Disadvantaged Children' held in Syracuse, New York, April 19-21, 1967. Reprinted with permission from *Developmental Medicine and Child Neurology*, 1970, IV, 5-17.

266

as does a child who has not been exposed to such conditions. Increasing opportunity for learning, though entirely admirable in itself, will not overcome such biologic disadvantages (Birch, 1964; Cravioto *et al.*, 1966).

There are two considerations with children who have been at risk of a biological insult. First, such children must be identified and not merely additional but *special* educational opportunities effective for them must be provided. As no socially deprived group can be considered to be homogeneous for any particular disability, groups of children from such backgrounds must be differentiated into meaningful subgroups for purposes of remedial, supplemental, and habilitative education. Secondly, if conditions of risk to the organism can be identified, principles of public health and of current bio-social knowledge should be utilized to reduce learning handicap in future generations.

Concern for the socially disadvantaged cannot in good conscience restrict itself to the provision either of equal or special educational and preschool opportunities for learning. It must concern itself with all factors contributing to educational failure, among which the health of the child is a variable of primary importance.

Such an argument is not new. The basic relationship between poverty, illness, and educational failure has long been known, as has the fact expressed by James (1965) that "poverty begets poverty, is a cause of poverty and a result of poverty." What is new is the nature of the society in which such an interaction occurs. As Galbraith (1958) has put it, "to secure each family a minimum standard, as a normal function of society, would help insure that the misfortunes of parents, discerned or otherwise, were not visited on their children. It would help insure that poverty was not self-perpetuating. Most of the reaction, which no doubt would be almost universally adverse, is based on obsolete attitudes. When poverty was a majority phenomenon, such action could not be afforded . . . An affluent society has no similar excuse for such rigor. It can use the forthright remedy of providing for those in want. Nothing requires it to be compassionate. But it has no high philosophical justification for callousness."

The pertinence of Galbraith's concern as it applies to the health of children, particularly those in the nonwhite segments of our population, is underscored by the fact that, according to then Surgeon General Stewart (1967), the United States standing with respect to infant mortality has been steadily declining with respect to other countries. Though we are the richest country our 1964 infant mortality rate of 24.9 per 1,000 live births causes us to rank fifteenth in world standing. Had we had Sweden's rate, the world's lowest, approximately 43,000 fewer infants would have died in that year. Of particular pertinence to the problem of social disadvantage is the fact that the mortality rate for nonwhite infants is twice as high as that for whites, with the highest rates for the country as a whole in the east south central states, Kentucky, Tennessee, Alabama, and Mississippi. Wegman (1966) notes that "Mississippi again has the dubious distinction of having the highest rate (infant mortality) . . . more than twice that of the lowest state." Most of this difference could be related to the higher Negro population of Mississippi.

The date on infant mortality have been extended to other features of child health by Baumgartner (1965) and by Densen and Haynes (1967), who have pointed out that although detailed and careful documentation of the "degree and magnitide of the Health problems" of the Negro, Puerto Rican, and Indian groups are not readily available, a strikingly dangerous picture may be pieced together as a montage from various public health statistics, research studies, and occasional articles. The picture is striking, not merely because it shows these minority groups to be at a significant health disadvantage with respect to the white segment of the population, but because it indicates that the disparity between white and nonwhite groups is increasing. Thus, while in 1930 twice as many nonwhite mothers died in childbirth, in 1960 "for every white mother who lost her life in childbirth, four nonwhite mothers died" (Baumgartner 1965). In 1940 the number of nonwhite mothers delivered by poorly trained midwives was 14 times that for white mothers, a discrepancy that rose to 23 times as great by 1960. Gold (1962) pointed out that while the over-all death-rate for mothers in childbirth had reached an alltime low of 3.7 per 10,000 live births, this change was largely due to the reduction of the mortality rate among white mothers to 2.6. Nonwhite mothers had a death-rate four times as great, 10.3, a rate characteristic of white mothers two decades earlier. In generalizing these findings Baumgartner believes "that the most advantaged nonwhite family has a poorer chance of having a live and healthy baby than the least advantaged white family."

In our concern with educational disadvantage we must therefore recognize the excessive risk of ill-health relevant to educational handicap that exists in the children with whose welfare and education we are concerned. To this end I shall discuss some selected features of health and how far they differentiate the population of socially disadvantaged children from other children in the U.S.A.

Prematurity and Obstetric Complications

Few factors in the health history of the child have been as strongly associated with later intellectual and educational deficiencies as prematurity at birth and complications in the pregnancy from which he derives (McMahon and Sowa, 1959). Although a variety of specific infections, explicit biochemical disorders, or trauma may result in more clearly identified and dramatic alterations in brain function, prematurity, together with pre- and prenatal complications, are probably factors which most broadly contribute to disorders of neurologic development (Lilienfeld *et al.*, 1955; Pasamanick and Lilienfeld, 1955).

A detailed consideration of health factors which may contribute to educational failure must start with an examination of prematurity and the factors associated with it.

Prematurity has been variously defined either by the weight of the child at birth, by the maturity of certain of his physiologic functions, or by gestational age (Coiner, 1960). Independently of the nature of the definition, in any society in which it has been studied prematurity has an excessive representation in the lower social strata and among the most significantly socially disadvantaged. Prematurity in any social group is simultaneously indicative of two separate conditions of risk. In the first place fetuses that are primarily abnormal and characterized by a variety of congenital anomalies are more likely to be born before term than are normal fetuses. Second, infants who are born prematurely, even when no congenital abnormality may be noted, are more likely to develop abnormally than are infants born at term. Thus, Baumgartner (1962) has noted that follow-up studies have "indicated that malformation and handicapping disorders (neurological, mental, and sensory) are more likely to be found among the prematurely born than those born at term. Thus, the premature infant not only has a poorer chance of surviving than the infant born at term, but if he does survive he has a higher risk of having a handicapping condition." One consequence of this association between prematurity and neurological, mental, sensory, and other handicapping conditions is the excessive representation of the prematures among the mentally subnormal and educationally backward children at school age (Drillien, 1964).

Baumgartner (1962) has presented the distribution of live births by birthweight for white and nonwhite groups in the United States for 1957 (Table 1).* For the country as a whole, 7.6 percent of all live births weighed 2,500 g. or less. In the white segment of the popula-

*All tables referred to in this chapter are shown after page 291.

tion 6.8 percent of the babies fell in this category, while 12.5 percent of the nonwhite infants weighed 2,500 g. or less. The frequency at all levels of low birthweight was twice as great in nonwhite infants. Baumgartner attributed the high incidence of prematurity among nonwhites to the greater poverty of this group. The studies of Donnelly, *et al.* (1964) in North Carolina, of Thomson (1963) in Aberdeen, Scotland, and of Shapiro *et al.* (1960) in New York suggest that many factors, including nutritional practices, maternal health, the mother's own growth achievements as a child, as well as deficiencies in prenatal care and birth spacing and grand multiparity, interact to produce group differences between the socially disadvantaged and more advantageously situated segments of the population.

It has sometimes been argued that the excess of low birthweight babies among the socially disadvantaged is largely a consequence of ethnic differences (*i.e.*, Negroes 'naturally' give birth to smaller babies). However, the high association of prematurity with social class in an ethnically homogeneous population such as that in Aberdeen, the finding of Donnelly, *et al.* that within the Negro group higher social status was associated with reduced frequency of prematurity, the findings of Pakter *et al.* (1961) that illegitimacy adds to the risk of prematurity within the nonwhite ethnic group, and the suggestion made by Shapiro *et al.* that a change for the better in the pattern of medical care reduces the prevalence of prematurity, all make the ethnically based hypothesis of 'natural difference' difficult to retain.

If gestional age is used instead of birthweight as an indication of prematurity, the nonwhites are at an even greater risk than when birthweight is used. In 1958-1959 (Baumgartner, 1962) 18.1 percent of nonwhite babies born in New York City had a gestational age of 36 weeks or less, in contrast to 8.5 percent for live-born white babies.

Both the date on birthweight and the data on gestational age leave little doubt that prematurity and its attendant risks are excessively represented in the nonwhite segment of the population. Moreover, an examination in detail of regional data such as that provided by Donnelly *et al.* for hospital births in university hospitals in North Carolina indicate clearly that in that community the most advantaged nonwhite has a significantly greater risk of producing a premature infant than the least advantaged segment of the white population.

For equal degrees of prematurity, nonwhite infants have a somewhat better chance for survival during the first month of life

(Erhardt, 1964). However, during the remainder of infancy this likelihood is reversed, particularly for infants weighing between 1,500 and 2,500 g. at birth. Baumgartner, reviewing these data, concludes "this observation strongly suggests that inadequate medical care, inadequate maternal supervision, inadequate housing and associated socio-economic deprivations are exerting unfavorable influences on the later survival of those nonwhite babies who initially appear the more favored. It is apparent that socio-economic factors not only influence the incidence of low birthweight in all ethnic groups, but greatly influence survival after the neonatal period."

If the low birthweight and survival data are considered distributively rather than categorically, it appears that the nonwhite infant is subject to an excessive continuum of risk reflected at its extremes by perinatal, neonatal, and infant death, and in the survivors by a reduced functional potential.

The Background of Perinatal Risk

Clearly, the risk of having a premature baby or a complicated pregnancy and delivery begins long before the time of the pregnancy itself. A series of studies carried out in Aberdeen, Scotland on the total population of births of that city (Thomson, 1963; Walker, 1954; Thomson and Billewicz, 1963) indicate that prematurity as well as pregnancy complications are significantly correlated with the mother's nutritional status, height, weight, concurrent illnesses, and the social class of her father and husband. Although the relation among these variables is complex, it is clear that the women born in the lowest socio-economic class and who have remained in this class at marriage were themselves more stunted in growth than other women in the population, had less adequate dietary and health habits, were in less good general health, and tended to be at excessive risk for producing premature infants. The mother's stature as well as her habits were determined during her childhood, tended to be associated with contraction of the bony pelvis, and appeared systematically related to her risk condition as a reproducer. In analyzing the relation between maternal health and physique to a number of obstetrical abnormalities such as prematurity, caesarean section, and perinatal death, Thomson (1959) (Table 2) has shown each of these to be excessively represented in the mothers of least good physical grade.

The finding of a relation between the mother's physical status and pregnancy outcome is not restricted to Scotland. Donnelly et al., in their study of North Carolina University Hospital births, has shown a clear distribution of height with social class. In Class I (the most advantaged whites) 52 percent of the women were less than 5 ft. 5 in. tall. In contrast in social class IV (the least advantaged nonwhites) 75 percent of the women were under 5 ft. 5 in. in height. The proportion of shorter women increased consistently from Classes I to IV and within each class the incidence of prematurity was higher for women who were less than 5 ft. 3 in. tall. Moreover, within any height range the least advantaged whites had lower prematurity rates than the most advantaged non-whites. Thus in the least advantaged whites less than 5 ft. 3 in. tall the prematurity rate was 12.1 percent as contrasted with a rate of 19.6 percent for the nonwhites in the same height range. In the tallest of the most disadvantaged whites the rate was 5.6 percent whereas in nonwhites of the same height range who were least disadvantaged the prematurity rate was 10.1 percent.

Dietary Factors—Pre-war and War-time Experience

The physical characteristics of the mother which affect her efficiency as a reproducer are not restricted to height and physical grade. As early as 1933, Mellanby, while recognizing that "direct and accurate knowledge of this subject in human beings is meagre," asserted that nutrition was undoubtedly "the most important of all environmental factors in childbearing, whether the problem be considered from the point of view of the mother or that of the offspring." It was his conviction that the reduction of a high perinatal mortality rate as well as of the incidence of maternal ill health accompanying pregnancy could effectively be achieved by improving the quality of the diet. Acting upon these views he attempted London antenatal clinics and reported a significant reduction in morbidity rates during the puerperium.

Although Mellanby's own study is difficult to interpret for a number of methodologic reasons, indirect evidence rapidly came into being in support of his views. Perhaps the most important of these was the classical inquiry directed by Sir John Boyd-Orr and reported in *Food, Health and Income* (1936). This study demonstrated conclusively that the long recognized social differential in perinatal death rate was correlated with a dietary differential, and that in all respects the average diet of the lower income groups in Britain was inadequate for good health. Two years later McCance *et al.* (1938) confirmed the Boyd-Orr findings in a meticulous study of the individual diets of 120 pregnant women representing a range of economic groups ranging from the wives of unemployed miners in South Wales and Tyneside to the wives of professionals. The diet survey technique which they used and which has, unfortunately, been rarely imitated since, was designed to minimize misreport. The results showed that there was wide individual variation in the intake of all foods which related consistently neither to income nor to intake per kilogram of body weight. But when the women were divided into six groups according to the income available for each person per week, the poorer women proved to be shorter and heavier and to have lower hemoglobin counts. Moreover, though economic status had little effect on the total intake of calories, fats, and carbohydrates, "intake of protein, animal protein, phosphorus, iron, and Vitamin B[1] rose convincingly with income." The authors of the study offered no conclusions about the possible outcome of the pregnancies involved, but the poorer reproductive performance of the lower class women was clearly at issue. For as they stated, "optimum nutrition in an adult implies and postulates optimum nutrition of that person as a child, that child as a fetus, and that fetus of its mother."

A second body of indirect data supporting Mellanby's hypothesis derived from animal studies on the relation of diet to reproduction. Warkany (1944) for example, demonstrated that pregnant animals maintained on diets deficient in certain dietary ingredients produced offspring suffering from malformation. A diet which was adequate to maintain maternal life and reproductive capacity could be inadequate for normal fetal development. The fetus was not a perfect parasite and at least for some features of growth and differentiation could have requirements different from those of the maternal host.

It would divert us from the main line of our inquiry to consider the many subsequent studies in detail. However, Duncan *et al.* (1952), in surveying these studies, as well as the wartime experiences in Britain, have argued convincingly that the fall in stillbirth and neonatal death rate could only be attributed to a reduction in poverty accompanied by a scientific food rationing policy. Certainly there was no real improvement in prenatal care during the war when so many medical personnel were siphoned off to the armed forces. Furthermore, the improvement took place chiefly among those deaths attributed to "ill defined or unknown" causes—that is among those cases when low fetal vitality seems to be a major factor in influencing survival—and these types of death "are among the most difficult to influence by routine antenatal practice." Of all the possible factors then, nutrition was the only one which improved during the war years (Garry and Wood, 1945). Thomson (1959) commented that the result was "as a nutritional effect" all the more convincing "because it was achieved in the context of a society where most of the conditions of living other than the nutritional were deteriorating."

While this National "feeding experiment" was going on in the British Isles, a more controlled experiment was being carried out on the continent of Europe (Toverud, 1950). In 1939 Dr.Toverud set up a health station in the Sagene district of Oslo to serve pregnant and nursing mothers and their babies. Though war broke out shortly after the station was opened, and it became progressively more difficult to get certain protective foods, an attempt was made to insure that every woman being supervised had the recommended amounts of every essential nutrient, through the utilization of supplementary or synthetic sources when necessary. In spite of food restrictions which became increasingly severe, the prematurity rate among the 728 women who were supervised at the station never went above the 1943 high of 3.4 percent, averaging 2.2 percent for the period 1939-1944. Among the unsupervised mothers the 1943 rate was 6.3 percent and the average for the period 4.6 percent. In addition, the stillbirth rate of 14.2/1,000 for all women attending the health station was half that of the women in the surrounding districts.

Meanwhile, even as the British and Norwegian feeding experiments were in progress, there were some hopefully never-to-be repeated starvation 'experiments' going on elsewhere. when they were reported after the war, the childbearing experiences of various populations of women under conditions of severe nutritional restriction were to provide evidence of the ways in which deprivation could negatively affect the product of conception, just as dietary improvement appeared able to affect it positively.

Smith (1947), for example, studying infants born in Rotterdam and the Hague during a delimited period of extreme hunger brought on by a transportation strike, found that the infants were shorter and lighter (by about 240 g.) than those born both before and after the period of deprivation. Significantly enough Smith also found that those babies who were five to six month fetuses when the hunger period began appeared to have been reduced in weight as much as those who had spent a full nine months in the uterus of a malnourished mother. He was led to conclude from this that reduced maternal caloric intake had its major effect on fetal weight beginning around the sixth month of gestation. Antonov's study of babies born during the siege of Leningrad (1947) confirmed the fact of weight reduction as well as Smith's observations that very severe deprivation was likely to prevent conception altogether rather than reduce the birthweight. Antonov found that during a six-month period which began four months after the start of the siege, there was an enormous increase in prematurity as judged by birth length—41.2 percent of all the babies born during this period were less than 47 cm. long and fully 49.1 percent weighed under 2,500 grams. The babies were also of very low vitality—30.8 percent of the prematures and 9 percent of the full-term babies died during the period. Abruptly, during the latter half of the year, the birthrate plummeted —along with the prematurity rate. Thus, while 161 prematures and 230 term babies were born between January and June, 1942, five prematures and 72 term babies were born between July and December. Where information was available it suggested that the women who managed to conceive during the latter part of the year, when amenorrhea was widespread, were better fed than the majority, being employed in food industries or working in professional or manual occupations which had food priorities. Antonov concluded that while the fetus might behave for the most part like a parasite, "the condition of the host, the mother's body, is of great consequence to the fetus, and that severe quantitative and qualitative hunger of the mother decidedly affects the development of the fetus and the vitality of the newborn child."

Long after the war, Dean (1951) was able to confirm the Smith and Antonov results with a careful analysis of a series of 22,000 consecutive births at the landesfrauenklinik, Wuppertal, Germany, during 1937-1948. It was apparent from this series that the small reduction in the average duration of gestation recorded was insufficient to account for the degree of weight reduction observed. The study demonstrated even more clearly than before, that severe hunger did not merely reduce the mother's ability to maintain the pregnancy to term, but could act directly through the placenta to reduce the growth of the infant.

Post-war Studies

These wartime and post-war analyses leave little doubt of an association between maternal diet and the growth and development of the child in utero. Moreover, they suggest that the nature of the diet is significantly associated with pregnancy course and complications.

It is unfortunate that most of the more recent studies of the relation of maternal nutrition to pregnancy course and outcome have tended to obscure rather than to clarify the issue. Most of these studies, such as the excellently conducted Vanderbilt Cooperative Study of Maternal and Infant Nutrition (Darby *et al.* 1953 *a* and *b*, McGanity, 1954) have produced confusing and equivocal findings because of patient selection. Since the women included for study have tended to be those who registered for obstetrical care early in pregnancy, the lowest class women were markedly unrepresentative of their social group. As a result, these studies have failed to include the very women who are most central to our concern. What is sorely needed is a detailed study of nutrition and pregnancy course in socially disadvantaged women who come to obstetrical notice far too late to be included in the usual dietary surveys in obstetrical services. The design of such a study and its conduct would not be easy. However, if conducted, it would have one virtue absent in most extant studies—pertinence.

Obstetrical Care of Lower Class Women

Obstetrical care, as suggested above, is markedly different in socially advantaged and disadvantaged segments of the population. A preliminary view of the obstetrical care received by lower-class pregnant women may be obtained from a consideration of Hartman and Sayle's (1965) survey of 1380 births, at the Minneapolis General Hospital. This hospital, which served medically indigent patients living in census tracts having notably high rates of infant mortality, delivered 43 percent of its patients with either no prenatal care or only one third trimester antenatal visit. Of the women who did attend the hospital's prenatal clinic, 3 percent made their initial visit during the first trimester, and 71 percent in the last trimester. Infant mortality appeared to vary according to prenatal care. The mothers having no prenatal care experienced fetal deaths at a rate of 4 percent, a rate considerably higher than the 0.7 percent fetal death rate for mothers having one or more visits to the prenatal clinic.

Boek and Boek (1956), in upper New York State, collected their sample through an examination of birth certificates. 1,805 mothers were interviewed and grouped according to social class as determined by the child's father's occupation. The amount and type of obstetric care correlated with social class. Mothers in the lowest social classes tended to seek health care later during pregnancy than higher class women. Lower class mothers tended to use a family doctor for both pre- and postnatal care, rather than the obstetric specialists and pediatricians heavily patronized by upper class women. More than twice as many upper class women attended group meetings for expectant parents than did lower class mothers. Lower class women tended to stay in the hospital fewer days than upper class women, and although the former paid lower doctor's bills, they tended to pay higher hospital bills since more higher than lower class families had hospital insurance. Three months after the birth of the child fewer lower class women had received postnatal checkups than upper class women and fewer mothers in the lowest social class had their babies immunized with a triple vaccine or planned to have this done.

The effects of a good, comprehensive health program on pregnancy losses was studied by Shapiro *et al.* (1960), in a comparison of the infant mortality rates for members of the Health Insurance Plan and the general New York City population. Obstetric-gynecology diplomates delivered 72 percent of the HIP babies. Only 24 percent of the general New York population received specialist care, and only 5 percent of nonwhite babies were delivered by specialists. Because of these radical differences in type of delivery care, the investigators compared the HIP prematurity and perinatal mortality rates only to those New Yorkers who were patients of private physicians. Socio-economic status was judged by the occupation of the father as recorded on birth and death certificates. The data on prematurity for a three-year period are presented in Table 3. The white patients who participate in the Health Insurance Plan had their prematurity rate reduced from the 6 percent characteristic for their group in the city as a whole to 5.5 percent. This reduction just missed statistical significance at the 5 percent level. In the nonwhite group the rate was reduced from 10.8 to 8.8 percent, a difference significant at the .01 level of confidence. Within each specific category of physician used, Shapiro found that white deliveries had a far lower perinatal mortality than nonwhite for the general New York City group. General service deliveries had a far greater mortality rate than private physician cases in hospitals for both the white and nonwhite groups. "Among white deliveries mortality was considerably higher for general service cases than for those under the care of private doctors in each occupation category . . . This raises the interesting question whether the greater mortality in general services is principally due to factors associated with type of care of the setting in which it is received, or whether the poorer risk women within each occupation class tend to turn to general service."

One example of the type of risk that careful prenatal attention can diminish is shown in Kass's study (1960) of bacteriuric pregnant women in the Boston City Hospital prenatal clinic. The investigators wished to see if treatment for bacteriuria during pregnancy would have any ill effects on the health of the fetus, but shifted emphasis when they found that bacteriuric women had a dramatically higher rate of infant mortality and prematurity than nonbacteriuric women. Patients diagnosed bacteriuric and adequately treated so that they were nonbacteriuric at term had a 14 percent lower prematurity rate than untreated women (Table 4). Since the incidence of bacteriuria was 6 percent of the pregnant women seen at the prenatal clinic, Kass predicted that "it should be possible to lower the total perinatal death rate by about 25 percent and the total prematurity rate by between 10 and 20 percent, simply by screening for bacteriuria and treating it properly."

In view of the potential importance of prenatal care on pregnancy course and outcome and the suggestion that such care is deficient in the lowest socio-economic groups it is important to examine the ethnic distribution of antenatal care. The study of Pakter *et al.* (1961) though restricted to New York is representative of conditions that exist on a national scale. His findings, reported in Table 5, can be replicated in any urban community having a significantly large nonwhite population. In rural areas the situation is equally bad. Approximately 30 percent of Puerto Rican mothers received no prenatal care during the first six months of pregnancy. In contrast, only 13 percent of white married mothers were subjected to a similar lack of care.

Postnatal Conditions for Development

Densen and Haynes (1967) have indicated that many types of illness are excessively represented in the nonwhite segments of the population at all age levels. I have selected one, nutritional status, as the model variable for consideration. A considerable body of evidence from animal experimentation as well as field studies of populations at nutritional risk (Cravioto *et al.*, 1966) have suggested a systematic relation between nutritional maturation and competence in learning.

At birth the brain of a full-term infant has achieved about one quarter of its adult weight. The bulk of subsequent weight gain will derive from the laying down of lipids, particularly myelin, and cellular growth. Animal experiments on the rat (Davidson and Dobbing, 1966), the pig (Dickerson *et al.*, 1967; McCance, 1960) and the dog (Platt *et al.*, 1964) have all demonstrated a significant interference in brain growth and differentiation associated with severe dietary restriction, particularly of protein, during the first months of life. In these animals the behavioral effects have been dramatic with abnormalities in some cases persisting after dietary rehabilitation.

The relation of these data to the human situation is made difficult by the extreme severity of the dietary restrictions. More modest restrictions have been imposed by Widdowson (1965) and Barnes *et al.* (1966) and the latter experiments indicated some tendency for poorer learning in the nutritionally deprived animals. Cowley and Griesel's work (1963) suggests a cumulative effect of malnutrition on adaptive behavior across generations.

The animal findings as a whole can be interpreted either as suggesting a direct influence of malnutrition on brain growth and development, or as resulting in interference with learning at critical points in development. In either case the competence of the organism as a learner appears to be influenced by his history as an eater. These considerations add cogency to an already strongly held belief that good nutrition is important for children and links our general concerns on the relation of nutrition to health to our concerns with education and the child's functioning as a learner.

Incidents of severe malnutrition appear rarely in the United States today, but there is evidence to suggest that the low income segments of the population suffer from subtle, subclinical forms of malnutrition which may be partially responsible for the higher rates of morbidity and mortality of children in this group. Brock (1961) suggests that "dietary sub-nutrition can be defined as any impairment of functional efficiency or body systems which can be corrected by better feeding." Since "constitution is determined in part by habitual diet . . . diet must be considered in discussing the aetiology of a large group of diseases of uncertain and multiple aetiology . . ." The relationship between nutrition and constitution is demonstrated by the fact that the populations of developed nations are taller and heavier than those of technically underdeveloped nations and that "within a given developed nation children from economically favoured areas are taller and heavier than children from economically under-privileged area."

In comparison to the vast body of data available on the diets of people in tropical countries, very little research has been done in recent years on the nutritional status of various economic groups in the United States. The effects of long term subclinical malnutrition on the health of the individual are not yet known, and little research has been directed at this problem since 1939. However, it is instructive to review the studies comparing the diets of low-income people with the rest of the population since these lay the basis for hypothesizing that nutritional differences may have some effect on the over-all differences in health and learning ability between groups.

The nutritional differences between lower and higher income individuals begin before birth and continue thereafter. In a study of maternal and child health care in upper New York State, Walter Boek *et al.* (1957) found that babies from low income families were breast fed less often and kept on only milk diets longer than upper income infants. In a study of breast feeding in Boston, Salber and Feinleib (1960) confirmed Boek's results and, "social class was found to be the most important variable affecting incidence of breast-feeding" (Table 6).

Social class differences in feeding patterns continue after weaning. Filer and Martinez (1964) studied 4,642 six-month-old infants from a nationally representative sample and found that "infants of mothers with least formal education and in families with lowest incomes are fed more milk formula . . ." and less solid foods at six months old than those from higher educational and economic groups. Class differences in the intake of most nutrients varied primarily according to the amount of milk formula consumed.

The researchers found that for "almost all nutrients studied, the mean intakes were well above recommended levels. The single exception was iron; more than half of infants do not get the lowest recommended provision—a finding that corroborates the results reported by a number of other investigators." Iron deficiency was most prevalent among infants of mothers with low educational and income levels. Infants whose mothers attained no more than a grade school education received a mean intake of only 6.7 mg. of iron a day, as compared to the 9.1 mg. mean intake of infants whose mothers had attended high school. Since "nutritional iron deficiency is widespread and most prevalent in infants in the low socio-economic group," and iron deficiency is the most common cause of anemia in infants during the first two years of life, malnutrition at least with respect to this nutrient is widely prevalent in lower class infants.

A study of Negro, low-income infants in South Carolina (Jones and Schendel, 1966) uncovered more extensive areas of malnutrition in this group; the death-rate for Negro infants in South Carolina was twice the national rate. Thirty-six Negro infants from low income families were tested when they visited a Well-Baby Clinic for routine examinations. The subjects ranged in age from four to ten months. "The bodyweights of 66 percent of the infants were below the 50th percentile in the Harvard growth charts, 34 percent below the 10th percentile and 9 percent below the 3rd percentile." Twenty-nine percent of the subjects had "serum albumin concentrations which have been associated with marginal protein nutrition" and serum globin concentrations below normal range. Sixty-one percent had total protein concentrations below normal and 33 percent had "serum ascorbic acid concentrations which have been associated with a sub-optimal intake of vitamin C." One infant's albumin concentration showed severe protein deficiency and "eight . . . infants had concentrations of serum ascorbic acid reflecting a severely limited dietary intake of vitamin C." The researchers concluded that "it would appear possible that malnutrition may be one of the many underlying causes for the high rate of Negro infant mortality in South Carolina." Since Greenville County, where the study was conducted, has a relatively small number of infant deaths, "it is possible that malnutrition may be even more severe and/or prevalent in many other counties of the state.

Since the sample used in this study is small (36 infants), the results must be viewed as suggestive rather than conclusive. But taken together with the findings on iron intake, a New York study which shows that anemia is common among Negro and Puerto Rican infants (James, 1966) and the recent finding of Arneil (1965) that "some anemia was present in 59 percent of Glasgow slum children," the suggestion is strengthened that poor diet may be partly responsible for the poor health of lower socio-economic class children.

The studies so far reviewed have dealt with populations that are in some way representative of the nutritional status of large groups of children. Since these studies are few in number and limited in approach, they cannot give a complete picture of the nutritional status of lower class Americans. Hints about areas of malnutrition which have not been thoroughly investigated can be drawn from studies of special groups within the American population. In a survey of the "Dietary and Nutritional Problems of Crippled Children in Five Rural Counties of North Carolina," Bryan and Anderson (1965) found that the diets of 73 percent of the 164 subject sample were less than adequate. The cause for the malnourishment of nine out of ten of the poorly fed children was poor family diet and in only one of ten cases was the malnutrition related to the physical handicap of the child.

Although all the children were from families in the low income group, the researchers found certain significant differentiations between the Negro and white families studied. Seventy-one precent of the Negro children and 35 percent of the white children's diets were rated as probably or obviously inadequate. Only a limited number of food items were used and "in many of the families . . . only one food was cooked for a meal and this would be eaten with biscuits and water, tea or Kool-Aid . . . For the most part, the diet of our low income families contained few foods that are not soft or that require much chewing." Suggestions of poor nutrition in infancy and childhood can also be drawn from studies of constitutional differences as well as from measurements of food intake.

A study of the nutritional status of junior high school children in Onondaga County, New York (Dibble *et al.*, 1965) compared subjects from broadly different economic groups. School 'M' was 94 percent Negro, while Schools 'L' and 'J' were overwhelmingly white. The schools were also differentiated on the basis of the occupation of the students' fathers: ". . . of the 58 percent of the employed fathers from school M, 52 percent were laborers, whereas only 10 percent from school L and 38 percent from school J were in this category." When the heights and weights of the subjects were compared, a greater percentage of students from the lower socio-economic class school fell in the short stature and low-weight zones. There was also a tendency for students from the predominantly Negro school to have less subcutaneous fat by ranking of skinfold than students from other schools.

Blood and urine samples were taken for all the subjects and the researchers set up criteria to determine the level of adequacy for the various nutrients. "Subjects from school M, (the Negro school) had a slightly lower average hematocrit, largely due to the greater number of female subjects from that school in the low classification (and) the average plasma ascorbic acid value for school M was about half as great as the average in school L." There was also a tendency for the Negro population to have low values for hexose and pentose when erythrocyte hemolysate transketolase activity was determined. Average urinary excretions of riboflavin and thiamine was above acceptable level in all groups, but data for folinic acid indicated lower levels of excretion for children from school M than for children in schools L and J. The question whether this observation was related to the lower ascorbic acid levels of these children indicates a need for further study in this area. The authors conclude that the differences between the schools show a relationship between nutrition and socio-economic status. These differences are greater than the differences between male and female students, and are related to each other on the various parameters of the study. "There was a slight indication that the growth of the male subjects in . . . school (M) had not been as great as that of the subjects in the other schools with whom they were compared. This fact was supported by somewhat lower average levels in the other parameters . . ."

Although the students at the predominantly Negro school in Onondaga County did not appear to suffer from gross nutritional deficiencies, their diets were significantly less adequate than the subjects from the white, middle-class schools. The investigators did not attempt to link dietary habits with health records, but the results of the study lead to speculations about the relationship between suboptimal diet, rates of infection, school absence, and academic performance.

Why Malnutrition?

Why, in a society with an abundant and often enriched food supply, are several groups of the population inadequately nourished. The answer appears to lie in two broad areas: money and information. Cultural differences in food habits and beliefs, though important, appear to lose their significance relatively quickly when adequate funds, higher general education, and sound knowledge of proper nutrition become available. Thus in an article on "The Nutritional Status of American Negroes," Jean Mayer (1965) finds that "the food habits of Negroes belonging to the higher socio-economic classes appear to be essentially those of their white counterparts, (however) it can be fairly stated that in general the state of nutrition of Negroes is inferior to that of whites in the same geographic areas. In some cases, it is vastly inferior." Just as poverty and lack of education breed poor eating habits among lower economic class Negroes, low income combined with a good education can produce adequate nutrition, as has been shown in a comparison of the dietary habits of students' wives with other low income groups (Jeans *et al.*, 1952).

In a detailed study of the "Eating Patterns Among Migrant Families" in Palm Beach County, Florida, Delgado *et al.* (1961) found that a combination of low income, lack of education, and lack of kitchen equipment and proper storage facilities contributed to dramatically poor diets in the migrant families.

When the family diets were analyzed in terms of the various

nutrients, only 20 percent of the families met the National Research Council calorie requirements. Thiamine, protein, Vitamin A, and iron requirements were not met by over 50 percent of the families. About 80 percent did not meet the requirements for calcium and riboflavin and 97 percent did not have enough Vitamin C. None of the families met stated requirements for milk, green and yellow vegetables; only a few had citrus fruits and tomatoes, potatoes or other fruits and vegetables and eggs; and only 43 percent of the families met the daily requirements for meat.

Negro migrant agricultural workers have "the highest proportion of malnourished individuals of any group in the country" and Mayer (1965) finds the "shortage of published data in this field striking." Although lack of money to buy nutritious foods is aparently the major reason for malnourishment, the lack of information about nutrition is also to blame for both the rural and urban Negro diet. A monotonous, limited diet is the rule for Southern rural Negroes and the inadquacy of the diet is exaggerated for Southern urban Negroes for whom the availability of green vegetables is decreased. "Consumption of fresh vegetables is low and consumption of citrus fruits negligible. Milk consumption is substantially lower than in white families . . . This is for a large part a reflection of lower income; but even at equal income, milk consumption may be lower for Negro families." Although calorie requirements are usually met in urban families, protein, calcium, thiamine, riboflavin, nicotinic acid, Vitamin A, and Vitamin C requirements are often inadequately met.

In the North "even as approximate a description of the nutritional status of the Negro population is impossible to arrive at." Mayer observes, however, that familiar Southern foods of minimal nutritional value, such as turnip, mustard greens, kale, okra, and plantains, are stocked by stores in northern Negro areas. "Careful perusal of the records available in large cities, as well as the collection of impressions of experienced physicians, dietitians, and health administrators, leaves little doubt that our Negro slums represent the greatest concentration of anemias, growth failures, dermatitis of doubtful origin, accidents of pregnancy and other signs associated with malnutrition."

Although the studies reviewed here are helpful for their indications and descriptions of areas of suboptimal nutrition in this country, a detailed and comprehensive study of the nutrition of the low income population is still lacking. Since suboptimal nutrition can have social and psychological ramifications, as well as constitutional and medical results, a more thorough knowledge of the ways in which nutrition can affect the daily life of the individual would be useful for all those who seek to improve the health and social well being of the poor.

Conclusions

In this review I have examined certain selected conditions of health which may have consequences for education. Other factors such as acute and chronic illness, immunizations, dental care, the utilization of health services and a host of other phenomena, perhaps equally pertinent to those selected for consideration, have been dealt with either in passing or not at all but in fact the studies of these factors that do exist reflect the same picture that emerges from those variables which have been discussed. In brief, though much of the information is incomplete, and certain aspects of the data are sparse, a serious consideration of available health information leaves little or no doubt that children who are economically and socially disadvantaged and in an ethnic group exposed to discrimination, are exposed to massively excessive risks for maldevelopment.

Such risks have direct and indirect consequences for the functioning of the child as a learner. Conditions of ill health may directly affect the development of the nervous system and eventuate either in patterns of clinically definable malfunctioning in this system or in subclinical conditions. In either case the potentialities of the child as a learner cannot but be impaired. Such impairment, though it may in fact have reduced functional consequences under exceptionally optimal conditions for development and education, in any case represents a primary handicap which efforts at remediation may only partially correct.

The indirect effects of ill health or of conditions of suboptimal health care on the learning processes may take many forms. Only two can be considered at this point. Children who are ill-nourished are reduced in their responsiveness to the environment, distracted by their visceral state, and reduced in their ability to progress and endure in learning conditions. Consequently, given the same objective conditions for learning, the state of the organism modifies the effective environment and results in a reduction in the profit which a child may derive from exposure to opportunities for experience. Consequently, the provision of equal opportunities for learning in an objective sense is never met when only the school situation is made identical for advantaged and disadvantaged children. Though such a step is indeed necessary, proper, and long overdue, a serious concern with the profitability of such improved objective opportunities for socially disadvantaged children demands a concern which goes beyond education and includes an intensive and directed consideration of the broader environment, the health and functional and physical well-being of the child.

Inadequacies in nutritional status as well as excessive amounts in intercurrent illness may interfere in indirect ways with the learning process. As Cravioto *et al.* (1966) have put it, at least "three possible indirect effects are readily apparent:

(1) *Loss of learning time.* Since the child was less responsive to his environment when malnourished, at the very least he had less time in which to learn and had lost a certain number of months of experience. On the simplest basis, therefore, he would be expected to show some developmental lags.

(2) *Interference with learning during critical periods of development.* Learning is by no means simply a cumulative process. A considerable body of evidence exists which indicates that interference with the learning process at specific times during its course may result in disturbances in function that are both profound and of long-term significance. Such disturbance is not merely a function of the length of time the organism is deprived of the opportunities for learning. Rather, what appears to be important is the correlation of the experiential opportunity with a given stage of development—the so-called critical periods of learning. Critical periods in human learning have not been definitively established, but in looking at the consequences associated with malnutrition at different ages one can derive some potentially useful hypotheses. The earlier report by Cravioto and Robles (1965) may be relevant to the relationship between the age at which malnutrition develops and learning. They have shown that, as contrasted with older patients, infants under six months recovering from kwashiorkor did not recoup their mental age deficit during the recovery period. In older children, ranging from 15 to 41 months of age, too, the rate of recovery from the initial mental deficit varied in direct relation to chronological age at time of admission. Similarly, the findings of Barrera-Moncada (1963) in children, and those of Keys *et al.* (1950) in adults, indicated a strong association between the persistence of later effects on mental performance and the age at onset of malnutrition and its duration.

(3) *Motivation and personality changes.* It should be recognized that the mother's response to the infant is to a considerable degree a function of the child's own characteristics of reactivity. One of the

first effects of malnutrition is a reduction in the child's responsiveness to stimulation and the emergence of various degrees of apathy. Apathetic behavior in its turn can function to reduce the value of the child as a stimulus and to diminish the adults' responsiveness to him. Thus, apathy can provoke apathy and so contribute to a cumulative pattern or reduced adult-child interaction. If this occurs it can have consequences for stimulation, for learning, for maturation, and for interpersonal relations, the end result being significant backwardness in performance on later, more complex learning tasks.''

However, independently of the path through which bio-social pathology interferes with educational progress, there is little doubt that ill health is a significant variable for defining differentiation in the learning potential of the child. To intervene effectively with the learning problems of disadvantaged children it would be disastrous if we were either to ignore or to relegate the physical condition and health status of the child with whose welfare we are concerned to a place of unimportance. To do so would be to divorce education from health; a divorce which can only have disorganizing consequences for the child. Unless health and education go hand in hand we shall fail to break the twin curse of ignorance and poverty.

Acknowledgments: The research reported was supported in part by the National Institutes of Health, National Institute of Child Health and Human Development (HD-00719); the Association for the Aid of Crippled Children; and the National Association for Retarded Children.

The background examination of the literature and the detailed spelling out of many problems was carried out in conjunction with Mrs. Joan Gussow and Mrs. Ronni Sandroff Franklin.

This paper was commissioned under United States Office of Education Contract #6-10-240 (ERIC). It was also used at the Conference on 'Bio-Social Factors in the Development and Learning of Disadvantaged Children,' held in Syracuse in April 1967 under the terms of United States Office of Education Contract #6-10-243.

References

Antonov, A. N. (1947) 'Children born during the siege of Leningrad in 1942.' *J. Pediat.*, **30**, 250.

Arneil, G. C. McKilligan, H. R., Lobo, E. (1965) 'Malnutrition in Glasgow children.' *Scot. med. J.*, **10**, 480.

Barnes, R. H., Cunnold, S. R., Zimmerman, R. R., Simmons, H., MacLeod, R., Krook, L. (1966) 'Influence of nutritional deprivations in early life on learning behaviour of rats as measured by performance in water maze.' *J. Nutr.*, **89,** 399.

Barrera-Moncada, G. (1963) Estudios sobre Alleraciones del Crecimiento y del Desarrollo Psicologico de Sindrome Pluricarencial Kwashiorkor. Caracas: Editoria Grafos.

Baumgartner, L. (1962) 'The public health significance of low birth weight in the U. S. A., with special reference to varying practices in providing special care to infants of low birth weights.' *Bull. Wld Hlth Org.,* **26,** 175.

——(1965) 'Health and ethnic minorities in the sixties.' *Amer. J. publ. Hlth,* **55,** 495.

Birch, H. G. (1954) 'Comparative psychology.' *In* Marcuse, F. A. (Ed.) Areas of Psychology. New York: Harper.

——(Ed.) (1964) Brain Damage in Children: Biological, and Social Aspects. Baltimore: Williams & Wilkins.

Boek, W. E., Boek, J. K. (1956) Society and Health. New York: Putnam.

——and co-worker (1957) Social Class, Maternal Health and Child Care. Albany, N. Y.: New York State Department of Health.

Brock, J. (1961) Recent Advances in Human Nutrition. London: Churchill.

Bryan, H., Anderson, E. L. (1965) 'Dietary and nutritional problems of crippled children in five rural counties of North Carolina. *Amer. J. publ. Hlth,* **55,** 1,545.

Corner-B. (1960) Prematurity. London: Cassell.

Cowley, J. J., Griesel, R. D. (1963) 'The development of second generation low-protein rats.' *J. genet. Psychol.,* **103,** 233.

Cravioto, J. DeLicardie. E. R., Birch, H. G. (1966) 'Nutrition, growth and neuro-integrative development: an experimental and ecologic study.' *Pediatrics,* **38,** 319.

——Robles, B. (1965) 'Evolution of adaptive and motor behaviour during rehabilitation from kwashiorkor.' *Amer. J. Orthopsychiat.,* **35,** 449.

Darby, W. J., Densen, P. M., Cannon, R. O., Bridgeforth, E., Martin, M. P., Kaser, M. M., Peterson, O., Christie, A., Frye, W. W., Justus, K., McClellan, G. S., Williams, C., Ogle, P. J., Hahn, P. F., Sheppard, C. W., Crothers, E. L., Newbill, J. A. (1953) 'The Vanderbilt co-operative study of maternal and infant nutrition. I. Background. II. Methods, III. Description of the sample data.' *J. Nutr.,* **51,** 539.

——McGanity, W. J., Martin, M. P., Bridgeforth, E., Densen, P. M., Kaser, M. M., Ogle, P. J., Newbill, J. A., Stockell, A., Ferguson, E., Touster, O., McClellan, G. S., Williams, C., Cannon, R. O. (1953) 'The Vanderbilt co-operative study of maternal and infant nutrition. IV. Dietary, laboratory and physical findings in 2,129 delivered pregnancies.' *J. Nutr.,* **51,** 565.

Davison, A. N., Dobbin, J. (1966) 'Myelination as a vulnerable period in brain development.' *Brit. med. Bull.,* **22,** 40.

Dean, R. F. (1951) 'The size of the baby at birth and the yield of breast milk.' *In* Studies of Undernutrition, Wuppertall, 1946-49. M. C. R. Special Report Series, No. 275. London: H.M.S.O. Chap. 28.

Delgado, G., Brumback, C. L., Deaver, M. B. (1961) 'Eating patterns among migrant families.' *Publ. Hlth. Rep. (Wash.),* **76,** 349.

Densen, P. M., Haynes, A. (1967) 'Research and the major health problems of Negro Americans. Paper presented at the Howard University Centennial Celebration, Wahington. (Unpublished.)

Dibble, M. F., Brin, M., McMullen, E., Peel, A., Chen, N. (1965) 'Some preliminary biochemical findings in junior high school children in Syracuse and Onondaga County, New York.' *Amer. J. clin. Nutr.,* **17,** 218.

Dickerson, J. W., Dobbing, J., McCance, R. A. (1967) 'The effect of under nutrition on the postnatal development of the brain and cord in pigs.' *Proc. roy. Soc. B.,* **166,** 396.

Donnelly, J. F., Flowers, C. E., Creadick, R. N., Wells, H. B., Greenberg, B. G., Surles, K. B. (1964) 'Maternal, fetal and environmental factors in prematurity.' *Amer. J. Obstet. Gynec.* **88,** 918.

Drillien, C. M. (1964) The Growth and Development of Prematurely Born Children. Edinburgh: Livingstone, Baltimore: Williams & Wilkins.

Duncan, E. H. L., Baird, D., Thomson, A. M. (1952) 'The causes and prevention of stillbirths and first week deaths. I. The evidence of vital statistics.' *J. Obstet. Gyncea. Brit. Emp.,* **59,** 183.

Erhardt, C. L., Joshi, G. B., Nelson, F. G., Kron, B. H., Weiner, L. (1964) 'Influence of weight and gestation on perinatal and neonatal mortality by ethnic group.' *Amer. J. publ. Hlth.,* **54,** 1,841.

Filer, L. J., Martinez, G. A. (1964) 'Intake of selected nutrients by infants in the United States: an evaluation of 4,000 representative six-year-olds.' *Clin. Pediat.,* **3,** 633.

Galbraith, J. K. (1958) The Affluent Society. Boston: Houghton Mifflin.

Garry, R. C., Wood, H. O. (1945-46) 'Dietary requirements in human pregnancy and lactation: a review of recent work.' *Nutr. Abstr. Rev.,* **15,** 591.

Gold, E. M. (1962) 'A broad view of maternity care.' *Children,* **9,** 52.

Hartman, E. E., Sayles, E. B. (1965) 'Some reflections on births and infant deaths among the low socio-economic groups.' *Minn. Med.,* **48,** 1,711.

Hunt, E. E. (1966) 'Some new evidence on race and intelligence.' Paper read at the meeting of the New York Academy of Sciences—Anthropology Section, Oct. 24, 1966. (Unpublished).

James, G. (1965) 'Poverty and public health—new outlooks. I. Poverty as an obstacle to health progress in our cities.' *Amer. J. publ. Hlth,* **55,** 1,757.

————(1969) 'New York City's Bureau of Nutrition.' *J. Amer. dietet. Ass.*, **48,** 301.

Jeans, P. C., Smith, M. B., Stearns, G. (1952) 'Dietary habits of pregnant women of low income in a rural state.' *J. Amer. dietet. Ass.*, **28,** 27.

Jones, R. E., Schendel, H. E. (1966) 'Nutritional status of selected Negro infants in Greenville County, South Carolina.' *Amer. J. clin. Nutr.*, **18,** 407.

Kass, E. H. (1960) 'Bacteriuria and the prevention of prematurity and perinatal death.' *In* Kowlessar, M. (Ed.) Transactions of the 5th Conference on the Physiology of Prematurity. Princeton, 1960.

Keys, A., Brozek, J., Henschel, A., Mikelsen, O., Taylor, H. (1950) The Biology of Starvation. Vol. 2. Minneapolis: University of Minnesota Press.

Lilienfeld, A.M., Pasamanik, B., Rogers, M. (1955) 'Relationship between pregnancy experience and the development of certain neuropsychiatric disorders in childhood.' *Amer. J. publ. Hlth,* **45,** 637.

McCance, R. A. (1960) 'Severe undernutrition in growing and adult animals. I. Production and general effects.' *Brit. J. Nutr.,* **14,** 59.

————Widdowson, E. M., Verdon-Roe, C. M. (1938) 'A study of English diets by the individual method. III. Pregnant women at different economic levels.' *J. Hyg. (Lond.),* **38,** 596.

McGanity, W. J., Cannon, T. O., Bridgeforth, E. B., Maring, M. P., Densen, P. M., Newbill, J. A., McClellan, G. S., Christie, A., Peterson, J. O., Darby, W. J. (1954) 'The Vanderbilt co-operative study of maternal and infant nutrition. VI. Relationship of obstetric performance to nurition.' *Amer. J. Obstet. Gynec., 67,* 501.

MacMachon, B., Sowa, J. M. (1961) 'Physical damage to the foetus.' *In* Causes of Mental Disorders: A Review of Epidemiological Knowledge, 1959. New York: Milbank Memorial Fund, p. 51.

Mayer, J. (1965) 'The nutritional status of American Negroes.' *Nutr, Rev., 23,* 161.

Orr, J. B. (1936) Food, Health and Income. London: Macmillan.

Pakter, J., Rosner, H. J., Jacobziner, H., Greenstein, F. (1961) 'Out-of-wedlock births in New York City. II. Medical aspects.' *Amer. J. publ. Hlth, 51,* 846.

Pasamanik, B., Lilienfeld, A. M. (1955) 'Association of maternal and fetal factors with development of mental deficiency. I. Abnormalities in the prenatal and perinatal periods.' *J. Amer. med. Ass., 159,* 155.

Platt, B. S., Heard, R. C., Stewart, R. J. (1964) 'Experimental protein-calorie deficiency.' *In* Muntro, H. N., Allison, J. B. (Eds.) Mammalian Protein Metabolism. New York: Academic Press. p. 446.

Salber, E. J., Feinleib, M. (1966) 'Breast feeding in Boston.' *Pediatrics, 37,* 299.

Shapiro, S., Jacobziner, H., Densen, P.M., Weiner, L. (1960) 'Further observations on prematurity and perinatal mortality in a general population and in the population of a prepaid group practice medical care plan.' *Amer. J. publ. Hlth,* **50,** 1,304.

Smith, C. A. (1947) 'Effects of maternal undernutrition upon the new born infant in Holland.' *J. Pediat.,* **30,** 229.

Stewart, W. H. (1957) 'The unmet needs of children.' *Pediatrics,* **39,** 157.

Thomson, A. M. (1959) 'Maternal stature and reproduction efficiency.' *Eugen. Rev.,* **51,** 157.

——(1959) 'Diet in pregnancy . III. Diet in relation to the course and outcome of pregnancy.' *Brit. J. Nutr.,* **13,** 509.

——Billewicz, W. Z. (1963) 'Nutritional status, physique and reproductive efficiency.' *Brit. J. Nutr.,* **28,** 55.

Toverud, G. (1950) The influence of nutrition on the course of pregnancy.' *Milbank mem Fd. Quart.,* **28,** 7.

U. S. Welfare Administration, Division of Research. (1966) Converging Social Trends—Emerging Social Problems. Welfare Administration Publication No. 6. Washington: U. S. Government.

Walker, J. (1954) 'Obstetrical complications, congenital malformations and social strata.' *In* Mechanisms of Congenital Malformations. New York: Association for the Aid of Crippled Children. p. 20.

Warkany, J. (1944) 'Congenital malformations induced by maternal nutritional deficiency.' *J. Pediat.,* **25,** 476.

Wegman, M. E. (1966) 'Annual summary of vital statistics, 1965.' *Pediatrics,* **39,** 1,067.

Widdowson, E. M. (1966) 'Nutritional deprivation in psychobiological development: studies in animals.' *In* Proceedings of the Special Session, 4th Meeting of the 'PAHO Advisory Committee on Medical Research, June, 1965. Washington: World Health Organization.

TABLE 1
Percentage Distribution of 4,254,784 Live-Births By Birth Weight and Ethnic Group, USA 1957

Birth weight (g.)	Total	White	Non-white
1,000 or less	0·5	0·4	0·9
1,001–1,500	0·6	0·5	1·1
1,501–2,000	1·4	1·3	2·4
2,001–2,500	5·1	4·5	8·1
2,501–3,000	18·5	17·5	24·5
3,001–3,500	38·2	38·4	37·2
3,501–4,000	26·8	28·0	19·6
4,001–4,500	7·3	7·8	4·8
4,501–5,000	1·3	1·3	1·3
5,001 or more	0·2	0·2	0·2
Total	100	100	100
Percentage under 2,501 g.	7·6	6·8	12·5
Median weight (g.)	3,310	3,330	3,170
Number of Live Births	4,254,784	3,621,456	633,328

From Baumgartner 1962

TABLE 2
Incidence of Obstetric Abnormalities in Aberdeen Primigravidae by Maternal Health and Physique as Assessed at the First Antenatal Examination. (Twin Pregnancies have been Excluded.)

	Health and Physique			
	Very good	Good	Fair	Poor; very poor
Prematurity* (%)	5·1	6·4	10·4	12·1
Cesarean section (%)	2·7	3·5	4·2	5·4
Perinatal deaths per 1,000 births	26·9	29·2	44·8	62·8
No. of subjects	707	2,088	1,294	223
Percentage tall (5 ft 4 in. or more)	42	29	18	13
Percentage short (under 5 ft. 1 in.)	10	20	30	48

* Birthweight of baby 2,500 g. or less (From Thomson 1961)

TABLE 3
Prematurity Rates by Ethnic Group, New York City, and HIP (Adjusted) 1955–1957

	Single Live Births Attended by Private Physician in Hospital			
	Prematurity Rate per 100 Live Births[1]			
Ethnic Group	New York City[2]	HIP Adjusted[2]	Standard Error of Difference	P[3]
Total (Excluding Puerto Rican)	6·2	5·7	0·23	0·04
White	6·0	5·5	0·24	0·06
Nonwhite	10·8	8·8	0·74	<0·01

1. *Prematurity rate*—no. of live births 2,500 gm. or less/100 live births. 2. N.Y.C. observed rates for deliveries of women of all ages except those under 20 & age not

stated. HIP rates adjusted to age of mother & ethnic distrib. of N.Y.C. deliveries (except those of women under 20 & age not stated). 3. 'P' represents probability that NYC-HIP difference is due to chance factors. (Shapiro 1960).

TABLE 4

Effect of Bacteriuria During Pregnancy on Occurrence of Pyelonephritis, Prematurity, and Perinatal Death

Patient Group	No. of Patients	No. with Pyelo- nephritis	Premature Infants (per cent)	Perinatal Mortality (per cent)
Untreated bacteriuric ..	48	20	24	14
Treated bacteriuric ..	43	0	10	0
Non bacteriuric	1,000	0	9	2

(From Kass, 1960)

TABLE 5

Obstetric Care in Different Ethnic Groups

	White		*Puerto Rican*		*Non-White*	
	married	*unmarried*	*married*	*unmarried*	*married*	*unmarried*
Private services	85·8	17·3	—	—	—	—
Ward services	12·2	81·0	90·4	97·5	82·1	97·4
Prenatal care in first six months	87·2	36·7	60·4	43·5	61·7	42·9

(Drawn from Pakter 1961)

TABLE 6

Incidence and Duration of Breast-Feeding Among 2,233 Mothers

	Social class of father		
	Students	*Class 1 and 2 (Warner's)*	*Class 3–7 (Warner's)*
Total Number	88	550	1,595
Number Breast-Feeding ..	61	219	217
Percentage Breast-Feeding	69·3	39·8	13·6
P For Difference in Proportion	< ·01	< ·01	< ·01
Mean Duration (Days) ..	123·0	111·7	98·5
P. For Difference in Means	> ·05	> ·05	> ·05

(Data drawn from Salber and Feinleib 1966)

22. Compensating, Remediating, Innovating, and Integrating: Illusions of Educating the Poor

Sol Gordon

Introduction

"Knowledge is increasing so fast, a recent ad said, that the problem of education is to find better ways to 'pack it into young heads.' This popular belief is wrong and causes much of what is wrong with our schools. For years, it is true, learned men used their brains to store and retrieve information. Today, the child who has been taught in school to stuff his head with facts, recipes, this-is-how-you-do-it, is obsolete even before he leaves the building. Anything he can do, or be taught to do, a machine can do, and soon will do better and cheaper.

What children need, even just to make a living, are qualities that can never be trained into a machine—inventiveness, flexibility, resourcefulness, curiosity, and, above all, judgment.

The chief products of schooling these days are not these qualities, not even the knowledge and skills they try to produce, but stupidity, ignorance, incompetence, self-contempt, alienation, apathy, powerlessness, resentment, and rage. We can't afford such products any longer. The purpose of education can no longer be to turn out people who know a few facts, a few skills, and who will always believe and do what they are told. We need big changes and in a hurry."[*]

—John Holt

The U.S. Riot Commission Report in 1968 warned that: "Without major changes in educational practices, greater expenditures on existing elementary schools serving disadvantaged neighborhoods will not significantly improve the quality of education."

Now, four years later, with some eight billion dollars of federal money invested in the education of the poor, as well as several significant federal injunctions forcing integration, are we any further

---

[*]"Why We Need New Schooling," *Look,* Jan. 13, 1970

along in the education of the so-called "disadvantaged"?

The evidence appears to be overwhelmingly in favor of the supposition that compensatory education is a failure.

—The school systems of almost every large metropolitan city in the country already have a majority of black (and other minority group) public school students or are moving in this direction.

—The Skelly Wright Decision, hailed by progressives as a landmark for integration in Washington, D.C., is probably an important factor in the District's school system approaching 100% black students.

—Virtually every large city school system has experienced a decline in reading scores for four years in a row.

—Of the 244 compensatory education programs reviewed in 1966 by E. W. Gordon and D. A. Wilkerson, hardly more than a handful were still in existence in 1971, according to a status report by Adelaide Jablonsky.[7]

—The following headlines appeared after October, 1971 in *The New York Times:*

SCHOOLS, NOT PUPILS, ARE FOUND AT FAULT IN READING FAILURES (October 29)
CHICAGO REPORTS SEGREGATION IS UP (November 28)
SURVEY SAYS SCHOOL MORALE ERODING (October 19)
O.E.O. ADMITS FAILURE IN TESTS OF COMPANY LEARNING PROGRAMS (Feb. 1, 1972)

The best way to waste billions earmarked for education of disadvantaged children is to expand existing services and practices such as:

—Hiring more remedial reading teachers, guidance counselors, psychologists, and social workers.

—Increasing and even mandating sensitivity training and human relations workshops.

—Continuing the practice of introducing and abandoning at least one new reading, math, or science program each year with plans for the following year to escalate to the introduction and abandonment of two new entirely innovative courses of study designed especially for disadvantaged children.

—Mandating busing from mediocre schools to interior ones.

—Continuing and accelerating the supposed "real" teaching of children who have not learned much during the school day in after-school programs.

—Using whatever small amount of funds allocated for research to evaluate programs in operation less than a few months or about to be abandoned. (Under no circumstances should federal money be used for serious long-range studies.)

—Quieting the "black" agitation by ordering a packaged $1,000 library of the forgotten books on Negro history.

—Introducing aides and paraprofessionals into the school with little or no training, purpose, or opportunity for advancement.

—Arranging for the big money to go for consultants (university professors), conferences, and workshops on every conceivable topic—but providing no funds for in-service courses for classroom teachers on how to teach basic reading and arithmetic to children who have not learned it by the end of the first grade.

The Current Report

Current state and federally funded educational programs seem to focus on four major themes: remediation, curriculum innovations, correcting racial imbalance by busing, and compensatory education. Compensatory education refers to educational programs which are designed to make up for deficiencies in a child's home environment.

I believe that we will never provide a meaningful school experience for the ghetto child until we stop placing the onus of his failure to learn on his mode of life, his economic condition, and his lack of motivation. My hypothesis is that school failure in urban ghetto neighborhoods need not be attributed to the existence of de facto segregated schools or to our failure to understand the perceptual or cognitive style of a particular subculture. Ghetto children can learn equally as well in all-black schools as in integrated schools. In fact, we might learn something if we studied the few all-black Southern public and private high schools of the 1920's which, despite terrible circumstances, seem to have graduated the majority of the black intellectual elite of their time.

Some False Assumptions

Schools first assume that the disadvantaged child (in fact, any child who is not learning) has a short attention span and poor auditory acuity, yet the short attention span is often a child's response to boredom and frustration. The same youngsters who appear hyperactive or unmotivated in the classroom stand at a pinball machine or watch television for hours.

If school is so unpleasant for disadvantaged youngsters, why don't we liven it up and make it fascinating, engaging, challenging, and enjoyable?

The answer is that schools assume that (1) before getting to the interesting stuff, the child must first learn the "simple basics," (2) minority groups cannot handle "abstract" ideas and must therefore learn from a "concrete," "relevant" curriculum, (3) educators must not waste time on "irrelevant" material since there is so much "basic" information which must be drilled in, and (4) we must wait until the child is "ready."

Regarding (1) and (2), there is little evidence that learning progresses directly from the simple and "concrete" to the complex and "abstract." The notion that minority groups cannot handle "abstractions" guarantees "stupidity." Speech, which is ordinarily grasped well before a child enters school, is one of the most abstract areas of learning. Yet, we do not *first* drill him in consonants and vowels. Rather, he expresses a concept with a rough approximation of the sound of the word first. *Later,* he refines this sound and, later yet, he is able to break the sound down into its component sounds. Learning does not start at the "bottom;" it starts in the "middle."

Focusing on (2) and (3), it's just those "irrelevant" things belonging to the imagination that excite and arouse children. Imagination can be one of the most potent allies in learning—provided it is nourished (or at least not stifled). It can be used to teach improvisation, self-reliance, and creativity. A child allowed freedom of imagination jumps at the opportunity to have fun—to express and give substance to his wishes, desires, impulses, and feelings. Innocent imaginations fuel effort and productivity like few other things. Children caught up in their imaginative exploits are excited, interested, and motivated—in what *they* are *doing.* The so-called academic tools they will need in the adult world—literacy and "numeracy"—are absorbed along the way by children who find the images and ideas provided by reading and arithmetic exciting, who want to know what Horton will do about the Who (but who could care less about whether or not Dick is black and urban). (Of course some of the new educational material is good. But it has little impact in schools that suffer from poor leadership and demoralized teachers. In fact, one index of a "bankrupt" school is a stockroom loaded with new materials that will never be used.)

Certainly part of life is coping with relevance and boredom. But children should be exposed to such experiences only in small doses. Certainly, some routines are good, but not too many, and only those designed for relatively unimportant areas of life. Yes, some exercises are necessary, but do not expect children to enjoy them. Drills are boring.

Regarding (4), just what is "readiness" anyway? I know many boys who were not "ready" to learn the multiplication tables until they got a paper route (or started playing poker), who could not be cajoled or browbeaten to add a row of figures and come up with the right answer—until they stood to lose money if they didn't. Certainly, most kids are not "ready" to learn calculus in the third grade. But in the *meantime* we could talk about spaceships and, incidentally, Newton's laws of motion and gravitation. The point is that, if he is treated creatively from the start, the child is continuously ready to learn. In other words, it is essential to give kids experiences that *make* them ready to learn.

Another factor must be recognized. Very often there is a conflict between the teacher's values and the child's, between those of the school and those of the surrounding neighborhood. The schools value hard work, a delay in reward and gratification, an emphasis on obedience and intellectual achievement—but these may often be at odds with a child's personal ambitions. Teachers must be brought to recognize that *the values of the school are goals rather than prerequisites for learning*.

The disruptive child is the focus of still another misconception. Though ghetto teachers and administrators are almost unanimous in criticizing the roles of psychologists, social workers, and remediators, educators still define the problem as not enough services. *New* models, not *more*, are needed.[5]

Teachers can usually identify maladjusted children in the elementary grades; subsequent tests and interviews confirm their opinions. Classrooms burst with behavioral and learning problems that teachers do not know how to handle. The school has concentrated on diagnosis and, instead of devoting its energies to creating a climate that fosters mental health, has relied on guidance clinics and other outside agencies to *change the child*. Unfortunately, many existing social agencies are still geared to service "maladjusted" children from middle-class families. They have not kept pace with rising social disintegration in the inner city.

Remediation: Exercises in Futility

Generally, the school has used mental health specialists ineffectively. The main leverage applied for intervention in crises has been remedial. In the case of learning disabilities, children are usually two years below the accepted grade level norm in achievement before referral. By that time many have become behavior problems, and it is difficult to sort out, diagnostically, which direction intervention should take.

The processes which determine an individual's mental and scholastic growth are established during the early formative years. As Benjamin Bloom[1] has suggested, the loss of intellectual development during this period may never be recovered. Hence, intervention should take place during early childhood and should involve the children in education by inseparably binding competence and achievement to feelings of well-being and constructive behavior. At the same time, early intervention should provide the tool skills of reading and arithmetic, thus negating "cumulative deficit," by which youngsters fall further and further below national scholastic norms with every passing year. (Once, of course, a child is blocked in reading, we should not magnify his problem by forcing a direct confrontation with his greatest area of vulnerability.)

A shocking percentage of children from urban ghettoes reach junior high school with the reading and writing skills of fourth graders. In effect they are illiterate. Their handicap will not only severely limit future educational and vocational opportunities but will make many everyday activities difficult. Despite the current emphasis on reading, the U. S. Office of Education reports that 24 million adults 18 years of age and older cannot read beyond a fourth grade level, and an estimated eight to 12 million school-age children have such serious reading problems that they are headed toward the same functional illiteracy.[8]

Recent years have seen a proliferation of methods for teaching reading. Yet the academic gap remains between ghetto and middle-class students. For example, in New York City, the reading ability of public school pupils fell back two months during the 1968-69 school year. One-fourth, or nearly 135,000 pupils, were two years below their grade level. The previous year, one-fifth of those tested were two years behind.[9] In Philadelphia, two out of five public school pupils perform "below minimum functioning levels," according to the latest standardized tests. "Minimum functioning levels" are defined by the tests' publishers as levels sufficient to cope with basic instructional materials, such as basal readers and textbooks.[13]

A big remediation push in a school sometimes results in an overall improvement. Yet careful analysis reveals that those who already know how to read improve, while those who do not remain as they were.

In addition, there is no impressive evidence that children learn better, or learn at all, when their educational environment is highly structured and free from "extraneous" stimulation. In fact, isolating, programmed routines reinforce dependency and feelings of inferiority. But somehow we find a simpler solution disconcerting. If a child is blocked in reading, we should not give him more reading; instead, we should teach him swimming, photography, or any other *ego-enhancing* activity. Similarly, I have seen whole fifth grade classes of children who could no longer be taught even simple arithmetic, but who grasped chess, checkers, or Monopoly.[2]

It is futile to try to unblock a block with a block. If a kid has arrived at a point where he hates reading for 15 minutes, an hour of "remedial" reading will only make things worse. The fact is he cannot read because his experiences with reading have been frustrating and humiliating. To put pressure on him to "catch up—or fail" usually means that he will fail. Sometimes it is better for us to lay off; if necessary, we should avoid teaching "reading" for a couple of years, until the child has had success in other areas of learning and feels more secure and confident.* Concentration on reading is doomed to failure because of blocking. Once motivated and unblocked, my experiences have shown that a child can make rapid headway and achieve a level that *theoretically* is supposed to take much longer.[3,4] (After all, millions of adult illiterates all over the world are now being taught to read successfully.)

We must acknowledge that relatively little statistical information has been *compiled* which would validate the assertion that success in learning one activity associated with school increases chances of success in learning other activities also associated with school, including reading and arithmetic.

Although my own short experiences as an educator in predominantly black schools strongly suggest to me that this assumption is valid, so few public schools have tried the strategy of creative learning that I have outlined, over an extended period, that there can be no appropriate statistical analysis. However, I certainly would suggest that this strategy is worth trying and evaluating.

In addition, educators hardly consider the patterns of behavior distinctive to specific stages of development and their effect on translating educational goals to classroom practices. For example, adolescents entering high school are antagonistic to adult expecta-

---

*Of course parents must be included in such a plan. The blanket assumption made by some educators that parents, especially from community schools, will not accept postponement of remediation is just another myth.

tion, confuse nonconformity with independence, and identify strongly with the concepts of "gang" and "team." Against this pattern, the schools become defensive. As a result, students spend their time trying to beat the system by cutting classes and cheating on exams. The school, in turn, talks about stiffening the curriculum and raising standards. For too many young people, high school is valueless in itself and important only in terms of the final result—the diploma.*

Another area in which I predict yet another failure is in the much sought after bilingual studies programs where there are large numbers of Puerto Rican or Mexican children. By offering these programs to Spanish-speaking kids, you might just as well be telling them, "You're inferior, you can't learn English, so why should we even bother to try?" But the fact of life is that these children have to survive in an English-speaking society and economic system! Why reinforce patterns that will guarantee failure? While cultural pluralism is a desirable and healthy aspect of American life, we should not assume that any group cannot learn English. Failure to teach English as an exciting, positive aspect of life in Amierca is an indication of an inferior school rather than an inferior individual.

The big questions concerning creative learning seem to be: What do we do about curriculum? How can we grade bowling and chess? My answer is that grading and concomitant deadlines should be abolished during the early years and only introduced, if at all, gradually and gently as the child gets older.

That does not mean that we need to be "permissive" and reject discipline. However, there are only a few rules that it is urgent for children to obey even before they can comprehend them. Like other learning, ethics, values, and morality are most meaningful and effective when the individual has learned them for himself. Self-discipline is the best discipline. Naturally, self-discipline is something the child gradually *teaches* himself.

Innovation: Curriculum Is Not Sacred

"Innovative" curricula are one of the most frustrating educational fads. Typically, an "innovative" program is introduced into an inner city school, only to be abandoned, in reality if not publicly,

---

*In *Psychology For You* (Oxford Books: New York, 1972), a text for high school youths, I included many ideas on how to turn on students; cf. especially the last two chapters.

before the year is out. In that period, a big chunk of grant money is spent, but not much else is accomplished.

As Albert Shanker puts it:

"Year after year, new programs are introduced in the schools—team teaching, ungraded schools, higher horizons, educational TV, computer assisted instruction, differentiated staffing, and so on, and on. To the public, the introduction of each program may signify an educational advance, but for the teacher the new program is more likely to be a replay of an old tune. The adoption of new programs and the abandonment of old ones can, by and large, be better understood in the light of the public relations needs of boards of education than of the educational needs of children. Small wonder, then, that teachers have become skeptical. The longer they teach, the wider—and more disillusioning—their experience with innovations. The "old ways" (last year's innovations) are always described in negative terms: the new programs are "doomed to succeed."

Thus, school districts throughout the country are busy ousting their school superintendents (who have failed) and replacing them with new ones. In their hunt for new school superintendents and new school programs, school districts are engaged in a game of educational musical chairs in which each district hails as new and innovative that which is being discarded as a failure in a neighboring area."*

In reality, it is the *child*—and the *teacher*—who should be (allowed to be) innovative—not the curriculum.

After all, teachers—90% or more of them—want to teach. Whatever other hangups they may have, they do want to teach. Many critics do not understand that the process of *not teaching* is as exhausting for teachers as the process of *not learning* is for the child. (Is it any wonder that after-school programs are generally not useful to the children for whom they are intended? Exhausted by the process of not learning during the school day, the child is unreasonably expected to "come alive" after school.) Teachers in ghetto areas are usually forced to teach under intolerable conditions. And they are powerless to effect changes in the schools where they work. Teachers are virtually unrepresented at all levels of educational planning, including federally supported projects for disadvantaged children.

No idea is as important as the person (teacher) implementing it, yet the teacher is usually not formally consulted in the planning of

---

*Excerpted from "Where We Stand—A Weekly Column of Comment on Public Education by Albert Shanker, President, United Federation of Teachers." The column appeared as a paid advertisement in the July 18, 1971 *New York Times*.

programs. The educational "think tanks" and the dozens of federally- and foundation-supported education panels rarely, if ever, include classroom teachers. Little wonder that not much, if anything, filters down to the classroom. Then, teachers are blamed and criticized for programs that fail, programs they had nothing to do with in the first place.

At the same time, however, teachers have not been vigorous enough in forging alliances with local community groups to effect change. Teachers have tolerated university programs that are not realistic in terms of the needs of teaching in today's schools, and they have let themselves be intimidated by boards of education into accepting programs that do not make any sense.

Integration: At What Price?

Integration of schools in the big cities—where most of the population resides—is not working. According to a 1971 survey by the Department of Health, Education and Welfare,[10] 17 large cities have a majority of black (and other minority group) public school students. The figures are: Chicago, 54.8 percent; Detroit, 63.8; Philadelphia, 60.5; Baltimore, 67.1; Cleveland, 57.6; Memphis, 51.6; Washington, 94.6; St. Louis, 65.6; New Orleans, 69.5; Atlanta, 68.7; Newark, 72.2; Kansas City, 50.2; Oakland, 56.9; Birmingham, 54.6; Richmond, 64.2; Gary, 64.7; and Compton, Calif., 83 percent. (According to a 1970 census by the New York City Board of Education, 57.2 percent of public school students are black and Puerto Rican.)[11]

According to the New York State Fleischmann Commission (1972), ninety-three percent of the state's public school pupils "are being educated in 676 school districts that are segregated" and the state's schools are more segregated today than they were in 1954.[12]

The HEW survey indicated that most of the cities studied showed an increase in black percentages from 1968. The whites are avoiding busing and fleeing to the suburbs. The assumption that middle-class suburban whites will "allow" the courts to impose busing on their children to inferior schools in the inner city or will "allow" their suburban school to become populated with even one-third inner city children is in my judgment unrealistic.

No amount of busing will significantly improve racial balance in cities where the majority of pupils are already black. At any rate, the "evidence" that forced integration can significantly improve the education of poor blacks is shaky, at best. The Coleman Report suggested that the differences between black ghetto schools and white suburban schools were not all that great.[6] While I could agree with many critics that suburban schools are generally depressing, they are still tremendously more successful than ghetto schools. The differences are enormous. Unfortunately, most of the schools that would have revealed these differences were not considered because 13 of the 15 largest cities refused to cooperate with the Coleman researchers.

Community Schools: An Opportunity

"Educational disadvantage," "lack of motivation," and all the other cliches are mostly due to the school's failure to instruct, rather than the child's failure to learn. Compensation, remediation, innovation, and integration will continue to be futile until this fact is acted upon.

What poor children need are good schools—places where children can enjoy the experience of learning. Black youngsters from the ghetto are quite as capable as white youths from the suburbs of being motivated to learn—to learn to read and write, even to use "abstract" ideas, and to become self-reliant.

In Washington, D.C., the Morgan Community School[14] has had a significant impact. In a recently completed study, I concluded that at the fourth grade level, Morgan Community School pupils registered impressive gains in reading and math. For the first time in recent history, its fourth grade pupils are achieving at national norm levels and have among the best scores in the city. Thus, the pupils who started out with the Morgan Community orientation in the first grade seem to have benefited greatly from the reading and math curriculum. (The Morgan School pupil population is relatively stable, and a large percentage of its fourth grade pupils were enrolled at the school from the beginning.)

The sixth grade reading and match scores present a reverse picture. Scores in both areas are among the worst in the city. I have no explanation for this extreme and uneven performance. Obviously, it is a trend that must be watched, and the crucial tests would be in the next couple of years when most of those sixth graders will have completed a full six years in the Morgan Community School.

We cannot be sure that community schools will be more effective than centralized schools. Community schools are not a solution; they are an opportunity. However, whether parents do a good job or not, it is still necessary—morally if for no other reason—that they build a political power base within their communities and that they have a real stake in the education of their children.

After all, as the situation stands now, the "educational establish-ment" tends to "meet its responsibilities" by instituting compensa-tory programs and by issuing pious pamphlets calling for integration and quality education. (What public educator, outwardly, isn't for integration these days?) When laymen have the tenacity to call these career administrators to task, the only responses are stock excuses couched in the latest professional jargon: "cultural deprivation," "short attention span," "nondeferred gratification," etc. Only a handful of exceptional principals have successfully met the chal-lenge and built a teaching school in the ghetto.

The current decentralized systems in New York, Detroit, St. Louis, and some other large cities provide an excellent opportunity for city planners and teachers to join forces with community groups to design neighborhood community schools in the context of urban renewal proposals. Urban planners and schools of education and architecture could assist with such things as site selection, building design, classroom organization, educational technology, developing and publishing curriculum materials, creation of community ser-vices within the schools, creation of new types of classroom furni-ture, etc. The common objective would be the achievement of a set-ting which facilitates learning and offers a full range of services to the community. It would offer unlimited opportunities to engineers, architects, artists, functional design experts, publishers, writers, etc. However, the parents, teachers, and administrators would be in control.

Ideally, a community school would serve all the people in a neigh-borhood. It would operate at some level twenty-four hours a day, all year round, and would include day care, recreation, health and wel-fare services, adult education and entertainment, and community self-help services. It would be an exciting community focal point—something the community would have a stake in. We should redirect the enormous sums spent on compensatory programs and busing into developing ghetto neighborhood schools that are so good and so exciting that white parents would *want* to send their children to these black schools.

Conclusions

The proposals outlined here are directed toward the existing ghetto neighborhoods, not because we have abandoned the principle of integration, but rather because we must acknowledge our obliga-tion toward the children who are *now* in the urban slum. We can no longer ignore the fact that many of our large city public school systems already have nonwhite enrollments which make up more than fifty percent of the entire student body. While many of us consider eventual integraton a necessary goal for our democratic society, the "black power" position makes a great deal of sense both politically and in terms of the black individual's self-image.

Programs designed to improve education in de facto segregated schools must aim at increasing the frequency of success and heightening the levels of aspiration of each child. Curriculum innovations, along with the many compensatory techniques which have been employed in ghetto neighborhoods cannot, by themselves, bring about the sought-after results. It is my contention that white and black children, separately or together, can learn in neighborhood schools which ideally would be developed as community schools.

Decentralized schooling offers an opportunity to mobilize educators, planners, and community residents for the purpose of upgrading education in their own decentralized school. Above all, it will make administrators accountable for what is happening in their institutions.

This is the challenge. Educators and city planners must take the initiative in forging hundreds of alliances with local community organizations and civil rights groups to achieve increased local autonomy and effect basic changes in the schools—beginning with every low-income, minority group neighborhood in this country.

Note

Since this article was written, a fair amount of material has been printed which adds dimension to the thesis presented here. What follows are some additional references of special interest.

1. The most important document is the "Fleischmann Commission Report on Quality, Cost, and Financing of Elementary and Secondary Education," which is a devastating review of the decline of public schools in New York State. While many of its findings are significant, the Commission makes the mistake of recommending more compensatory programs.

2. Christopher Jencks' *Inequality: A Reassessment of the Effect of Family and Schooling in America* (New York: Basic Books, 1972) is a crucial book because of the controversy that it has raised over the effectiveness of schooling as it relates to either equal opportunities *or* equal incomes. Rather than being the conclusive work on the subject, it poses new questions for researchers. For instance, if schooling has little effect on cogni-

tive skills, what factors account for the higher incomes that come with increased schooling.

3. The latest Census report *(New York Times,* Dec. 8, 1972) shows a sharp rise in schooling over the last 32 years. The data indicates great gains for blacks too, although blacks as a group lag two years behind whites. The census reported a clear relationship between schooling and income, but not between income and achievement. As Jencks pointed out, income is affected by certification and the "survival" skills and attitudes learned with more and more years of schooling.

4. New York City School Chancellor Harvey B. Scribner reported that the reading ability of N.Y.C. pupils has declined steadily. His comment was that the problem "defies simple solutions." Albert Shanker, President of the United Federation of Teachers, blamed the decline on lack of money, and Professor Kenneth B. Clark attributed the failure to the ineffectiveness of decentralization, citing the poor performance of teachers and unions, and the educational "establishment." (*New York Times,* Nov. 19, 1972, Nov. 30, 1072, and Dec. 3, 1972, respectively.)

5. Perhaps a more telling verification of my thesis is a report recently issued by the Ford Foundation called "A Foundation Goes to School." The report is a self-examination and review of the 30 million dollars that Ford granted to various educational projects. They found most of the programs designed to improve education to be failures.

6. As predicted, more and more of our urban schools are becoming overwhelmingly black (*New York Times,* Nov. 26, 1972).

7. The New York State Legislative Commission to study the causes of educational unrest reported that extensive busing failed to integrate schools (*New York Times,* Jan. 7, 1973).

References

1. Bloom, B.S., *Stability and Change in Human Characteristics* John Wiley: New York, 1964.
2. For other specific suggestions and techniques, see *Signs,* by S. Gordon, a series of three booklets focusing on a nonreading approach to reading, New Readers Press, Syracuse, New York. See also S. Gordon, *Primary Education in Urban Slums,* in *The Urban R's,* R. Dentler, *et. al.* (Eds.), Frederick A. Praeger: New York, 1967. Also, Ronald, S. Horowitz, Teaching Mathematics to Students in Learning Disabilities, *Academic Therapy,* No. 1, 1971, p. 17.

3. Gordon, Sol, "Education and the Impulse Life of the Child," *Canada's Mental Health,* January 1967.
4. Gordon Sol, "Quality Education in De Facto Segregated Schools," *Changing Education,* Fall 1969.
5. Gordon, Sol, and Martin Berlin, "Planning for Mental Health in the School," in *The Pyschology of School Adjustment,* Bernard D. Starr (ed.), Random House: New York, 1970.
6. Guthrie, J.W., What the Coleman Reanalysis Didn't Tell Us, *Saturday Review,* Education, July 22, 1972, p.45.
7. Jablonsky, Adelaide, Status Report on Compensatory Education, *IRCD Bulletin,* Vol. 7, No. 1 & 2, Winter/Spring 1971.
8. *New York Times,* February 15, 1969.
9. *New York Times,* October 11, 1970.
10. *New York Times,* June 18, 1971. HEW canvassed every school district in the nation with 3,000 or more pupils and made sample surveys of the rest.
11. *New York Times,* June 18, 1971. A separate article from that referenced above.
12. *New York Times,* Jan. 30, 1972.
13. *Philadelphia Evening Bulletin,* Feb. 12, 1970.
14. *The Morgan School/Washington, D.C.,* (April, 1971). A publication of the Center for Urban Education, 105 Madison Avenue, New York, N.Y. 10016.

Part Five

THE CONCEPT OF "INTELLIGENCE"

How applicable to minority group children are conventional intelligence and achievement tests? Are the tests biased against these groups? And should their administration to minority group children be discontinued? These questions demand earnest examination. The lawsuit of Diana vs. the California State Board of Education was settled in behalf of Diana and some 22,000 Mexican-American students trapped in classes for the mentally retarded because they were given allegedly culturally unfair IQ tests in English instead of Spanish." Legal suits are under way which allege misplacement in special classes of Black children based on intelligence tests.

Who shall be tested? Does psychological testing help or hinder? Clinical child pasychologists' concern with these questions is reflected in this section.

23. Intelligence Testing of Minority Group Children: A Symposium

I
Danger: Testing and Dehumanizing Black Children*

Robert L. Williams

Two of the most thoroughly researched concepts in psychology
are those of intelligence and achievement testing. Yet they are two
of the most ill-used and grossly abused procedures employed in the
assessment of intelligence and school achievement of Black children. Conventional ability tests improperly label and classify Black
children. Thus, if a Black child scores low on a test that is biased
and if he is placed (or misplaced) in an "educational tracting" program because he scored low, then that child is trapped in a vicious
circle known as the "Rosenthal Effect" or the self-fulfilling prophecy (Rosenthal, 1968). The self-fulfilling prophecy refers to the
extent to which a teacher's expectancy influences her responses as
well as the direction of the behavior she expects to occur. That is, if
she predicts certain behaviors, e.g., poor performance in the
classroom based upon I.Q. and achievement test results, then the
mere prediction and expectation of that behavior will influence her
actions in such a way as to increase the likelihood of her predictions
actually occurring. Ability tests, then, not only label Black children
unfairly; they may create unfair teacher expectancies as well.
According to the self-fulfilling prophecy, placing a Black child in
one of the lower levels based upon an unfair test appraisal may significantly reduce that child's chances for a higher education.

Rosenthal (1966) and Burnham and Hartsough (1968) present an
impressive array of data suggesting that in addition to creating
expectancies by tracting, other factors such as sex, age, and face of
the teacher may affect the performance of children and the teacher's
appraisal of those children. A teacher may respond more positively
to a child in Tract I than to a child in Tract III and vice versa.

---

*Reprinted from the Clinical Child Psychology Newsletter, 1970. IX 1.

Rosenthal (1968) reports that children who are labeled as "intellectually blooming" were rated by teachers as more appealing, better adjusted, and more likeable than children labeled as "intellectually non-blooming."

At the 1969 annual meeting of the Association of Black Psychologists in Washington, D.C., the following statement on psychological testing of Black people was adopted as the Association's official position:

> STATEMENT ON TESTING
> The Association of Black Psychologists fully supports those parents who have chosen to defend their rights by refusing to allow their children and themselves to be subjected to achievement, intelligence, aptitude and performance tests which have been and are being used to A. Label Black people as uneducable. B. Place Black children in "special" classes and schools. C. Perpetuate inferior education in Blacks. D. Assign Black children to educational tracts. E. Deny Black students higher educational opportunities. F. Destroy positive growth and development of Black people.

The Association of Black Psychologists is calling a moratorium on this continuing abuse of Black people. We expect help from others who are concerned about stopping injustice toward Black people. An old African proverb gives a message to the onlookers:

> "When you see the vultures eating the carcasses, do not say 'leave them alone.' Instead you should say 'Leave us alone.' "

It is appalling that psychologists have not addressed themselves sufficiently to this abuse of ability testing and subsequent misplacement of Black students. Eels, Davis, Havighurst, Herrick and Tyler (1951) pointed out almost two decades ago this inequity in ability testing. Later, Davis and Eels (1954) developed the "Davis-Eels Games Test," an instrument reportedly less culturally biased than conventional paper and pencil tests. A study by Williams (1955) showed essentially that Black children do better on the Davis-Eels Games Test than on the culturally-unfair tests.

It is unfair to assume that Black and White cultures are so similar that the same tests can be properly used in psychological testing and placement. America is a schizophrenic society: one Black and one White. Since ability tests tend to favor the White middle-class, thereby penalizing low-status Blacks (and low-status Whites as well), it is now incumbent upon Black psychologists to develop (1) intelligence tests which select test items from Black culture for representation on ability tests, (2) develop tests that are drawn entirely from Black culture or (3) validate Black responses to White-oriented tests. For example, the author developed the BITCH Test (Black Intelligence Test Counter-balanced for Honkies) to be used for testing both White and Black populations. All items were drawn entirely from Black culture. Preliminary results indicate that Whites systematically score low or in the defective range of intelligence on the test; Blacks systematically score in the superior range. Studies have been developed to determine whether the BITCH Test will predict academic success for Blacks.

In summary, conventional intelligence and ability test scores are unfair to Black children and can endanger their futures. They have supported the phenomenon of the self-fulfilling prophecy. Black children are tracted by the schools on the basis of these inappropriate tests. Teachers develop expectancies based on essentially meaningless test scores which, in turn, influence their behavior toward Black children. A vicious circle is created in which the Black child is the victim. Ability tests may do a service to school children, or a disservice. The raw fact is that until these tests are more equitable for children in American schools, they should be considered not only as merely unfair but invalid in predicting academic success for Black children. The use of test scores derived from conventional intelligence and achievement tests should be discontinued immediately with Black children!

References

Rosenthal, R. Self-Fulfilling Prophecy, *Psychology Today*, Vol. 2, No. 4, 1968, pp. 44-51.

Rosenthal, R. *Experimenter Effects in Behavioral Research*, Appleton-Century-Crofts, 1966.

Burnham, J.R. and Hartsough, D.M. Effects of Experimenter's Expectancies (The "Rosenthal Effect") on Children's Ability to Learn to Swim, Paper presented at the meeting of the Midwestern Psychological Association, Chicago, May, 1968.

Eels, K., Davis, A., Havighurst, R., Herrick, J., and Tyler, R. *Intelligence and Cultural Differences*, Chicago: The University of Chicago Press, 1951.

Williams, R. L. An Investigation into the Effects of Social Class on Intelligence, *An Unpublished Masters Thesis*, Wayne State University, Detroit, 1955.

II
Danger: Chauvinism, Scapegoatism, and Euphemism
Norman A. Milgram

In the Spring 1970 issue of the *Clinical Child Psychology Newsletter,* Robert Williams made a passionate statement denouncing the use of intelligence and achievement tests with Black children. He criticizes these tests on the grounds that (1) a Black child is likely to score lower than a white child because these tests are based on a middle class white culture with which the Black child is unfamiliar; (2) if a Black child scores low, he will be misplaced in an inferior educational tract which imposes minimal expectations and requirements upon his learning ability and thereby reduces his opportunity to obtain higher education. Williams proposes that we immediately discontinue using these tests in the conventional manner with Black children and that we develop response norms for Black children to the original tests and/ or develop new tests based wholly or in part on Black culture.

I am also very concerned about the proper use and misuse of conventional tests, but am more concerned about the proper education of Black children than about the proper use of tests. What arouses me and should arouse Dr. Williams is not the low test scores of some Black children on conventional tests, but their poor academic performance in conventional school learning experiences. I am convinced that the chief problem confronting *some* Black children in the schools today is our failure to provide appropriate educational programs for them. *Some* Black children because, while all children in our society today would profit from changes in the educational enterprise, children from lower class families have the most urgent need for the most drastic changes, and within the lower classes, Black and other non-white children most of all.

Children of middle-class or upwardly mobile lower-class parents, regardless of color, make a fair to good adjustment to conventional schooling on the average. Children from impoverished families— whose parents have recently arrived in the urban centers from rural backgrounds, who cannot cope effectively with the demands of urban life, who neither aspire to higher education nor hold forth high aspiration levels for their own children—do not. These are the children with whom we must be primarily concerned. Any child who matches this description has one strike against him in the conventional school system and any Black child matching this description has two strikes against him because of the legacy of racial persecution which compounds his struggle and that of his family and community to cope effectively with the demands of the larger society. Poor prenatal or postnatal nutrition, material poverty, illegitimacy and broken homes, and the quality and quantity of cognitive and linguistic stimulation which are the lot of many Black children are significant barriers to their optimal development and adversely affect their ability to learn in school. These factors and not conventional tests are the important problems with which we should deal. We will not deal intelligently and effectively with the problems of these children if we delude ourselves as to the nature of their difficulties and if we waste professional rhetoric and energy on scapegoat issues such as the use or misuse of conventional tests or if we extol the virtues of the Black ghetto as some militants have indeed done, even as we are asked to alter the conditions under which the ghetto came into being and continues to exist. The advantages accruing to the impoverished Black child from living in the contemporary ghetto do not outweigh the disadvantages. It is to these disadvantages that we must turn our attention if we are to help Black children to develop to their more full potential.

Conventional achievement and intelligence tests do exactly what they are supposed to do, namely to predict scholastic achievement, and they do it rather well. Children who have accumulated the knowledge and skills tapped by these tests do better in school than children who have not. If this correlation follows from the fact that both these tests and the criterion school performance are based on the same norms, e.g., white middle class norms, then so much the better. Predictive validity would be weak or nonexistent if predictor and criterion variables did not share a common cultural base.

If the preschool experiences of the lower class Black child are different from those of the middle class child, Black or white, then what is needed is a change in curriculum and teaching approach for these Black children, not the devising of new tests or new norms for existing tests while retaining the original curriculum and instructional methods. In my opinion, teachers today provide inferior or inappropriate education to many lower class Black children for a number of reasons including, but not restricted to, prejudice and the associated negative expectations about the ability of lower class Black children; discouragement because of their own lack of success in teaching such children; lack of knowledge of any alternative educational approaches; and circumstances prevailing in the Black community, e.g., the gang structure imposed by young Blacks on themselves in some cities (Philadelphia) which disrupts orderly and predictable life experience and saps energies that could be directed to academic pursuits. Abolish the tests and these other reasons still persist. These factors persist, moreover, despite the fact that the majority of teachers of lower-class Black children are themselves Black whether in the urban north or in the south. There is no evidence, moreover, that Black teachers, themselves middle-class, have greater understanding and more positive expectations of the learning ability of lower class Black children than white teachers. Color is no guarantee of Soul.

There is a grain of truth in the Rosenthal notion of teacher expectancies, but only when expectancies are backed up by appropriate behaviors over a significant time span. To claim that teachers who fail to bring ghetto children along at the same rate of progress as more favored white or Black middle-class children are derelict is to do a disservice to the teachers and to the children. Even when expectations are positive, appropriate teaching behaviors do not necessarily follow. Good intentions are no substitute for the drastic changes in educational approach that are necessary.

One major innovation is the recognition that the pre-school home environment is a major determinant of the preparedness or lack of preparedness of the child for the formal school experience. Middle-class or upwardly mobile and middle-class striving parents, regardless of race, handle their children differently than lower-class parents. These differences are in the quality and quantity of verbal communication, in the informal teaching and correctional experience, and a host of other cognitive transactions between adult and child that have nothing to do with maternal love and affection, but a great deal to do with preparing the child for the school experience. I am *not* extolling middle-class practices as a model pattern in promoting mental health and the fostering of self-reliance and other important social and emotional dimensions. I am merely saying that the middle-class parent adopts for himself the role of teacher, while the lower-class parent does not. From this differential handling follows the differential performance of lower class children whether Black or white, not merely on intelligence and achievement tests, but on their performance in school. The involvement of parents and of other adults in the Black community, drastic changes in teacher training programs, and in teaching methods, are essential ingredients in helping lower class Black children to learn according to their genuine abilities.

My remarks are intended to convey a very strong objection to the tone of Dr. Williams' article and to his failure to identify, what are in my opinion, germane problems. His reference to the BITCH test, the Black Intelligence Test Counterbalanced for Honkies, reflects a frankly racist attitude. The BITCH test may be a useful device for building Black pride, but is useless as a predictor of success in the majority culture. Morever, the term "honky" is as degrading to the Black user as the term "nigger" to the White. My genuine concern about the education of disadvantaged children prevents me from remaining silent on these controversial issues, even at the risk of being myself called racist.

III

Danger: Attacks on Testing Unfair

Richard L. Wikoff

An article by Robert L. Williams appeared in the Spring 1970 *Clinical Child Psychology Newsletter* titled, 'Danger: Testing and Dehumanizing Black Children." Dr. Williams attacks the use of standardized tests for placement of Black children. Similar articles have frequently appeared in the literature. I am bothered by articles of this type because I believe the attacks are misdirected and many of the statements made are either in error or lack supporting evidence. I would like to reply specifically to some of the statements made by Dr. Williams.

Dr. Williams admits that testing of intelligence and achievement is based upon thorough research. Yet, he states, "Conventional ability tests improperly label and classify Black children." He gives no supporting evidence. Any test used for placement is good only if it has predictive validity. While indiscriminant use of standardized tests may misplace some Black children (as well as White children) there are many good tests which if properly used have high predictive validity for both Black and White children. The reason they are good predictors is that many children come from a culture that is quite different from the culture experienced by most school children. Because of this difference in their cultural background they do not score high on the tests, but they also do not do well in the typical classroom. Instead of attacking the tests, psychologists should be attacking either the early culture or the typical classroom, perhaps both.

Dr. Williams makes much of the "Rosenthal Effect" (Rosenthal, 1968). He gives as an example predicting "poor performance in the classroom based upon IQ and achievement test results" and indicates that predicting such poor performance influences the teachers' expectations. While this may be true, this was not shown by Rosenthal, since Rosenthal created expectations of good performance only. Related criticism of the work by Rosenthal is contained in a review of *Pygmalion in the Classroom* (Rosenthal and Jacobson, 1968) by Robert L. Thorndike (1968). However, generalizing from other studies, let us assume that the "Rosenthal Effect" holds for both good and poor performance. It is still true that Rosenthal gave the teachers "misinformation." That is not the way tests are supposed to be used. It is possible for teachers to get wrong impressions about some children from tests but they also get true impressions about many children from tests which can be very helpful. The important point to be made is that teachers will get impressions about children from some source, if not from tests from other sources. If they do not have valid, objective information they will use subjective information. They will react to a child on the basis of color of skin, socioeconomic class, cleanliness, kind of clothing, or other invalid criteria. The Rosenthal Effect will not be eliminated by eliminating tests. In fact, fewer errors of placement will be made by properly using tests than by not using them.

Instead of attacking testing, psychologists and educators should consider testing as a very valuable tool for diagnosing needs of individual children with an emphasis upon meeting the child's needs. Tests should never be used alone and teachers should be trained to recognize not only the importance but also the limitations of testing. We need to help teachers to see that valid tests, properly used, give an indication of a child's current level of ability and achievement but that they do not give accurate indications of innate ability. A low score on an IQ test does not necessarily mean an inherent lack of ability. It does mean that there is a problem that needs attention, regardless of its cause. With special attention to his individual needs, a child's ability and achievement levels may be changed.

Proper attitudes need to be developed concerning special education classes, also. Instead of considering children in special classes as "dummies," or inferior, it should be recognized that these are children with special needs which cannot be met in a regular classroom. The child who needs additional help is fortunate if he can be placed in a learning situation where these needs can be met. In the special education class, the teacher-student ratio is small enough that the children can be given individual attention and can progress at their own rate. They should be reevaluated every year and when they are able to return to the regular classroom, they should be moved back.

Dr. Williams stated, "It is unfair to assume that Black and

White cultures are so similar that the same tests can properly be used in psychological testing and placement." It is also unfair to assume that Black and White cultures are so similar that children from both cultures can be placed in the same classroom and be expected to compete with one another. For some it is possible, but for many it is not. If a child, whether Black or White, comes from a culture that has deprived him of the opportunities to develop readiness for scholastic activities, he should be given special help to develop the proper foundations. In my opinion, it is worse to place a child in a situation where he cannot succeed, where he constantly experiences failure, than to place him in a special group, because in the special group he can receive positive reinforcement and can develop according to his own ability.

I have administered the Stanford-Binet Intelligence Scale to several hundred children (most of them White). A large number of these children have scored between 85 and 100 on the deviation IQ scale used in the test. Their ability is now low enough to place them in the typical special education class, but they are unable to achieve adequately in the regular classroom. I am sure that many Black children would also be so classified. Instead of eliminating testing, special education classes should be developed for these children. This need not be done at the expense of integration since many White children have the same needs as many Black children.

Dr. Williams mentioned the use of so-called culture-fair tests, specifically the Davis-Eels Games Tests and stated that Black children do better on this test than on "culturally-unfair tests." Once again, no test measures innate ability. The usefulness of any test for school placement depends upon its correlation with success in school. Culture-fair tests in general have been found to have little predictive validity for academic work. The Davis-Eels Test, specifically, is neither as reliable nor as valid as the more usual type of test used in predicting school achievement (Freeman, 1962). Furthermore, according to Doppelt and Bennett (1967, p. 4), "The preponderant weight of evidence indicates that nonverbal tests do not measurably benefit disadvantaged groups."

In summary, the problem of providing a proper education for Black children is much greater than the problem of misplacement on the basis of testing and the solution is not to do away with tests. On the contrary, objective, valid tests correctly used can be a real help in meeting the needs of Black children. To quote from a recent Test Service Bulletin (Doppelt and Bennett, 1967, p.5),

"The rejection of measuring instruments which register the consequence of . . . deprivation is merely a modern version of killing the messenger who brings bad news."

The solution to the problem includes giving attention to the following: (a) further research and validation of tests is needed to improve predictive ability, (b) the culture of Blacks needs to be improved and enriched in order that Black children will acquire the foundation needed for school success, (c) the typical elementary school needs to be reorganized to better meet the needs of individual children, and (d) the attitudes of teachers concerning the use of tests and the potential achievement of children need to be improved. I sincerely hope that the time will come in our schools when each individual child will be carefully evaluated and the curriculum developed to meet that child's needs without reference to his skin color, his father's socioeconomic position, his religion, or any other unrelated factors.

References

Doppelt, Jerome E. and Bennett, George K. Testing Job Applicants from Disadvantaged Groups. *Test Service Bulletin,* No. 57, May, 1967, pp. 1-5.

Freeman, Frank S. *Theory and Practice of Psychological Testing* (3rd ed.). New York: Holt, Rinehart, and Winston, 1962.

Rosenthal, Robert. Self-Fulfilling Prophecy. *Psychology Today,* Vol. 2, No. 4, 1968, pp. 44-51.

Rosenthal, Robert and Jacobson; Lenore. *Pygmalion in the Classroom.* New York: Holt, Rinehart, and Winston, 1968.

Thorndike, Robert L. Book review in *American Educational Research Journal,* Vol. 5, No. 4, November 1968, pp. 708-711.

Williams, Robert L. Danger: Testing and Dehumanizing Black Children. *Clinical Child Psychology Newsletter,* Division of Clinical Psychology, American Psychological Association, Vol. 9, No. 1, Spring, 1970, pp. 5-6.

IV

Testing Minority Group Children

T. Ernest Newland

I write in regard to the article "Danger: Testing and Dehumanizing Black Children" by Dr. Robert Williams published in the Vol. IX, No. 1 Spring 1970 issue of the *Clinical Child Psychology Newsletter.*

It is unfortunate that the point which Dr. Williams seeks, quite properly, to make is so weakly, and in spots inaccurately, made. Specifically, his support for his important position is at fault in the following respects: (1) "Ability tests" do not label any children or adults. The adults who use them do that on the basis of scores earned on tests. Human beings do the labeling, as well as the selecting of the tests used to obtain scores in terms of which any such labeling is done. (2) The citing of the "Davis-Eels Games Test" was unfortunate, since considerable research, conducted just after that instrument was published, showed that the results obtained by means of it were more biased culturally than were the tests which Davis and Eels implicitly were criticizing. (3) Citing the Rosenthal research on the role of expectancy (as reported presumably in *Pygmalion in the Classroom*) was analogous to seeking a ride on a sunken ship—as evidenced by the criticisms published regarding the quality of that research.

That the phenomenon of expectancy has operated to the disadvantage of many Blacks I in no way debate, even though it has not yet been adequately researched. Too often have I seen the pernicious operation of white teacher expectancy for Blacks. Too often have I seen psychological test data misused, not only with respect to Black pupils but also with respect to different kinds of handicapped children, by psychometrically oriented, rather than psychologically competent, persons.

It is understandable that there might be a desire to construct learning aptitude tests with items more reflective of Black culture (more rational than the Chitlins Test), but the results on such a test would, in my opinion, become as difficult and potentially misleading to interpret and use socially and educationally in constructive ways as the tests about which so much complaint has risen. What is needed, however, is the use of tests which now exist and which can be developed in terms of valid psychological constructs, which sample behavior in terms of the psychological processes by means of which children learn, as contrasted with using tests which sample what has been learned and inferring from that the *capacity* to learn.

In standardizing a test of learning aptitude for use with blind children (BLAT), I had occasion to obtain data on both Black and white blind children in three southeastern states. In addition to getting performances on BLAT, I obtained Hayes-Binet and WISC Verbal scores on the same children. While I found differences between the racial groups on the Hayes-Binet and the WISC Verbal tests to be quite similar to most published findings of this sort, I found no differences between the two groups, across age, on BLAT.

The data for 12 states showed a similar picture, although, for this whole group, there were slight (but I suspect insignificant) differences on BLAT. While this picture results from data on blind children, the underlying concept explanatory of this difference between differences is broadly applicable. This concept, now being flirted with by numerous persons — inadequately by Jensen, factorially by Cattell and Horn, and sketchily by Vernon, for instance, is developed in my paper entitled, perhaps over-optimistically, "Cognitive Capability of Exceptional Children."

I do not desire to be perceived as just "joining the battle"; I've been in it, clinically, for over thirty years, and with respect to many kinds of children, not just Black children.

V

From Dehumanization to Black Intellectual Genocide: A Rejoinder

Robert L. Williams

The purpose of my first article, "Danger: Testing and Dehumanizing Black Children"[1] was to expose the white pimp and hustler type psychologists who have been agents in the abuse and dehumanization of Black people by employing an instrument called the psychological test. The purpose of the present article is not only to respond to Milgram, Newland and Wikoff's criticisms but to posit a stronger indictment against the use of tests: Black intellectual genocide.

Two of the three critics (Milgram & Wikoff) imply that psychologists must get to the root of the problem (namely, improving early Black culture and the poor education programs) rather than hacking away at the branches of the problem (namely, culturally biased intelligence tests). It is axiomatic that the best method of killing a tree is to attack its roots. While preferred, this method, however, is not always practicable. Other strategies exist. For example, one could amputate a sufficient number of the tree's branches and it would die. The Association of Black Psychologists proposes precisely to hack away at the branches of the tree of racism until it dies or screams "Uncle." We realize, of course, that while psychologists have a major vested interest in psychological

---

[1]*Clinical Child Psychology Newsletter*, Spring, 1970.

tests, and even more importantly that the testing industry in the United States is a big business. It is reported that a recent budget of one of the large testing corporations was 30 million dollars!

We are not objecting to psychologists testing white children on whom the tests were standardized, but we boldly and strenuously oppose testing Black children who were not included in the normative groups. In 1944 David Wechsler clearly warned that his I.Q. test norms were to be used exclusively for the white population:

> . . . We have eliminated the 'colored' vs. 'white' factor by admitting at the outset that our norms cannot be used for the colored population of the United States. Though we have tested a large number of colored persons, our standardization is based upon white subjects only. We omitted the colored population from our first standardization because we did not feel that norms derived by mixing the populations could be interpreted without special provisos and reservations.[2]

In addition, three of the most popularly used intelligence tests (the Sanford-Binet, the Wechsler Intelligence Scale for Children and the Peabody Picture Vocabulary Test) deliberately and systematically excluded Black children from the normative samples. The 1937 Stanford-Binet, standardized on 3,184 "American-born white children" was in use twenty-three years before being replaced by its racist twin, the 1960 Form L-M Revision. The latter used 4,498 subjects in the normative sample. The WISC was standardized on 2,200 white children, the Peabody Picture Vocabulary on 4,012 white children. No Black norms exist for any of the three tests, but yet Black children continue to be tested and mislabeled. A white female psychologist told me recently that since conventional I.Q. tests underestimate Black ability, she had been encouraged to add ten points to every test score for Black children!

With regard to the issue of predictive validity, one of my critics, Milgram, states: "Conventional achievement and intelligence tests do exactly what they are supposed to do, namely predict scholastic achievement, and they do it rather well." For my critic's information, I, Robert L. Williams, Ph.D., have an I.Q. of 82 as measured by a popular conventional intelligence test, and the instrument is reported to be a good predictor of scholastic

[2]Wechsler, D. *The Measurement of Intelligence, Baltimore:* The Williams & Wilkins Company, 1944, P. 107.

achievement. Because of my dull normal I.Q., I was counseled not to enter college. But having finished high school at the early age of 16, I was a misfit. After missing one semester in college, I finally decided to make an effort, despite the bad advice of the counselor. While "struggling" through college, earning all A's and B's except 3 C's, I barely managed, with my 82 I.Q., to compile a 2.35 GPA on a 3.0 scale, to graduate with academic honors, to win distinction in my field and to rank 6th in the graduating class. My critics are, perhaps, yelling in unison, "Yes, but you are an exception." My contention is that I am not the exception. Countless numbers of Black children have been and continue to be extruded from the educational system because of the unfair tests. Consider a few of the higher uneducated Black mental giants: Eldridge Cleaver, Malcolm X, Huey P. Newton, Claude Brown and thousands of unknowns who were tested out of the system because of the racist instruments.

Another one of the critics, Wikoff, states, "Because of this difference in their (black and white children) cultural background, they do not score high on this test, but they also do not do well in the typical classroom." Both the criterion variables and the conditions under which the Black child performs are unfair. An example is necessary here. Let us take two track stars, Runner A and Runner B. In the 100 yard dash, the results show that Runner A is clocked at 10.0 seconds with the help of a twenty-five mile per hour tail wind. Runner B is clocked at 10.2 running against a twenty-five mile per hour wind. Who is the better runner? When we talk about achievement, it is necessary to consider the conditions under which the learner is performing and the judges as well. It is conceivable that a judge unaware of the conditions of Runners A and B would consider Runner A a faster runner.

The Black child performs "poorly" in the typical classroom due to a number of reasons, chief among which is the lack of validation of Black culture and the Black cognitive learning style. For many years the myth existed that Black children are poor in their expression of verbal skills. The Black verbal style does differ from the white verbal style. This difference in verbal style does not mean that the Black child is inferior. It means that the Black experience produces unique verbal skills found mainly in the typical Black community and that these skills are not validated or accepted in the middle-class oriented classroom. To push the point further, many Black children "play the dozens" and play them rather well. I hope my critics understand "the dozens" which simply refers to a kind of verbal insult in reference to another's parents. I have known Black children who were masters at playing dozens. These same children could not read and did not enjoy school. They could, however, phrase their dozens in iambic pentameters with ease and create such an emotional stir in their listeners that no questions ever arose in the Black community regarding lack of verbal skills. In addition, the average Black child learns with ease rather long poems such as the "Signifying Monkey" and the "Pool Shooting Monkey."

Black children are not inarticulate. They simply are not permitted to bring their cognitive learning and expressive styles into the classroom. They are forced to leave their Black culture and verbal skills on the outside. Thus, it is not surprising that Black children are turned off by the "Look Dick, Look Jane" cognitive style of learning.

Finally, the current ability and achievement testing serves as a tool for promoting Black intellectual genocide. For the Black child the tests, together with the white middle-class styles and the sterile classroom, constitute a giant Skinner box in which the child receives aversive reinforcement for evincing the Black cognitive style of learning. Black children do not receive positive reinforcement for "emitting" their natural language style; rather they receive either aversive reinforcement or none at all. Thus, the Black style may be extinguished before the child reaches the sixth grade. At that point he is called a "drop-out." A better term is a "push-out" or a "squeeze out." As Thomas Gray so succinctly stated in his *Elegy Written in a Country Churchyard:*

> Full many a flower is born to blush unseen
> And waste its sweetness on the desert air.

In conclusion, I make one simple proposal to my critics: It is either time now to halt the dehumanization and genocide of Black minds using psychological instruments as tools, or Black psychologists have no alternative but to develop our own strategies. One possibility is the publication in the Black community of answers to all ability and achievement tests.

VI

Clinicans must Listen!

Florence C. Halpern

When psychologists, and particularly clinical psychologists, fail to hear what is being said to them, then I think we are truly in a bad way. Reading the Fall 1970 issue of THE CLINICAL CHILD PSYCHOLOGY NEWSLETTER was therefore a particulary disturbing experience. This issue of the NEWSLETTER was devoted largely to the controversy raised in the Spring 1970 NEWSLETTER by Dr. Robert Williams in regard to the testing of Black children. From the responses that appeared in the NEWSLETTER, one might infer that Dr. Williams did not appreciate the predictive value of tests. Yet I feel quite safe in saying that he is surely as aware of their function in this regard as those who feel compelled to spell out what standard intelligence and achievement tests do. But Dr. Williams goes further, recognizing not only the predictive value of tests but their social and emotional impact both on those who give them and those who take them. Surely this is something about which clinicians should be concerned. What I hear Dr. Williams saying is, "Stop testing Black children because the tests you use and the uses to which you put the test findings only serve to humiliate the child and add fuel to the disease of racism."

Abolishing test programs is of course no panacea and will not in any way solve the problem of the Black child. But the continued use of inappropriate tests reflects an insensitivity to the way Black people feel as well as an unwillingness to recognize that, despite all good intentions, test results are frequently misinterpreted and misused. True concern about the education of Black children must take into account how the Black child experiences himself and those who are supposedly educating him. If the community is angry about the testing program, the child is not very likely to have a positive feeling toward the school or the teacher; and under such conditions learning will go by the board. Similarly, suggesting that criticism of tests should be replaced by attacks on the various depriving cultures in our society also causes the hackles to rise among the Black people. Such statements are made over and over by educators, psychologists and sociologists, but strangely enough very little of constructive order takes place.

How sincere can the Black people feel we really are when we become unduly concerned about a lack of cognitive skills but do nothing about the child who comes to school hungry, who lives in a crowded vermin-infested flat and has no place to sit down and study and whose mother does not know where the rent money is coming from or even money for food and clothes?

Of course Black children do badly on standard intelligence and achievement tests just as most of us would do badly if we were presented with tests in Sengalese or Hindu! And we do not need tests to tell us that Black children will not do well in school unless there is a change, not only in the current school set-up, but also in the overall attitude of the white community that controls that set-up. Yet none of this means that the Black child is stupid or that he cannot learn. Every day of his life, in everything he does, the Black child gives clear indication of his ability to learn and adjust. If he had not been able to learn and use what he has learned appropriately for his particular circumstances, he would not have survived. I am reminded of a ten year old Black girl I have come to know. Her mother had gone to Chicago and left her alone to cope with an eight year old sister and an eleven month old brother. She carried her brother several miles to a Health Center she had heard about but had never visited because she thought he was sick. He was; he had pneumonia. How many middle-class White children of ten, with high I.Q's, would have the initiative, the judgment, the determination and the strength to make a trip like that, to an unfamiliar institution, in search of help for an ailing sibling? This little girl had learned from her family and her neighbors what must be done to stay alive. She is certainly not stupid, but I seriously doubt she would score well on a formal intelligence test.

If psychologists who emphasize tests, statistical findings and prediction were truly scientific they would recognize that their procedure in giving and using test results, with no Black children in the standardization population, is highly unscientific. Furthermore, the *APA Code of Ethics* distinctly states that using tests in ways that are detrimental to the subject is unethical. Administering inappropriate tests to Black children and then publishing the results of such tests is exactly what supplies the ammunition that such high powered researchers as Jensen and others employ in their "scientific" investigations.

Let clinicians recognize that intelligence and cognition do not comprise the total human being! Surely this recognition is our special contribution to the understanding of human behavior, including learning. As part of this understanding, let us not be so self-righteous about the anger that Black psychologists feel and express in relation to testing programs. Surely they have every right to be angry! And if that anger appears to take the form of racism, from whom have they learned it?

24. Social Responsibilities and Failure in Psychology: The Case of the Mexican American[1]

Manual Ramirez III

A survey[2] recently conducted by the Association of Psychologists for La Raza revealed that there are only thirteen Mexican-Americans who hold the doctorate in psychology. Of this number, only nine have full time teaching appointments in colleges and universities. These findings emphasize the fact that Mexican-Americans are vastly under-represented in psychology.

The shortage is particularly critical because so many of the issues brought to light by the Mexican-American Civil Rights Movement require the expertise and skills of psychologists. For example:

1. Many Chicano school children are being mistakenly placed in classes for the mentally retarded because they are not sufficiently familiar with the English language or well enough acquainted with information peculiar to mainstream American middle class culture.

Evidence for this was obtained in a study conducted under the auspices of the California State Department of Education (Chandler and Plakos, 1969). A group of Mexican-American pupils, who were enrolled in classes for the educable mentally retarded (EMR) in school districts throughout California, were retested in Spanish to determine if they had been incorrectly diagnosed because of difficulty with the language when the test was originally administered in English. The children were retested with the *Escala de Inteligencia Wechsler Para Ninos* (with some minor modifications), the Spanish translation of the *Wechsler Intelligence Scale for Children*. Results showed that the average gain between the testing in English (which resulted in placing the children in the EMR classes) and the testing in Spanish was 13.15 I.Q. points (the mean score for the test-

[1] Reprinted from *Journal of Clinical Psychology*, 1971-72, I, 1, 72, 5-7.
[2] The author would like to thank Alex Gonzales, a student at Pomona College, for his help in conducting the survey.

ing in English being 68.61, and that for the testing in Spanish 81.76). It can be concluded from the findings of this study, then, that many Mexican-American pupils are being placed in EMR classes solely on the basis of depressed performance due to unfamiliarity with the language in which the test is usually administered.

Furthermore, most standard intelligence tests require familiarity with information which is peculiar to mainstream American middle class culture. Most Mexican-Americans, and specially those from poor homes, have never been exposed to this information.

A study by Jensen (1961) highlighted this particular weakness of intelligence tests. A series of tasks, which assessed ability to learn independently of culturally biased content and language, were administered to Anglo and Mexican-American students who were divided into two groups (high and low) based on scores obtained with the California Test of Mental Maturity. The results of the study showed that Mexican-American children who had obtained low I.Q. scores on the California Test of Mental Maturity, performed significantly better than the Anglo-Americans with low I.Q.'s; thus, indicating that they had been misclassified. Furthermore, it was found that the Mexican-American children in the low group performed as well on the learning tasks as did Mexican-Americans and Anglos in the high group. Jensen's conclusion, then, was that tests like the California Test of Mental Maturity are culturally biased, and thus, invalid for assessing Mexican-Americans.

Some steps are being taken to forbid the use of culturally loaded test instruments with Mexican-American children. As a result of a suit filed in Monterey County, in 1970, *California against the California State Department of Education,* the Federal District Court ruled that all children whose primary home language is other than English must be tested in both languages. The case prompted the State Legislature to pass a law requiring that children be tested in their home language. This is clearly only a most superficial consideration. Chicano psychologists are needed for developing new instruments which not only reflect the communication style of the Mexican-American child, but his cognitive and incentive-motivational styles as well.

2. Mexican-Americans are being misdiagnosed as pathological because of many of our instruments of personality assessment contain items which are culturally loaded. Research with the Child Manifest Anxiety Scale (Ramirez, in progress) showed that Mexican-Americans scored significantly higher than the Anglo-American normative group. An item analysis, however, revealed

that the high scores obtained by Mexican-American were primarily due to items which reflected Mexican-American cultural values such as concern for approval and well-being of parents, and also concern over bodily functions. Thus, while high scores on these instruments may be indicative of pathology in Anglo-American, they may merely be reflective of close identity with traditional Mexican values in Mexican-Americans. Since the items of the CMAS are based on those of the Manifest Anxiety Scale, and many of these items, in turn, were derived from the MMPI, this finding makes all of these instruments questionable for assessing Chicanos as well.

3. Most theories of psychological developments are culturally exclusive, thus frequently leading social scientists and educators to the conclusion that Mexican-American culture interferes with the intellectual and social development of Chicano children. For example, research with the Rod and Frame Test (Ramirez, Price-Williams, and Beman, 1971) showed that Chicano children are, in general, more field dependent than Anglo Children. Most researchers, however, place a good deal of emphasis on the presumed advantages of field independence and the disadvantages of field dependence. Field independent socialization or child rearing styles, have generally been described in more favorable (value-laden) terms than those characteristic of field dependent child rearing styles. It is only a short step from such descriptions to conclude that some cultures are pathological because they interfere with the development of field independent characteristics in children. In fact, Witkin's concept of psychological differentiation presumes field dependent mode may indeed be more appropriate in certain cultural settings and for a variety of activities in many social and cultural settings.[3]

4. Research by Kagan and Madsen (1971) has uncovered evidence of unique incentive-motivational styles in Mexican-American children. They compared the performance of Anglo, Mexican, and Mexican-American children in cooperative and competitive settings. When rewards could only be achieved if two children working on a task were asked to cooperate with each other, Mexican and Mexican-American children achieved the most rewards; on the other hand, when the children were instructed to compete with each other, Anglo children achieved more rewards than either Mexican or Mexican-American children. These findings suggest cultural differences in motivational styles. Anglo middle-class culture rein-

---

[3] For a more extensive discussion, see Ramirez and Castaneda, "Cultural Democracy in Education: The Case of the Mexican Child." To be published by Seminar Press.

forces children for competitive behavior whereas Mexican and Mexican-American cultures reward children more for cooperative behavior.

As was mentioned above, research on cognitive styles (Ramirez, Price-Williams, and Beman, 1971) has shown that Mexican-American children consistently score more in the direction of field dependence than Anglo-American children on the Rod and Frame Test. Yet, preliminary data on cognitive styles of teachers, and orientation of curriculum and other aspects of the learning environment of schools, indicate a bias toward field independence. These findings have also been supported by Cohen (1969). She has identified two cognitive styles, analytic (similar to field independence), and relational (similar to field dependence), and has found that the analytic style is favored more by the schools. She states.

"A new observation that emerged from this study of the literature on cognitive styles was that not only test criteria, but also the overall ideology and learning environment of the school embody requirements nor many social and psychological correlates of the analytic styles. This emphasis can be found, for example in its cool, impersonal, outercentered approach to reality organization . . . so discrepant are the analytic and relational forms of reference that a pupil whose preferred mode of cognitive organization is emphatically relational is unlikely to be rewarded in the school setting either sociallyor by grades regardless of his natural abilities and even if his information repertoire and background of experience are adequate."

There is great need for Mexican-American psychologists to develop educational programs which are consonant with the cognitive styles of Chicano children. Most bi-cultural, bilingual programs being developed are based on the more superficial aspects of culture and are, thus, resulting in superficial changes in educaitonal system.

5. Mexican-Americans are being inadequately served by mental health institutions because few mental health personnel speak Spanish and are familiar with the value system of Mexican-American culture. Edgarton and Karno, (1969), for example, have found that many Mexican-Americans do not make use of mental health facilities because of a complex of social and cultural factors, the most critical of these factors being the cultural insensitivity of institutional practices and personnel. They state,

" . . . Clinics and hospitals which offer psychiatric services do not operate in ways which fit the needs of Mexican-Americans and hence are little used by them. For example, the cost is too high, the distance too far, the hours are inappropriate and the staff do not demonstrate respect, promote self-dignity, nor evidence cultural sensitivity . . . Moreover, the majority of Mexican-Americans speak only Spanish, or prefer to or can only communicate in Spanish concerning intimate or affectively charged matters, there are very few or no personnel in mental health facilities who speak Spanish."

While Mexican-Americans, who are being served either directly or indirectly by psychologists, are falling victim to their biased tests and theories and the insensitivity of their institutions, those Mexican-Americans who are seeking to gain entry into the profession are being turned away because of similar practices in graduate and undergraduate training programs. Evidence for this was obtained in a survey conducted with Mexican-American college students in Southern California.[3] Students were sampled from junior colleges, state colleges, a private University, and two campuses of the University of California. Most responses given to questions regarding reasons for their abandoning psychology as a major identified the following weaknesses in training programs:

1. Introductory courses in psychology were dull and tended to alienate them. The math and scientific apsects of the field were overemphasized and most professors exhibited the attitude that, "If you don't like statistics and laboratory psychology then you shouldn't major in psychology."

Overemphasis on the science-math aspects of the field is incompatible with the expectations of Chicanos because Mexican-American culture emphasizes the importance of interpersonal relationships, thus giving its members an interest in personality, social and abnormal psychology. In addition, the needs and problems which have been highlighted by the Civil Rights Movement emphasize the importance of applied psychology.

2. Very few professors were willing to serve as models, i.e. take a personal interest in Chicano students. Almost all students interviewed felt that having a close friendship with a psychology professor was critical to their continued interest in psychology.

3. Many students interviewed felt that tests required for admission, such as GRE and Miller Analogies, are so culturally loaded that they have very little chance of obtaining scores which are high enough to qualify them for admission.

4. Students had little hope of obtaining sufficient fellowship money to make it possible for them to stay in graduate school. Because of the value of identity with the family in Mexican-

American culture, many Chicanos feel responsible for helping to finance the schooling of their younger siblings.

5. Teaching styles of professors, and content and structure of curriculum materials and tests were not consonant with the cognitive styles of Mexican-Americans. Complaints most frequently voiced were that professors were too aloof and impersonal, that test and lecture materials were too heavily slanted in the direciton of middle-class values and problems and that tests were too oriented towards regurgitation of facts.

There is little hope that the shortage of Chicanos in psychology can be alleviated quickly, because there are no Chicano institutions of higher learning. While NIMH has awarded training grants to three Black universities, there are none as yet available for Chicanos because there is presently no university where such a program could be instituted. The only hope, then, is that the following changes will be made in existing colleges and universities:

1. Professors in introductory courses should make attempts to personalize relationships with Chicano students and make a special effort to teach experimental methodology in a personality-social-abnormal context.

2. Professors should make attempts to change their teaching styles and after curriculum and test materials to maximize the Chicano students' chances for success. Examples of these are: small group discussions, translating exams into Spanish, and allowing students to write papers or conduct research projects (This would give them the opportunity to display abilities and skills which may not show up in exams structured in a traditional manner).

3. Use criteria for acceptance to graduate schools which are not culturally biased as are the GRE and Miller Analogies.

4. Establish cooperative arrangements between universities and public service institutions in the community which could offer jobs to Chicano students and in this way, help them to supplement their fellowship money.

It can no longer be ignored that the field of psychology has been injurious to Chicanos, as well as to other minority ethnic groups. It is also clear that at this time in history, psychology can play a major role in the Civil Rights Movement. Opportunities must be made available to Mexican-Americans in psychology so that they might help make the field more sensitive to cultural differences, and at the same time, assist in getting psychology to play a major role in the struggle for the social betterment of peoples of the minority ethnic groups.

References

Chandler, J.T., and Plakos, J., Spanish-Speaking Pupils Classfied as Educable Mentally Retarded, *California State Department of Education,* 1969.

Cohen, Rosalie, Conceptual Styles, Culture Conflict and Non-Verbal Tests of Intelligence, *American Anthropoligist,* Volume 71: 828-856, 1969.

Edgarton, Robert B., and Karno, Marvin, Perception of Mental Illness in the Mexican-American Community, *Archives of General Psychiatry,* February, 1969, Volume 20.

Jensen A. R., Learning Abilities of Mexican-American and Anglo Children, *California Journal of Educational Research,* 12: 147-159, 1961.

Kagan, S., and Madsen, M.D., Mexican-American and Anglo-American Children of Two Different Ages Under Four Institutional Sets, *Developmental Psychology,* 1971.

Ramirez, M., Price-Williams, D.R., and Beman, A., *The Relationship of Culture to Educational Attainment.* Center for Research in Social Change and Economic Development, Rice University, Houston, Texas, 1971.

Ramirez, M., Anxiety in Mexican-American Children, research in progress, University of California, Riverside.

Witkin, H. A., Psychological Differentiation and Forms of Pathology, *Journal of Abnormal Psychology,* 1965, Vol. 70: 317-336.

25. Exit IQ: Enter the Child

Constance T. Fischer

Efforts to assess a child's over-all competnece as well as his future possibilities traditionally have focused on his IQ. It is IQ that has been viewed as most determinative of success. For example, its improvement is a key criterion of progress in Head-Start programs; children are placed in different tracks according to it; compensatory programs are devised for children low in it; journals engage in controversy over whether blacks are genetically deficient in it; and whether a child is working to his potential is judged by it.

Recent protest by black psychologists has finally questioned whether IQ is indeed the core of intelligent being. And now a changing public consciousness is making way for more radical questioning. In this paper, that questioning is grounded in a rejection of scientism—the view that all scientific projects must follow the methods and assumptions of the pre-Heisenberg natural sciences. From this border perspective, it is possible to ask what in practice has been meant by "intelligence" and then to examine how that conception has been both limited and limiting. From there it becomes possible to formulate a fuller conception of intelligence and to develop methods of assessment that are specifically appropriate to humans (as more than merely objects of nature).

IQ as Only One Variation of Intelligence

Definition of Test-Intelligence

In psychological practice, intelligence has become synonymous with test-intelligence. Test-intelligence (quantified as IQ) *"refers to the effectiveness, relative to age peers, of an individual's approaches to situations in which competence is highly regarded by the culture"* (Fischer, 1969). At present, *the most valued competence is that involving facts and logical problem-solving.*

The general usefulness of this definition is that it demystifies the

333

IQ score by referring to the natures of the score and test themselves. Moreover, the definition is phrased so that it creates room for new ways of viewing old conceptions. Each component of the definition also helps to bring "IQ" down to earth:

(1) "Effectiveness relative to age peers" is a reminder that IQ is in fact a mathematical formulation, one based on the actual performances of a particular sample of people on concrete test items. Remembering this makes it clear that comparison of some one individual with that particular sample is not always appropriate. Also, thinking of IQ as similar to, say, a spelling grade based upon the class curve strengthens our sometimes weak understanding that IQ is not a measurement of an entity; it does not indicate how much one has, but instead, reflects how well one did on a particular test at a particular time in comparison to a specific group of people. This recognition serves as a further reminder that a person's effectiveness, or IQ in this case, may increase with practice and training. Similarly, speaking of "effectiveness" instead of ability points to the importance of observing *how* a person earns a score in contrast to the usual focus on *how much* score was earned.

In addition, highlighting the mathematical, test-related character of IQ also throws light on the consistency of scores. That is, only those items that proved to be highly similar to one another and to school tasks were retained in the final versions of any intelligence test. No wonder that test-intelligence seems to have a "general factor" running through it, and that test-intelligence predicts school success. This consistency is manmade rather than a law discovered in nature. Indeed, as will be seen below, "g" is an artifact of limited values.

(2) The phrase "competence highly regarded by the culture" thematizes the fact that the test items were selected and standardized by real-life psychometrists whose values were those of the middle class at the time that the test was constructed. Perpetuating Binet's legacy, the items express the emphases in our socializing institution, the educational system. That is, they stress exposure to predetermined and single-perspective truth, memorization of facts-as-facts, and application of the given facts to logical problem-solving. This recognition suggests the following questions: Don't we value more than effectiveness with facts and logical problem-solving? Are not other sorts of competence, other styles of relating to this many-faceted world, valued in our culture and indeed essential to its survival? Thinking in this way allows IQ to be seen as representing success in only one, limited (but admittedly very important) area of human functioning. Other forms of competence

can be affirmed also. And it becomes conceivable that low IQ *may* point to rich differences rather than to over-all deficiency.

(3) Finally, the phrase, "the individual's approaches to situations" can imply that a total person is always participating in a particular situation that has personal meanings and possibilities for him. Here, levels of effectiveness do not, after all, have to be seen as *caused, mediated,* or *typified* by an underlying IQ. Rather, the *person moves toward* the world, participating in and contributing to its meaning, even when his concern is with what we call "objective facts." Hence, it becomes important to observe and have dialogue with the person rather than merely measure his level of performance. Understanding the experienced environment and the styles through which the person approaches things is critical for going beyond measurement to, say, advising teachers of ways to reach a student and to help him to move further.

In short, looking at test-intelligence in terms of what the test is all about demystifies IQ and places it in the psychologist's service rather than the other way around. Harking back to the beginnings of the "IQ movement" in psychology, we can see that this content area evolved from application of the only research method then available: psychophysical measurement. The phenomenon of IQ was a product of preexisting method rather than a natural state for which appropriate methods were devised. It was by further circumstances, rather than by scientific plan, that tests which were originally devised to predict academic success came to be called intelligence tests, and that ever since we have been locked into a circle of equating the goals of education with the criteria of IQ (effectiveness at manipulating predetermined categories and memorizing facts-as-facts). But IQ is *not something* which determines or typifies a person's level of behavior; rather, it is the person's approaches toward the world which bring him to varying levels of achievement.

Intelligence as More than IQ

Then what, besides IQ, might "intelligence" mean? It can refer to the *ways a person is in effective touch with the world.* Indeed, prior to scientizing, "intelligence" does not exist except as someone's perception of how well another person can carry out a variety of projects; it is an *inter*-personal phenomenon, something going on among people, not *in*side a person. This is not to deny the relevance of brain-related processes and previous experience, but only to stress that these are *not in* a person and that they do not of themselves constitute intelligence. Furthermore, intelligent behaviors always occur in specific situations: the effective approach is always to something in particular and always within a given context. Intelligence is not something which one *has,* but is rather one's *way of moving, of approaching.* Returning to its original sense, then, intelligence is akin to the layman's sense of "personality." Both "intelligence" and "personality" point to typical styles and modes of openness to life's possibilities, to the ways a person moves through his lived world. "Intelligence," however, emphasizes the *effectiveness,* in specified situations, of these approaches. "General intelligence," then, would refer to a person's multiform styles and modes of openness through which he deals effectively with new and varied phenomena. This view of intelligence as effectiveness of multiple approaches is quite consonant with recent definitions of intelligence as "ability to learn" (cf, Cox, 1970), although it does not limit learning to so-called cognitive functions.

Nonetheless, even though there is a certain generalizability about effectiveness in similar contexts, *intelligence is better located through described approaches, situations, and outcomes than designated by a number.* Where we are concerned with a particular effectiveness, we should seek to identify the specific approach *and* context; it usually is inappropriate to characterize an over-all level of achievement or type of personality. It is also inappropriate to separate such abstractions as motivation, emotion, biography, or attitude from a situated approach. These are simply subfused aspects of both intelligence and personality; they comprise the approach—the varieties of lived bonds with the world—which is what is pointed to by both the terms "intelligence" and "personality."

Note that "effectiveness" can refer to more than productions and immediate endpoints. Certain approaches can be effective in that they bring the person into new worlds, ones which in turn support constructive visions and valued ways of life. For example, certain approaches allow ambiguity, appreciation of differences, recognition of multiple reality; these in turn support a democratic orientation.

Similarly, this presentation is *not* merely acknowledging a "process" as well as "product" aspect of intelligence. Intelligence *is* situated process with its particular success. To wrench level of success from that situated process and to treat it as though it were predictive (if not determinative) of success in general is naive, misleading, and obstructive to individual growth.

In summary, while the one-truth/analytic criterion of IQ is indeed a major and essential component in our scientistic, mechanized society, it is only one component. Especially in our growing awareness of the destructive potential of technocracy, including social divisiveness, the salience of multiple approaches to life and tasks becomes apparent. Perhaps ways can be found to equate the goals of both education and personal growth with this fuller sense of intelligence, rather than with its partial aspect, IQ.

Exit IQ: Toward a Method Appropriate to the Child

If above formulations are valid, at least in spirit, then it is clear that the prevailing use of IQs hides and restricts more of the child than it reveals and foster. Indeed, the psychometric tradition has concerned itself with the individual only insofar as he contributed to (or fit) statistical, categorical generalizations about all persons. Ironically, the field of "individual differences" addresses neither the individual nor differences per se. Historical happenstance must now give way to development of theories and methods specifically designed to fit the child. Our imperative challenge is to promote child welfare in a way that *addresses the child* instead of reducing him to physicalistic constructs and measures. To do this, we must forego the security and prestige of our scientistic certification. Specifically, *there must be a moratorium on testing for scores*. But this step does *not* imply an overthrow of the old for chaos, for loose humanism, or for new esoterica. The avenue proposed here is a *human science* (Giorgi, 1970), one which acknowledges that man is not merely an object but also participates in his actions.

Explanatory System: Radical Structuralism

A theory through which the humanness of the child can be met more comprehensively is that of a radical structuralism. It is structural in that it presents explanation of a phenomenon in terms of its interrelated parts (its structure). No one part is more essential than any other; a change in any component transforms the phenomenon. A behavior, then, is explained by describing *what* it is rather than looking for something behind it (the past) or beneath it (traits, etc., e.g., IQ). The past is, nevertheless, taken into account in the form of its present participation.

For example, to explain Jan's poor grades in algebra, we describe her *doing* of algebra (*what* it is). It turns out that Jan typically approaches problems by circling around them first and then zeroes in through concentric potshots. Thus, she scored quite high for her age on the WAIS vocabulary by first giving a vague generalization, then tossing out closer and closer approximations until (with the exmainer's patience) she earned full credit. Algebra, however, requires not only an overview but then a step-by-step linear approach. In doing an algebra story-problem, however, Jan lists the necessary numbers, shifts her attention among them for a while, and finally produces an answer that "feels right"(usually a close approximation). During this process, Jan finds herself feeling uneasy, anticipating failure in ambiguous territory. Rather than attempting to specify formulae and then experiment with written solutions, she finds herself thinking of such topics as her English theme (where her "circling" style works well).

This description of Jan's doing algebra *explains* her failure: it presents its "if—then" conditions, and in a shareable, repeatable way. It also affords intervention and control. But it does not fall back on attributing failure in algebra to constructs such as poor motivation, lack of abstract ability, or traumatically induced fear of failure. Thus, a tutor was able to work with Jan, teaching her how to adapt her concentric approach to mathematics. Together, they found ways for her to circle around both the numbers *and* the available equations until she zeroed in on an appropriate fit between them. In this now familiar terrain, Jan could linger and calculate without feeling uneasy or out of place.

The *radical* aspect of this structural explanation is that it includes a fundamental (*radicalis*: at root) relational unity between person and world. Man behaves in accordance with the world as he experiences it. Hence, the unit of study is man-in-his-world rather than man affecting world or world affecting man. This structuralism is radical also in that it deals with the mutuality of components as they exist prior to scientistic (physicalistic) categorizing. That is, what we call affect, intellect, reality, and so on, are not separate things which have impact on one another, but rather are abstractions out of the whole. But the abstraction necessarily distorts the integrity of the whole and its dimensions; we are falsely led into talking of *distinguishable* components as though they were separate, actual, and interactive. To avoid this distortion of human phenomena it is, then, necessary to describe as best we can the child-in-his-world rather than measure presumed independent variables such as IQ, social maturity, vocational interest, etc. Thus, it was advisable to describe Jan's doing of algebra instead of measuring her achievement, aptitude, motivation, etc., and then trying somehow to combine them.

Clinical Method: Contextualizing of Behavior[1]

Another way to speak of the example with Jan is to say that we *contextualized* her difficulty with algebra. That is, its whatness (structure) was described in a way that included the full situation (matrix or context). Context, then, may include the behavior or event, the approach (style and mode of moving) which led into and through it, body contributions, surrounding events, persons, and objects, consequences for self and others; all these from both the child's and outsiders' perspectives. "Affect" and "meaning' participate in all components. Indeed, "experiaction" (Von Eckartsberg, 1969) is a more accurate term than "behavior plus experience."

In addition to the fullness of the problem, its *when-not* should also be described. That is, the context of a phenomenon is thrown into relief by contrast with occasions when it does not occur. Where it is a difficulty that is focal, its when-not is the ground for developing solutions. Hence, with Jan, we saw that she did not "have" a pervasive deficiency of arithmetical ability, but that *when* solutions required a linear, deductive approach her concentric approximations were inadequate. However, this approach was not problematic until after she had already identified the relevant variables of an algebra story-problem. This, then, was the point of intervention from which she was helped to expand her effectiveness. The contextualizing of *when-nots* in addition to the *whens* also undercuts notions about traits, abilities, and defectiveness as being "in" a person, as constant, just waiting to be tapped.

All of this contextualizing begins with the referral itself. In my own work, I inquire directly of the referring person about the specific behaviors and situations out of which the referral arose. Together with the child, we work to identify the whens and when-nots of the troubled or troubling behaviors. In the process I often follow along into the classroom, cafeteria, playground, bedroom, backyard, and so on. In a sense, I try to step into the child's shoes for awhile. In this way there is no need for resort to explanation via IQ or other traits; I simply describe the structure, the context, of the focal behavior. Right there within the everyday life of the child, concrete and realistic recommendations are readily available. Further, this assessment necessarily already has been therapeutic in that the child and his adults experience themselves as able to resolve

---

[1]Greater detail about contextual practices may be found in Fischer, 1972a & b.

the difficulty by themselves. They see that the difficulty lies not in "native ability" or in "personality make-up," but in the ways the child approaches particular situations; and these "ways" are expandable.

Another fortunate effect of assessing within the child's own environment is that often we discover aspects of that setting which are particularly adverse to, or supportive of, flexibility of approach for all the children or adults. Hence, school system or family life, for example, may be restructured following assessment. Similarly, traditional values and practices are less likely to be applied unthinkingly. That is, description of a situated behavior confronts us with the "so-what?" principle: values for child, institutions, and society at large must be questioned and chosen anew with each situation. Diagnosis and classification can no longer substitute for responsible thought.

Still, I do make frequent use of test materials, usually when circumstances have not allowed sufficient exploration of the child's everyday world. But even then I have established a degree of common ground with him through familiarity with some of the people and objects of his life. From there, I use test materials with three purposes: (a) to allow me to watch the child firsthand in a situation familiar to me; I observe not only what he accomplishes but *how* and *with what further consequences:* (b) to share activity that goes beyond spoken description; and (c) to find springboards into the child's everyday life. To these ends, objective administration and scores take second place. Sometimes I present parents, teachers, or hospital staff with test productions and ask them to add to the child's recollections of similar behaviors (and situations) in his everyday life.

Data: Shareable Everyday-life Behavior[2]

The data of a contextual method, then, are not dynamics, mechanisms, causes, traits, x-rays, deficiencies, pathologies, or even abilities or habits. The data are situated life events. For example: *When Rolf experiences himself as commanded to perform in unfamiliar territory, he does not approach the task in his more usual carefully systematic manner; instead he throws himself into a rushed rendition of something similar but familiar. For instance, when told to solve a word problem out loud, he instead recited the relevant times tables.*

---

[2]Explicit philosophical and ethical grounds for everyday-life events as data are presented in Fischer, 1970 and 1972.

Granted, these data are mundane and commonsensical; this is their strength. With life data, including the child's experimental participation in them as the focus, the psychologist encourages the child's active participation in the assessment. Insofar as they are available, the child's accounts and views are what is central, not his productions and scores in themselves. Use of the latter has allowed the psychologist to remain in a realm of language and constructs inaccessible to the child and most of his involved adults. Although the life data method still necessitates that the adult professional be in charge, in the sense of guiding the assessment, the effects are quite different. Here, the child learns that he can examine his situations himself, that he can be responsible for his own development to a remarkable extent. He is not merely living out "native ability," "level of motivation," "that stage he's going through," etc. He also discovers that while not more real, his experience is as real and valid as that of authorities and theories. While the psychologist attempts to help the child and his adults to find new perspectives, he does not interpret among levels of reality. In short, where the data to be collected are life events, the child can participate in evaluating his progress and in trying out new ways of being effective. This is already a major step toward child welfare.

If psychological reports are to continue these steps, they must be merely interim accounts of how specific behaviors have been situated and redirected. The report contains no jargon, constructs, or diagnoses. Preference is given to the child's own language and world. The assessor refers to himself in the first person, and in other ways includes himself as part of the picture that emerged. Hence, all readers recognize that the psychologist's contributions are always limited to his own situated, perspectival view of the fuller structure. His views may open up new horizons, but they do not invalidate others' views, nor render his own more really real. Later notes may somewhat alter the initial understanding as additional components and nuances unfold. Indeed, the psychologist's report may simply provide an orientation from which the child and his involved adults can observe and interact more sensitively. In the process, they often develop broader understandings as well as new ways of carrying out the intent of the recommendations.

In addition, because the report is structural, there are no villains. Each person in the write-up appears in specific contexts and with his own experience respected. For example, rather than being presented as "intimidating," a mother might be described as "firm in her decisions about household matters unless *directly* and openly presented with specific alternatives." Each participant is reached in a constructive manner, if not immediately, then through readers' subsequent interactions with him.

Since life-data reports contain no esoterica or secrets, the child and his parents may have access to them. Indeed, they *should* add a postscript clarifying any misemphasis, misunderstanding, or difference of opinion. With this access, child and parents then can decide to whom they will give permission to read the report. As in the initial contextualizing of the referral, the problem is often resolved at the time of the request.

As with psychological reports, the data of school records ought also to be life data. The child's records, then, are an account of which actual experience and behaviors are available *under specified circumstances*. Among test scores, achievement-test performances could come to be seen as the most useful and valid (closely related to situated life performance). Intelligence test, personality test, and even interest test scores would become demystified as being temporary, uncompleted starting places for investigating the child's actual, situated experience and behavior. Instead of being viewed as measurements of the 'real' internal child, they would be seen as probably helpful but definitely incomplete. There would be no place for stark IQs or other mathematical quotients. Intelligence would be reported as effectiveness with particular goals via specified ways of moving toward and through them. And "data" that do not meet the "so-what?" criterion of relevance to everyday life intervention would never be entered in the record.

The above, of course, sounds more like a general psychological assessment than an evaluation of effectiveness. But it is both. From a structural/contextual perspective, intelligence is the effectiveness of ways of approaching, or of moving through, particular situations. By shelving IQ, we can shift focus from *how much does the child have?* to *what can he do, when?* The structure of that *what* and *when* necessarily includes what we call affect, meanings, style. Moreover, it indicates where expansion toward greater latitudes and effectiveness might be initiated.

Implications for Some Professional Issues

General

If clinical child psychologists are to be advocates for child welfare, then they are obliged to counsel not only children but also society and its educational system. They must continually question the relations between education and the child's (as well as society's) wellbeing. Specifically, they should insist vocally that the "right to education" implies the right of each child to an education that is suited to him personally. To the same end, psychologists could assist educators and the public to see that actuarial-based teaching programs and class assignments are geared to some previous "average child" rather than to present individuals; hence they are as limiting as they are helpful. Simultaneously, the IQ-education circularity should be clarified so that schools and families could set a broader goal of education: fuller intelligence—getting the child into working touch with the world through many modalities and perspectives.

In the remainder of this paper, only one representative professional issue will be explored in detail: the "genetic inferiority" controversy. Hopefully some of the implicatins for other issues also will be aparent in this discussion. Among these issues are: rescinding of statutory IQ criteria for admission to special programs; development of nonstatistical criteria for successful teaching; extension of teaching roles to parents, fellow students, and community volunteers; revision of referral practices from requests for categories to requests for behavior description and suggestions; support for heterogeneous and smaller classes; valuing ways of being rather than level of having (ability); establishment of recommendation-diagnosis to replace defect- or achievement-diagnosis; challenge to the assumption of necessary brain defect or deficiency in learning disability; deprofessionalizing of psychologists (giving psychology to all people); etc.

"Genetic Inferiority"?

The controversy as to whether blacks (in particular) are inherently deficient in intelligence has, of course, utilized IQ as its criterion. However, neither side has questioned the historical notion that IQ is an estimate of a general ability underlying all scholastic success; nor whether academic skills are the major ones of value to our society; nor, indeed, whether there might exist noncognitive components, if not nonanalytic modes and styles, of being effective, even in scholastic endeavors.

A moratorium on IQ-testing could allow *qualitative* research into the learning and living styles of humans in general and subcultures in particular. Similarly, only after having described black approaches in a variety of circumstances could the issue of genetic components of intelligence be raised. In short, the genetic inferiority controversy as it exists today is an artifact of the American psychometric movement, which has limited intelligence to being what its methods could already measure.

What approaches might there be other than one-truth/analytic? In *The Hidden Dimension*, Hall (1963) speaks of the ways members of different cultures experience and move in their environment. Eskimos, for example, use fewer of the visual and cognitive signs we depend upon; instead, they rely on bodily and sensory relationships with their ecological system. In our own culture, perhaps articulation of nonanalytic intelligence may emerge from the subgroups currently intrigued with altered states of consciousness, Eastern religion and states of being, and the human potential movement (sensitivity training, body wisdom, etc.). More likely, the European philosophical tradition may provide existential-phenomenological perspectives on effective consciousness and action, e.g., the body-subject, the chiasm of visible and invisible, and dialectical restructuration of phenomenal perception (Merleau-Ponty, 1963; 1968).

Labov's (1969) analysis of the structure of "nonstandard negro English" provides a more immediate example. It is, however, about a variation of logical form. He documents the ways in which the speech of black children *does* preserve the inherent logic of standard English. He also points to the consequences of teachers and psychologists not understanding that the black child speaks a *dialect* of, not a *deficient form* of, English. For example, projects like Head Start have been judged as failures when black children have not responded to a "compensatory" environment adequately enough to score higher on measures of intellect. Presumably, then, Head Start's intention has backfired: if environment does not make a difference, then black deficiency must be genetic. Or: black children should be removed from their homes still earlier in order to be adequately stimulated by a white environment. The black child's *difference* from the white child has been reduced to either environmental deprivation (deficiency) or genetic limitation (still deficiency).

Head Start's outcome might be transformed if its acculturation exercises were formulated as translation lessons or as enrichments intended to exist alongside those of the native culture. Surely, a strong, trusted homebase is essential to maximal exploration of new territory. Besides, the "whatness" of black modes, styles, and areas of effectiveness, to whatever extent they exist as "different," could thus emerge. This openness to difference as difference rather than as assumed deficiency might then extend to children in general—a major step toward promoting child welfare.

The above discussion throws light, if not extinguishing water, on the genetic controversy recently rekindled by Jensen (1969) and Hernstein (1971). Jensen concluded from experimental studies that blacks are skillful at rote memory but inherently inferior at higher-order thinking. In large part this latter conclusion was based on the statistical finding that, although black children improved their short-term class standing, their IQ's did not also jump. But an alternative conclusion can be derived from this article's analysis of IQ and intelligence: If black students improved by classroom criteria (school achievement), they *did* make progress in what the schools label as (higher-order) intelligence. Further, when intelligence is conceived as including the person's approaches to the particular tasks in question, it becomes apparent that more than a couple of semesters is required to make a middle-class schoolroom a thoroughgoing aspect of the black child's own world, so that the child can develop the additional approaches necessary for more generalized success such as on its IQ tests.

Hernstein (1971), too, concludes that statistical evidence supports the existence of black genetic intellectual deficiency (IQ as 80% inherited). His particular concern, however, is that as our governments provide increasingly comparable housing, education, and medical opportunities for the lower classes, our meritocracy will ensure that blacks remain at the lowest level of socio-economic status. According to Hernstein, our meritocracy rewards (scarce) intellectual ability with the lucrative and prestigious jobs. He argues, thus, strictly within the prevailing technocratic cultural values and "formidable" data accumulated via psychometrics.

Indeed, only from a psychometric approach could personal effectiveness be said to be made up of separate parts. The Aristotelian tradition of exclusive classes underlies the scientistic measurement of "independent variables," and has precluded investigation of the mutuality of structural dimensions. From a structural perspective, no aspect of effectiveness is more essential than any other since all are necessary for its existence. Hence, from this orientation it is meaningless to attribute percentages of participation to environment and heredity. While it is nevertheless true that a given genetic structure together with a given life situation limits any child's range of possibilities, we do not yet know which genes together with which situations allow what sorts of effectiveness. Moreover, our society might reward differently, perhaps not even competitively, if it recognized the importance to the quality of social life of (situated) acquiescence, artistic perspective, resistance, folk wisdom, and other as yet unnamed approaches. Structurally speaking, each is necessary, and hence in its way and place is as important to the whole as any other approach. We do not yet know much about that "way and place" of non-Aristotelian approaches.

It should be noted that, from the perspective outlined in this paper, the currently growing demand by blacks for black norms and for informed use of intelligence tests with black children is misguided. That is, it continues to focus only on one-truth/analytic effectiveness, and that only in terms of number of correct test items. This statistical approach to the child limits understanding to already existing categories. Insistence on competing with whites on standardized tests restricts all participants to existing middle-class, objectivistic, one-truth/analytic criteria.

To repeat, the genetic inferiority controversy is an artifact of psychometric totalization of intelligence. Investigation of genetic aspects of intelligence must await further understanding of the nature of multiform approaches as well as their role in going beyond technocratic society.

Summary: From Scientism to Child Welfare

IQ has been illuminated here as being an artifact of psychology's traditional commitment to imitating the physical sciences. This scientism has necessarily restricted its methods and content by pursuing human "nature" through belief in Aristotelian exclusive classes, linear causality, nonperspectival truth, mechanical interaction of cognitive and affective process, lived experience as only epiphenomenal, and, of course, in the psychologist as external objective observer. Hence, intelligence (IQ) has been restricted to problem-solving of the truth/analytic variety. It has also been seen as determinative of future success. Our scientistic heritage has imposed limited (and limiting) values on our schools and children.

If clinical child psychologists are to promote the growth and well-being of children, then we must institute a moratorium on IQ-testing. In its place we must address the child's fuller intelligence—his multiple styles and modes of being effective in a wide range of circumstances. From here we can develop systematic methods and content *appropriate* to children specifically and to humans in general.

Such a *human science* has been proposed here in the form of radical structuralism. That is, the whatness (including experiential aspects) of an event is its own explanation. Scientistic constructs are bypassed as the child is understood and supported through the method of contextualizing everyday-life events—the data of the child-advocate.

To Child Welfare

This focus on everyday-life data undercuts the statistical curve approach to education and child-rearing. It assures that *each child* will be met in his own concreteness and situatedness. *His* perspectives and realities must be respected as necessarily there and as powerful—he must be understood within *his* territory before he can be aided to move on. Such practices, if open and frequent, would also enhance growth by encouraging children to both respect the inevitable situatedness of others' perspectives, and to question the "truths" of established education, psychology, religion, science, etc.

Similarly, when we stop totalizing a child's effectiveness in terms of IQ, then we can begin to construct educational systems that encourage breadth, diversity, openness toward not just "problem-solving," but toward nature, cultures, persons, and styles of life. Surely promotion of child welfare and the foundations of a viable democracy are inextricable. And as the individual child's everyday behaviors become the starting point for expansion, that child and his involved others participate actively in assessing and redirecting his progress. There are no secret files for the school or mental health expert; any records are *for the child,* who can knowledgeably initiate specific assistance from others (including nonprofessionals). The child thus participates in a community of cooperation, innovation, and mutual respect.

Finally, as we deal with *each child,* we are confronted ever anew with the issue of values. Now we must continuously ask: What could this child (and mankind) become? We can no longer merely apply (impose) old labels and formulae; we must ask instead: Where is *this* child going? What might be the consequences? With the exit of IQ and related scientisms, clinical *child* psychology can become a positive science/service for maximal well-being of the *individual child* and hence of society.

References

Cox, F. *Psychology*. Dubuque: Wm. C. Brown, 1970.

Fischer, C. T. Intelligence defined as effectiveness of approaches. *Journal of Consulting and Clinical Psychology* , 1969, *33*, 668-674.

Fischer, C. T. The testee as co-evaluator. *Journal of Counseling Psychology*, 1970, *17*, 70-76.

Fischer, C. T. Contextual approach to assessment. *Community Mental Health Journal*, 1972a (in press).

Fischer, C. T. Theme for the child-advocate: Shareable everday life data of the child-in-the-world. *Journal of Clinical Child Psychology*, 1972b, I, No. 3, 23-25.

Fischer, C. T. Paradigm changes which allow sharing "results" with the client. *Professional Psychology* (in press).

Giorgi, A. *Psychology as a human science*. N.Y.: Harper & Row, 1970.

Hall, E. T. *The hidden dimension*. Garden City: Doubleday, 1963.

Hernnstein, R. I. Q. *The Atlantic*, 1071, *228*, 43-58; 63-64.

Jensen, A. How much can we boost IQ and scholastic achievement? *Harvard Educational Review*, 1969, *39*, No. 1, 1-123.

Labov, W. The logic of non-standard English. *The Florida Reporter*, Spring/Summer 1969, 60-74; 169.

Merleau-Ponty, M. *The structure of behavior* (A. Fisher, Trans.). Boston: Beacon Press, 1963.

Merleau-Ponty, M. *The visible and the invisible* (A. Lingus, Trans.). Evanston: Northwest University Press, 1968.

Von Eckartsberg, R. On experiaction ecology. Unpublished manuscript, Duquesne University, 1969.

Part Six

YOUTH IN PERSPECTIVE

Traditional clinical child psychology has been isolated from the mainstream of youth; we professionals have communicated primarily with each other. This section offers a spectrum of approaches demonstrating how we can share ideas, work, and responsibilities with youth.

26. Why Use Comic Books to Teach about Sex?

Sol Gordon and Roger Conant

Current approaches to sex education are being thwarted by three major barriers to communicating the knowledge that adolescents need to protect themselves:

1) The mistaken notion held by many adults that the less an adolescent knows about sex, the less chance he will "get in trouble."

2) Another mistaken idea held by many adults that the best way to keep kids in line is to "scare the pants off them."

3) The fact that most people, especially teenagers, don't much like to read.

On the first point, we comment: Keeping silent has never kept people "moral." In our experience, the less people know about something as important to them as sex, the greater the chance that their resulting confusion and frustration will lead to all sorts of inappropriate and usually damaging behavior.

Anyway, these days, as it has been in reality all through history, a great many adolescents will engage in premarital sex no matter what adults think they should not do. How can we ask our young people to be responsible for their behavior—sexual and otherwise—if we allow, and even guarantee, their ignorance?

Our response to the second point: Kids, like other people, resent overscare tactics. When they are fed a diet of scare lectures they quickly learn to tune out. If we are truly interested in helping our youth and if we really believe we have some valid things to say, then we must first approach them in such a way that they are willing to listen.

On the third point, we must understand that comic books are the only source of reading pleasure for huge numbers of young people. Hundreds of millions of comic books are sold annually in the United States.

Occasionally someone will claim that the cartoons are in poor taste. However, what constitutes good taste for such a critic is simply not read by most young people. And, although a lot of so-called tasteful literature has been written about sex, most of it is generally not very effective—because it is boring. Additionally, humor helps reduce the anxiety that turns people away from reading about what they really need to read about.

By the end of 1973, 600,000 copies of the comic book which follows have been distributed to social action groups, health departments, government agencies, and Planned Parenthoods throughout the United States and Canada. It is interesting to note that in our observation *whenever an adult staff meets in advance to decide whether to use one of the comics, they invariably decide against it.* However, *whenever an individual adult distributes copies on his own, his organization can't keep up with the demand.* Again and again, groups have begun by ordering a few and are soon ordering by the thousand.

The comic book, *Ten Heavy Facts About Sex,* was developed after reviewing some 10,000 questions submitted anonymously by teenagers in an unselected sample of high schools throughout the country. (The youngsters were asked to write one question that they had about sex.) The "heavy facts" are based on the ten most frequently asked questions.

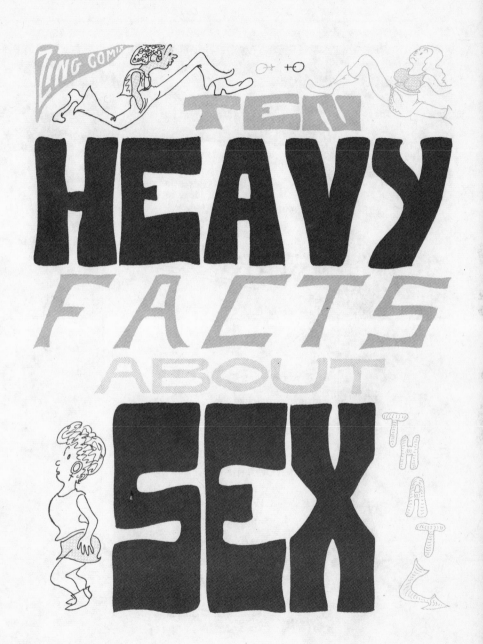

ZING COMIX

TEN HEAVY FACTS ABOUT SEX THAT

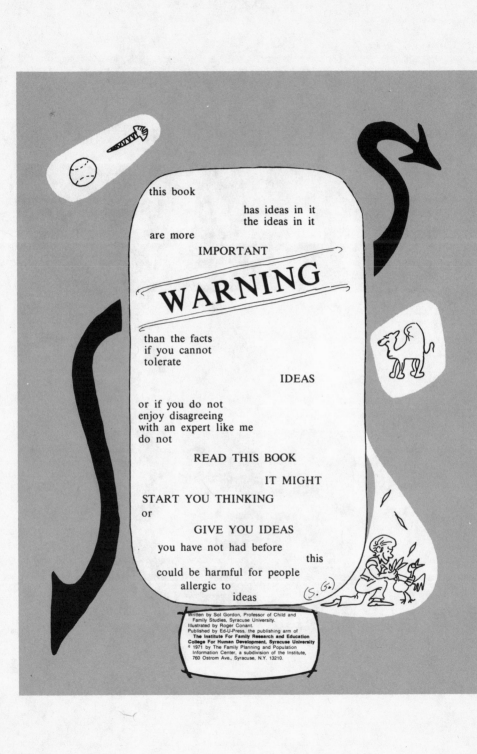

this book

has ideas in it
the ideas in it

are more

IMPORTANT

WARNING

than the facts
if you cannot
tolerate

IDEAS

or if you do not
enjoy disagreeing
with an expert like me
do not

READ THIS BOOK

IT MIGHT

START YOU THINKING
or

GIVE YOU IDEAS

you have not had before

this

could be harmful for people
allergic to
ideas

Written by Sol Gordon, Professor of Child and
Family Studies, Syracuse University.
Illustrated by Roger Conant.
Published by Ed-U-Press, the publishing arm of
The Institute For Family Research and Education
College For Human Development, Syracuse University
© 1971 by The Family Planning and Population
Information Center, a subdivision of the Institute,
760 Ostrom Ave., Syracuse, N.Y. 13210.

THAT...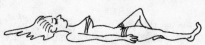

YOUR FRIENDS DON'T KNOW

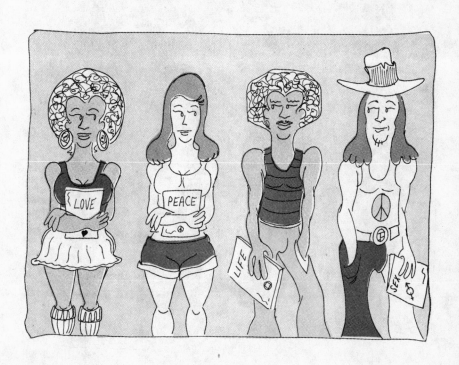

THAT... YOUR PARENTS DIDN'T TELL YOU

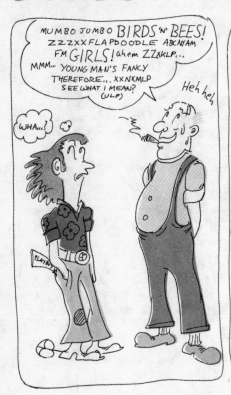

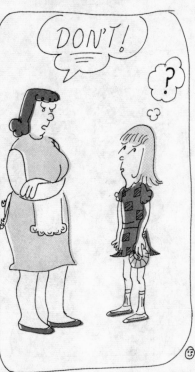

THAT... YOUR DOCTORS & COUNSELORS AIN'T TALKIN' ABOUT

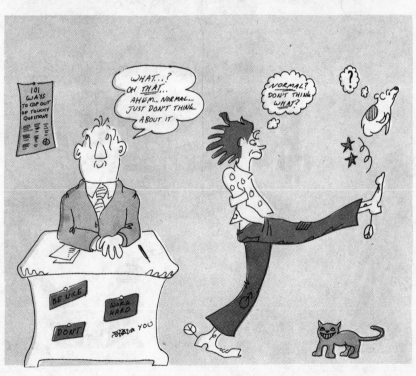

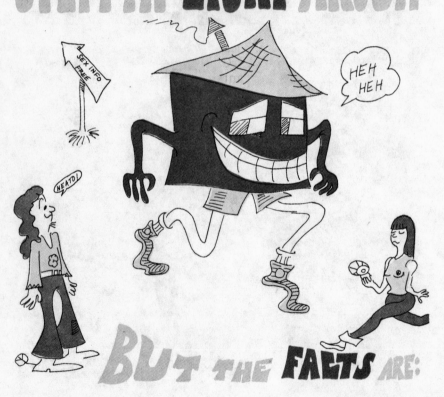

1 ALL THOUGHTS ARE NORMAL

Sexual thoughts, wishes, dreams, are normal -- no matter how far out. Only your actions count. Thoughts, images and fantasies cannot, in themselves, injure you.

If your fantasies make you feel guilty, you probably won't be able to avoid having them. Realizing that *all* thoughts are normal will let you have, for the most part, the ones you want. The thoughts you don't like will occur less and less.

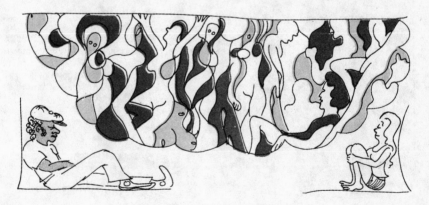

2 MASTURBATION

Masturbation is a normal expression of sex for both males and females. Enjoy it. There's no harm in masturbation no matter how often you do it.

Masturbation is a sign that something is wrong *only* when it is compulsive -- when you "can't help it." Compulsive

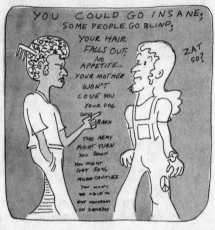

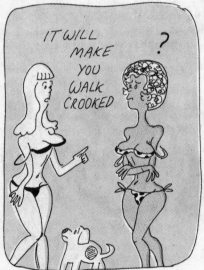

behavior is almost always related to feelings of guilt. If masturbating makes you feel guilty, it becomes a form of self-punishment.

Psychologically, masturbation is fine as long as you want to masturbate and as long as you enjoy it.

HOMOSEXUAL

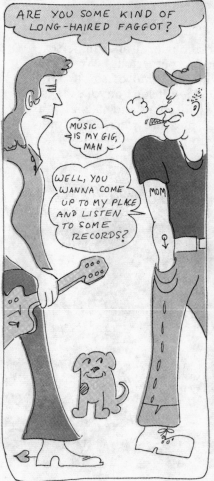

Most people, men and women, have occasional homosexual thoughts and many people have had homosexual experiences.

This doesn't make them homosexuals. A homosexual is a person who in his adult life prefers and has sex relations with members of the same sex.

Homosexuality is not biological or hereditary. Neither homosexual thoughts nor actual homosexual experiences during adolescence need influence the rest of your life. So choose the sexual life you want. Ninety per cent of the population prefer heterosexuality. That's their business. Ten per cent choose homosexuality or bisexuality. That's their business.

Letting yourself be bothered by fears of homosexuality is a waste of time.

Any sex, hetero, homo, or auto, can be considered "abnormal" if it is involuntary and exploitive. That's when sex is an expression of a problem rather than an enrichment of a relationship.

4 'PERVERSIONS'

A lot of people wonder about oral and anal sex, and some people think it is "perverted." We think there is nothing wrong with any kind of sex if both partners are mature and it doesn't hurt anyone. It is, for some, a normal part of foreplay and it is also a way to have intense sexual pleasure when you don't want to have sexual intercourse.

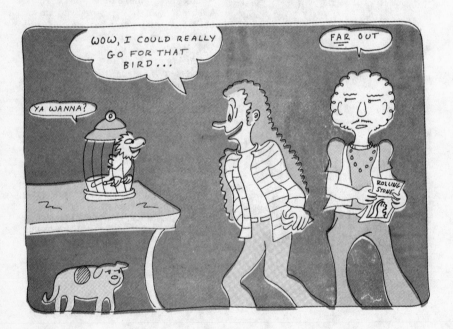

5 VD

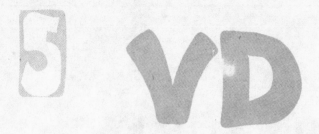

Venereal disease (V.D.) is spread by having sexual contact (heterosexual or homosexual) with someone who has it.

Males who use rubbers (condoms) greatly reduce chances of catching it themselves or of unknowingly giving it to someone else.

A fairly good way to cut down chances of getting V.D. is to urinate and wash with soap and hot water right after sex relations. This, however, is *no guarantee* against V.D. (Girls using contraceptive foam should not douche until six hours after relations.)

The two most common forms of V.D. are gonorrhea and syphilis. First signs of gonorrhea are pus and "burning" while urinating. First sign of syphilis is a sore on the penis, or in the vagina, mouth or rectum. Girls may not notice any signs when they have V.D.

Signs of V.D. go away by themselves without medical treatment. But the disease is still doing damage. You just don't know you have it.

You cannot get cured without treatment from a doctor. Many states have sensibly revised their laws to permit teenagers to be examined and treated without parental consent or knowledge. For instance: New York, New Jersey, Connecticut, California, Texas, Pennsylvania, Illinois, Oregon, Florida -- among others.

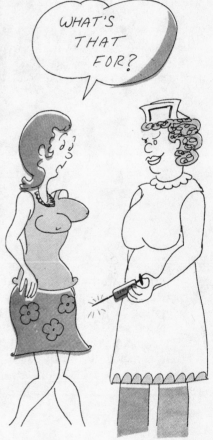

6 PENIS SIZE

Boys often wonder about the size of their penis and girls help them worry by making remarks. But no matter how big or small, the sexual pleasure -- for either sex -- is not determined by penis size.

Besides, you can't tell the size of a penis by looking at it when it is not erect.

PORNOGRAPHY

Pornography is harmless.
After awhile it gets
boring. If porno is your
bag, you don't have
much of an imagination
of your own.

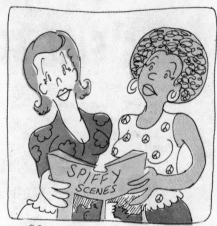

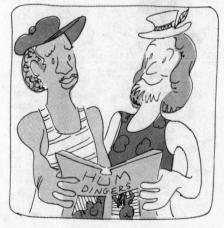

8 WHEN
CAN A GIRL GET PREGNANT?

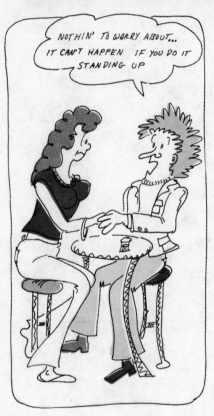

There is no 100 per cent safe time when a girl can have intercourse without risking pregnancy. But, in general, most girls are not able to get pregnant during menstruation or in the two or three days after menstruation.

A girl can get pregnant the first time she has sexual intercourse. She can get pregnant if she has sex standing up, sitting down, or in any other position.

Two ways of avoiding unwanted pregnancies: self control or birth control.

9 BIRTH CONTROL
~PILLS & RUBBERS~

The Pill -- still the most effective. Take heed: just taking one or two is no help. Females must take their pills regularly under a doctor's care. (The Pill has not yet been proved safe for adolescents who are in the early stages of their physical development.)

Other good medical birth controls are the IUD (intrauterine device) and the diaphragm.

The best birth control available without prescription is a combination of the rubber for the boy and the foam

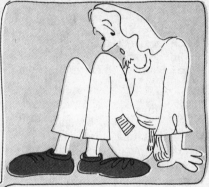

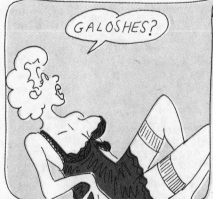

GALOSHES?

(which is inserted before sex) for the girl. When buying rubbers, ask for a brand name, such as Trojan. Delfen and Emko are two names of contraceptive foams. They are available in drugstores.

Douching (washing out the vagina) -- no matter with what -- and the rhythm method are not trustworthy ways to prevent pregnancy. The same goes for withdrawal of the penis before "coming" (ejaculation) -- although this is better than no protection at all.

WARNING: The Pill does not prevent V.D. If you have intercourse with someone who has V.D. and he does not use a condom, your chances of getting it are almost 100% if you are on the Pill.

10 ABORTION

Medical abortions are now legal in all States for women in the first 12 weeks of pregnancy. (In any case, if you are pregnant and want to avoid giving birth or if you are having sexual relations and want to avoid pregnancy, contact your local Planned Parenthood, Family Planning, county, or hospital clinic.)

We think having an abortion is more moral than bringing an unwanted child into this world. Having a medical abortion before the twentieth week is safer than giving birth -- so don't let anyone tell you it is a dangerous operation.

During the early stages of pregnancy a medical abortion is safe, brief and relatively painless. It is *very dangerous,* however, when it is *not done by a physician.*

Some people consider abortion immoral and they have a right to think this way. Most people, as well as the majority of religious groups, believe that women should have the right to make their own decisions about their unintended pregnancies -- whether to give birth (keep the child or put it up for adoption) or have an abortion.

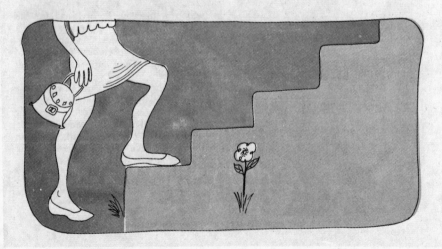

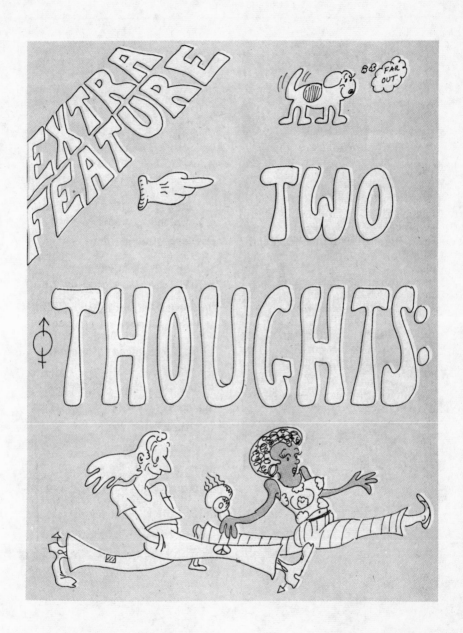

SEX 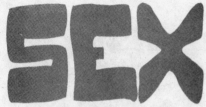 IS A DRAG WHEN...

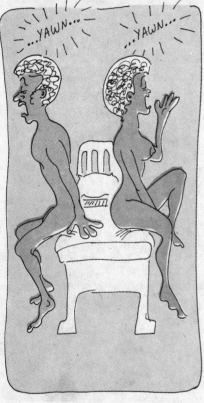

● You don't care about, much less love, your partner.

● It is compulsive. You do it a lot when you really don't want to and you get very little pleasure out of it.

● It is exploitive. You use sex against people as a way of trying to "prove" that you're not inadequate. (Frequency of sex has little to do with its meaning or importance in the lives of people).

SEX IS COOL WHEN...

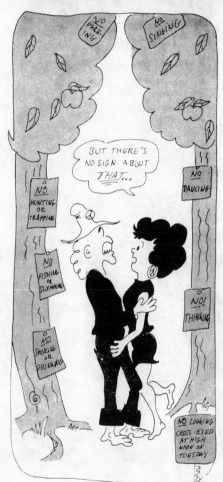

- You are ready for it. (It is even normal to wait until marriage.)

- You are in love.

- You want a baby or, if you don't,

- You use birth control.

Remember: The first few sexual experiences are not always enjoyable or satisfactory. That doesn't mean anything is wrong with you.

Some men may find that they are impotent -- unable to have an erection when they want to have intercourse -- or they may have a premature ejaculation -- "coming" before the penis goes into the vagina. Some women are "frigid." They don't enjoy sex, or even if they do, they don't get an orgasm. For both men and women, this may be a temporary situation. It could be due to guilt, inexperience of either partner, or unfavorable conditions often associated with first experiences of sex. For the woman it can also be the result of the man not being sensitive enough about her sexual needs. Sexual difficulties of this kind are usually solved in time when two people work at their problems with sympathy and understanding for each other. If problems persist, professional help should be obtained.

MORALITY IS GOOD FOR YOU

FOR GUYS:

- No sex unless you are ready for it.

- Protect your lover; wear a rubber.

- Don't reveal your sexual inadequacy by boasting about your sexploits.

- Don't go around hurting girls because you feel insecure. (A guy who is always on the make basically hates women.)

- *Machismo* is when you're man enough to take care of the family you started.

FOR GIRLS:

- No sex unless you are ready for it. (Don't fall for lines like: "If you don't have sex with me, we might as well stop seeing each other.")
- No sex without birth control.
- No sex with a guy who isn't your long-time lover without a rubber. (If the guy is too cheap to spend 35 cents for a condom, he shouldn't be allowed in.)
- No sex with anyone who doesn't really care about you. (Test by finding out if he'll go out with you even if you won't have sex with him.)
- Don't judge your adequacy by such things as breast size, which are not indicators of your sexuality.
- Join Women's Liberation NOW!

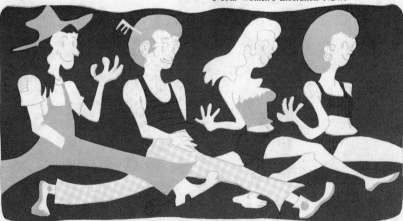

IF YOU WANT TO KNOW MORE:
Facts About Sex For Today's Youth
By Sol Gordon (John Day Paperback, $1.90)

IF YOU WANT TO KNOW MORE THAN THAT:
Understanding Sex - A Young Person's Guide
By Alan F. Guttmacher (Signet paperback, 95 cents)

IF YOU WANT TO KNOW ABOUT THE COLLEGE SCENE:
Sex In A Plain Brown Wrapper by
The Student Committee on Sexuality at Syracuse University
(760 Ostrom Ave., Syracuse, N.Y. 13210, $1.20)

27. Alternatives to the Family: An Open Letter to Clinical Child Psychologists*

Thomas Linney

We youth don't exist to be studied and yet we are all concerned with how people learn, how we can be creative, and how changes get made in society. At the same time, it is difficult for me to explain how we are different because I feel we are and yet we are struggling with issues that are universal in America in 1972; and how do I talk about this place as being both different and similar from all of that at the same time? I don't feel like I have any answers to any of those questions, but you should think about them as you read what follows.

So last night I'm reading, as I do voraciously when I'm evading work, and there is an article in *Newsweek* about Robert Coles. Coles, who is a friend of people in this house (Jared), writes about his work saying it "can be called an application of the clinical method, which assumes that an intensive study of a relatively small number of individuals can shed some light, a little light on matters that many of us are concerned with in one way or another, the emotions and purposes and beliefs that make us human beings."

Right on, I think to myself; that is something I want to say about this place in this article and those are the kinds of things I want to talk about, to any audience whatever. Whoever it is we are and whatever it is we are engaged in, we are human, trying, struggling to understand ourselves, where we came from, how we got to where we are, and how to build a new vision of people living together, taking up where we are, guided only by the assumption that we are unhappy with the dominant American ideal of family, even given that it may not in fact exist except as an abstraction.

We are products of the American culture, most of us of the post-

---

*Slightly revised version of an article "On Alternatives to the Family," *Journal of Clinical Child Psychology*, Vol. I, No. 2 (Spring, 1972).

war baby-boom, educated in public schools and colleges, destined
for success—leaders, cheerleaders, and student body presidents.
Somehow in ways that none of us quite understands, we were
unhappy and began to ask questions and not get answers. Civil
Rights and Vietnam were probably the first for most of us, although
Michael and Deborah remember McCarthy times and Caryl Chessman. The answers were not forthcoming and so we moved into politics and at the same time, as happens to nearly everyone (you, too, I
bet) fell in love with Pat and Paul and Sandy and our philosophy
professor. We made love, learned about sex (somewhat painfully in
most cases), and learned again—and oh how hard it was!—that love
and sex and marriage and kids were not all that we had been taught it
would be. So here we are. Twelve adults and three children in
America, 1972. We tried most of what the culture said we should do
to be happy, and we were not; and so we are trying some new ways
of looking at what it means to be a person living in America and
attempting to be happy.

Tonight Mahler's "Tragic" symphony plays as Orson, the dog,
sits curled up against the clear January cold (even in California) outside the back door waiting for me to go to bed where he usually joins
me unless there is something more exciting going on. Howie sits in
his room drinking coffee and writing in his journal while a friend
watches. Richard plays the recorder in his room and prepares to
leave us and go to live in the country. Jared calls from Oregon, courtesy of Ma Bell, and tells us it took him a week to get unspeeded
from living in the city and that folks in the country talk of going to
San Diego next summer to make another try at confronting this
country with the reality of itself. Sally puts Graham to sleep, while
her lover waits and talks with Leisa, just back from living a week
with her mother in Marin. Next door, Michael learns about fixing
cars, and Lorca sleeps while Karen is away for a week observing the
ritual of her 30th birthday, alone in the mountains with Bull, Orson's
father, and a truck she has just learned to drive. Ronnie plays in the
city with her new lover who plays guitar at all the old places I
remember from an earlier time in San Francisco, while Chris and
Jim-from-Santa-Fe walk—because all the cars are broken—to the
University to check the ride boards for a ride for him back to Santa
Fe. Upstairs, Sky studies for her Masters Degree, while Debbie,
her daughter, sleeps or watches TV.

A quiet night in the commune. Earlier, after dinner (as Graham
and Irena from down the street play with the tape recorder), we
talked of children and acid and making love, experiences of the
recent past that have freaked us out. We flash during the conversa-

tion that what we are talking about might be important for the drug study that we are all working on to get money, since we had just found out today that we have to do five group interviews about drug experiences. But the media co-opts the conversation, so Graham and Irena sing the ABC song and we have coffee and some cigarettes and talk about what to do when Graham asks Chris to take her pants off, being particularly conscious of our own sexual difficulties and from where they came.

Chris comes in—surprise! For we are apart after living together this past year—and takes my recorder and instruction book next door and puts water on for me to have coffee. I come to the kitchen. It's late, 12:30. Richard is fixing a peanut butter, banana, and mayonnaise sandwich, an Alabama special, he calls it. I fix a hot dog to go with my coffee. My weight matters not when I am trying to write, rationalize I. I fix coffee in a 39c cup with boiling water from the kettle that was from Chris' home with her former husband, stir it with a spoon lifted from TWA and protect my hand from the heat of the stove with a crocheted potholder made by Chris' grandmother, now partially paralyzed with a stroke in a hospital in Oklahoma. I flash on all of that in an instant and decide to include it now as I sit writing in the kitchen as Richard reads what I have written so far.

I have this strange sense of history, increased by acid and other perceptions of how old the struggle is that we are going through. But what to do with it? Write, says my mind sometimes, for we are a vanguard and our struggle is relevant for all the people. Bullshit, says my mind other times, for there is an inifinite gap between my experience and that of every other person, and we have not the technology to build bridges. Tools—maybe: Analysis, Freud, Jung, Acid, Yoga, Meditation, Sexuality, Rolfing, Gay Liberation, Primal Therapy, Sufi. Lenses all to look at patterns of culture, but viewed together as we are trying now to do, with a new synthesis as goal— difficult, maybe impossible, however. Embarked as we are on a journey as old as our consciousness and as young as the newest amongst us.

Click—snapshot. For those of you who know us, a look at our commune group as we appear on a typical—I hesitate to say normal —night. For those of you who don't, I feel like that was a quick look through the lens of my words. Now to be responsible I ought to give you the background to hold that brief picture up against.

We think of ourselves as a family. This place is three years old, first conceived of as an "alternative learning place" in an essay written by Michael as part of a strategy to attempt to give direction to what was then called rather smugly the "educational reform movement.'' Four of us have been here the entire three years, others have drifted in and out, and our newest member has been with us since last August. We live in three adjoining houses, pay rent in common and buy food mostly together. Between us there are four kitchens and five baths, and while we have three or four meals a week in common, there is a concern here for private space such that each person has his or her own room, including the children, and we live together and yet privately at the same time.

At the moment there is one married couple amongst us and they have a child a year and a half old. Somewhat proudly I add that they are not legally married in the eyes of the state but were married in an elaborate three-day ritual participated in by most of us and a thousand others nearly three years ago. The rest of us, now, are single, although several of us have lived as couples here and in other places. Two others of us have been married and there are two other children aged 5 and 12 living here now. We have one television set, six cars, mostly broken, five stereos, two dogs, four cats, two bicycles, and many lovers. Most of us have been to college, from an almost Ph.D. to one day. The three biggest issues that I guess we spend most of our time working on in one way or another are sex, work, and children, not necessarily in that order.

Sex

With the exception of the children, and even there I am not sure, none of us is a virgin. All of us have had significant interpersonal relationships, and most of us have very active sex lives. One of us is actively gay, and many of us are in the process of confronting our bisexuality. Several couples live here although at this moment almost everyone is living separately. Sexuality is a topic that we spend a great amount of time talking about. Many of us have worked with it in some fashion, in groups, in therapy, and in respect to what is popularly called men's and women's and gay liberation. While many of us have been each other's lover over the course of three years, that has mostly been confined to various couple relationships and almost none of those has gone on simultaneously. Serial monogamy has been the norm here up to this time. The sexual energy level here is high as befits our age group, and perhaps half of the people who now live here together came together because they were lovers with someone who lived here. We never have had any group sex although there has been some talk. We are open and extremely frank with each other in respect to sexual matters. Most of us know each other's lovers as friends, and again perhaps 50 percent of our relationships with other people have some sexual connection or implication. It has not been easy, and there is as much personal pain as there is personal pleasure around sexual relationships here, particularly between the couples/noncouples. Each of us is struggling with his or her identity, and sexual identity plays a large part in that struggle. For most of the couples, separation has come as a response to issues like dependence and domination, sometimes related to work and other times related to personal space/time difficulties. All of us are in similar spaces relating to sex, and in many ways sex is the issue where we come the closest to unanimity in our ways of dealing with it.

Work

From the beginning of this place, work has been a significant issue that we struggle with. For a long time we tried to find some common work we would all do together. At first, it was "educational reform," and we tried to assemble a group of people of similar interests such that local and statewide organizing would be possible. Then, we thought of ourselves as a group of people with varying skills, who could on occasion work on projects together. Neither of those models worked very well. For a time nearly nobody here worked, except at staying alive. Later we went through times of people doing individual work to get money. This work ranged from manual labor to topless dancing and included some people still working in politically-oriented work. We were unable to do much work collectively during any of this time, and money was for the most part treated as individual income to be spent by individuals. Recently, we have decided to try and work together although that does not yet include everyone who lives here. We are presently working on a project to study "drug use in the counter-culture," and while individual salary allotments are made with the money from that project, gradually people are coming to share their income and resources freely. It has always been a struggle for us to pay rent, which is $600 a month, but there has always been a free exchange of money on a "loan" basis. Now the need to loan or borrow money is falling away, and we are starting to look at both our income and expenses as a collective problem. We have come, in this process, to begin to drop distinctions between work and life though at different paces for different people. While few people here have detailed visions of their life's work, many have been deeply involved in specialized work that commanded professional wages and salaries. All of us have been unhappy and most have left those fields they may have been trained in. That collection of skills remains, and we are in the process of finding new ways to make those skills useful collectively and to move toward a greater synthesis of work and play and life.

Children

There are three now and likely to be more. They have made a great difference in all of our lives. We watched, directly and indirectly, through pictures, the birth of the youngest, Lorca. All of the mothers live their lives separately rather than being totally devoted to their children, though in varying degrees. We struggle with the issues around collective parenthood. Mothers want time alone without their children, and collectively we are finding ways to make that happen. Responsibility for meals is shared, and child care happens when needed, sometimes grudgingly. Several parents near us share responsibility for a "playgroup" so some days there are three more children here. Generally, we try to relate to the children as real, if slightly smaller, people with the same rights and responsibilities individually and collectively as we all try to have for each other. We are conscious of adult chauvinism. We are all learning, sometimes very deliberately, from each other. Having children around makes us all conscious of our own childhood, how we were reared with so many of our parents' expectations and hangups embedded deeply within us. Of late, this has enabled many of us to have significant conversations with our own parents in respect to what they did with us at various stages of our development. We are very aware of how quickly children learn from our examples and are both cautious and playful as a result. We are free with our bodies and spend a fair amount of time without clothes inside our home.

Children and how they are perceived and treated is a two-way problem. Sally and Karen each talk of feeling some guilt asking others to take care of Graham and Lorca, while the rest of us feel some guilt at not doing more to share the job of childcare. Sally and Karen need to feel more comfortable in asking others to help out, and others of us have to learn to offer more of ourselves without waiting to be asked. Children add to the atmosphere around here. People talk of them giving feelings of permanence and stability to this place and to us as a group of people, particularly as we all grow to have relationships with the children. Children are also seen as part of the work we do together. The decision to have more children here (one has been with us from the beginning) relates to our process of decision-making. There is no central authority. Decisions that are made are made collectively, usually by consensus in house meetings that sometimes stretch on for hours. There has been, on occasion, much conflict between individuals, some of it directly related to child-bearing practices. The lack of any central authority, except for the entire group itself, for everyone including the children (although parents still play major authority roles with their children), makes for difficult but also exciting patterns of dealing with problems of authority and authority figures. It has been difficult for all of us to adapt to a model of consensus conflict resolution. There is something childlike about all of us. We like to play and are trying to learn how to support each other as we struggle to *be* in ways that are spontaneous and creative. Most people here still see themselves as learners and are still trying to grow. Our relationship to children reflects these inclinations.

· At some point all of our concerns over work, sex, and children merge. There is great stress here on the creative, both in a personal and group sense. In the complex, there is a darkroom and potter's studio. Many work at crafts, and at least one person earns a living through jewelry-making. Work roles are flexible, everyone does the dishes, men cook as much or more than women, women fix cars and handle money. We all take care of children and see it as work.

  Change happens here. People see themselves as learners and everything we do is related to working and growing and changing, not without stability, but with a dedicated deliberateness. We are starting to be able to make plans for the future after many attempts and many shattered individual expectations. That is important and is an example of our decision-making, authority, and learning. We have come from a place where we all tried to fit each other into our personal view and expectations of the future. We have been unable to create unanimity around a single vision of future planning, in part because up to this time all of those visions tended to be designed around an individual or a couple. Now we are trying to create as a group a vision of our future that we can all relate to, make individual plans around, and move toward cooperatively, aware both of our group responsibility and our responsibilities as individuals. For some time, we have all had visions of having land some place, sometime, if for no other reason than that it makes more economic sense than to spend as much as we do renting places to live. Previously, we mostly thought of how each of us might move toward buying land, but now, having discovered that that is a common interest of so many of us, we are finding ways to view that process collectively, which has implications in all of the areas with which we concern ourselves. The feeling of permanence that the children bring, our moving toward income sharing, our increasing ability to work together, and our molding of group visions of the future, all come together in thinking about buying land. This allows us to see how far we have come and how far we have to go as a group.

There is a sign on the wall of the kitchen of the largest house: "Mommy, teach me how not to be afraid." Graham said it one night as we sat around the table after dinner, and Jared made a sign of it and put it on the wall in a process that is somewhat of a ritual around here. Each of us is saying that to ourselves and to each other. Does that make us an "Alternative to the Family?" I don't know. I know we are different and yet the product of the culture we grew up in. We have reached the point of being on our own, growing independently and learning to nurture ourselves. The implications for the future are potentially significant. Greater communal living in alternatives to the conventional family structure implies great changes in child rearing, sexual roles and attitudes, work roles, distribution of economic resources, private property, and authority relationship in the society as a whole. Changing those values would have a great effect on American culture as it exists today. The future is unclear, but change does seem to be in the air, and we are learning how not to be afraid each day.

28. Higher Learning in the Ignorant Society*

Michael Marien

If we are to survive as a viable global community with some degree of genuine democratic control, we must begin to consider seriously the learning needs of all age groups. And with some rough approximation of these needs, we can better appreciate the emerging patterns of where and how we shall learn.

There is a widespread assumption that we Americans are well-educated and well-informed. No nation in history has ever had such a high proportion of college graduates, and there is a massive distribution of knowledge through television, paperback books, information banks, telecopiers, conventions, etc. Thus, it is widely felt that Americans today are better informed than in the past, and this complacent view of the present is complemented by the image of a leisure society of the future, where everyone will play at the liberal arts.

A strongly opposing viewpoint is offered here: I believe that our learning needs are rapidly outdistancing our attainments, and that we are becoming increasingly an ignorant society where our failure to obtain necessary learning is becoming a threat to national—or even global—survival.

How can ignorance be increasing in the midst of more formal education and better communications?

1. As our society becomes more complex, the minimum skills necessary continue to rise. Bare literacy no longer suffices. We now require an increasingly higher level of literacy. In the future the standards of multi-media literacy and/or social literacy undoubtedly will rise higher. By raising standards, we define increasing proportions of our population as ignorant, and therefore as a society we become increasingly ignorant.

---

*Reprinted with permission from THE FUTURIST, April 1972.

2. The ignorance of our educated elite is also increasing. Despite the growth of our knowledge, the problems that we face appear to be outstripping our capacity to understand them. Our structure of knowlege is still largely fragmented into the traditional non-problem-oriented academic disciplines. More knowledge is not necessarily better knowledge, or to cite an advertisement for a major news-magazine, "Today you can be over-informed without being well-informed." Indeed, one might say that we increasingly suffer from mind pollution. New knowledge does not necessarily alleviate our ignorance, but may increase our ignorance by contradicting that which had been "known" or by pointing out further areas of ignorance.

3. As our society changes, knowledge acquired at other times and for other purposes becomes obsolete. We still employ the antedilu-vian figure of speech that one becomes educated by graduating from a purportedly educating institution, when, at best, one may thus be equipped for a lifetime of necessary learning and unlearning. As Peter Drucker points out, we are increasingly a knowledge society, in which, by the end of the 1970s, half of the labor force will be somehow involved in the production and distribution of knowledge. But this does not necessarily make us more knowledgeable, or bet-ter equipped to deal with the world macroproblem of population, ecology, governance, etc., as described by Willis Harman and his associates at the Stanford Research Institute's Educational Policy Research Center.

Greatest Need Is Among Post-School Population

The necessary adaption of our ignorant society involves improve-ment in the quality and distribution of our knowledge, as well as the capacity of our population to utilize large quantities of conflicting and changing information in our roles as workers, citizens, parents, and individuals. We cannot attain a desirable society with incompe-tent manual and mental workers, ill-informed citizens, primitive parents and their turned-off children, and future-shocked individu-als. More learning and different learning will be necessary not only for the young, but especially for the old. Indeed, our most important priorities for learning are not pre-school populations—where inter-ventions may be dramatic but nevertheless have a long term payoff —but among post-school populations that will continue to have a major influence in shaping our future during the turbulent decades ahead.

Three Paths to New Educational Institutions

Despite the ignorance that characterizes our era, our age-graded institutions of higher education face a serious financial crisis that may even reduce the present levels of service. The financial crisis has spurred a search for new institutions to promote higher learning, not only to provide a desirable array of options for the young, but— far more important—to handle the largely unacknowledged learning needs of the old. This search follows three interrelated paths: (1) new forms of learning sponsored by existing institutions, (2) new institutions that may compete with the old, and (3) new ways of recognizing, if not legitimatizing, other formal and informal learning.

Path One: Extensions of Present Institutions

The contemporary university now is extending itself in a variety of ways. The university extends itself upward to graduate and post-doctoral study, and downward to junior colleges and to high schools through various curriculum projects launched by the various academic disciplines. The other extensions are far less common but of far greater importance in ministering to an ignorant society. Several dozen institutions conduct campus-abroad programs (although we have yet to see a foreign university with a U.S. campus). A few institutions conduct courses on the premises of local employers, and many colleges broadcast courses on television. So far there has been little effort in the U.S. to extend degree-credit services to the older age groups. The University of London has offered an adult degree program for many years, and similar programs are well-established in Australia and Russia. In the U.S., adult degree programs are offered by 18 institutions, but such programs could hardly be considered widespread.

Legitimating off-campus learning experiences is a final dimension of institutional extension. Dozens—or perhaps hundreds—of campuses now give credit for such activities as tutoring poor children or participating in a political campaign. Academic credit is perfectly reasonable insofar as such activities enhance individual development and relate the academy to the real world, but the practice raises serious questions about equity in granting degree-credit for real-life experience. Is it proper for the university to collect tuition fees for a "course" toward which the university itself contributed almost nothing? Is it proper to equate a person who acquired the knowledge equivalent of a college education while he was gainfully employed with another who did without such earnings so that he could attend a university?

Path Two: Creation of New Institutions

The most dramatic developments of the 1970s will occur in the new multi-campus programs and non-campus organizations.

Multi-campus programs, sponsored by state university systems, or consortiums of institutions, provide a far greater array of resources to learners than does an individual campus. The State University of New York's Empire State College, which opened in September 1971, encourages students to utilize the resources of the entire SUNY system, in various combinations, combined with independent study. New Jersey's Thomas Edison College will parallel the Empire State College. Eight additional states are presently considering external credit plans that will utilize the resources of public institutions to some degree. They are California, Connecticut, Illinois, Maine, Maryland, Massachusetts, Oklahoma and Wisconsin.

The best-known consortium of institutions is the Antioch-based University-Without-Walls, also opened in September 1971, which coordinates local UWW programs at 20 widely differing institutions throughout the United States. Students, ranging in age from 16 to 60, enroll at one campus, but can take courses at any of the cooperating campuses. The students also can study independently and receive credit for various work experiences.

New organizations independent of existing campuses have the greatest potential for profoundly influencing higher learning. These non-campus organizations can be divided into three groups, depending on whether they offer (1) both guidance and degree credit, (2) only courses, or (3) only credit.

Guidance plus Credit. England's Open University, starting in January 1971 with an initial enrollment of 25,000 (and a planned enrollment of 100,000 by 1976), is an entirely new and independent institution, utilizing weekly BBC programs on television and radio, correspondence packages, and the services of 3000 part-time tutors and counselors at 250 study centers throughout the nation. Although presently limited to students aged 21 and over, the British government is increasingly interested in services for the college-age population, because the cost per student in the Open University is about one-third of conventional campus-based services. Litttle wonder, then, that inquiries have come in from more than 100 nations!

In the United States, where education is still organized at the state level, 50 different programs would result in considerable duplication, and proposals for regional cooperation—if not a national system—would surely occur. Already, Alexander M. Mood of the University of California at Irvine has proposed a national "Video University"; Lawrence E. Dennis, provost and director of the Massachusetts State College System, has proposed a University of North America, and the Academy for Educational Development has suggested an International University for Independent Study.

One continental experiment—which may prove to be most significant of all educationally—is already in operation. Campus-Free College (Box 161, Arlington, Mass. 02174) utilizes a network of almost 200 Program Advisors, each one responsible for admissions and the creation of a highly individualized learning program that employs any combination of formal and informal experience. Small private liberal arts colleges not already involved with the University-Without-Walls consortium may come to employ CFC as a supervisor of the non-campus learning of their students, similar to the functions performed for state systems by New York's Empire State College and New Jersey's Thomas Edison College.

Courses Without Credit. Several U.S. organizations that offer no degrees (e.g., Futures Resources and Development, Inc., 49 John St., Southport, Connecticut) are developing course packages that may be used on traditional campuses or by individual students in external degree programs, which may thus be able to save the cost of hiring additional professors.

Credit Without Courses. Just as there now are programs that offer courses but give no credit toward degrees, there are also programs that give credit but do not offer courses. These credit-only programs provide legitimation for designated areas of knowledge that has already been acquired, regardless of where, how, or when. The New York State Education Department's College Proficiency Examination Program has been administering examinations for course credit since 1963. On the national level the College-Level Examination Program, sponsored by the College Entrance Examination Board, was quietly introduced in 1967. In the next two years, both programs expect their workload to be more than double that of 1970 levels. This year, the New York State Regents will offer an

External Degree by examination. The expansion of external courses and examinations will surely be furthered by many of the above-mentioned programs, as well as new credit-only institutions such as the regional examing universities proposed in the first Newman report (or, more formally, the *Report on Higher Education*, published by the U.S. Department of Health, Education and Welfare in Spring 1971; an additional report is due in Spring 1972), the National Baccalaureate Examinations proposed by Bernhardt Lieberman and Deborah Wycoff of the University of Pittsburgh, or the National University proposed by Jack Arbolino of the College-Level Examination Program and John Valley of the Educational Testing Service.

This plethora of proposals, plans and programs will surely change the structure of higher learning in only a few years. But the ultimate shape of higher education remains quite uncertain. State and regional electronic universities may eventually consolidate into national and international universities. Or one or more world universities, offering credit and/or courses, might obviate the neeed for more parochial institutions. Or we may find a wide assortment of electronic universities, perhaps intercontinental universities.

Eventuallly, perhaps, there may be a Global Electronic University, contributing to world harmony, the widespread sharing of knowledge, and equality of opportunity, while competing with conventional institutions on traditional criteria such as cost, choice, and quality of instruction. The idea of a world university is, of course, hardly new; globalist-educator Harold Taylor has estimated that more than a thousand such proposals have been made since World War I. But the fact of a globalizing society and new enabling technology could soon translate this longheld sentiment into reality.

Although profound changes in structure are underway, these changes will not necessarily result in change in the content, or that which is learned. Yet, in the heady rush to create new institutions, this distinction is virtually ignored. Many of the new programs, such as CLEP, merely provide a new means of acquiring credit for the traditional fragmented curriculum. England's Open University has reformed the curriculum into general courses, but learning acquired is nevertheless packaged. It is the nonstandardized programs such as the University-Without-Walls, Empire State College, and most notably Campus-Free College that truly individualize programs and place much—but by no means all—of the determination of "an education"in the hands of the student, thereby encouraging independent learning in the deepest sense. Such programs are amenable to a holistic focus for organizing one's learning—futuristics, general systems, theory, policy science, ecology, etc. Indeed, Campus-Free

College is considering the possibility of offering scholarships for futures studies!

Path Three: Legitimation of Other Kinds of Learning

Up to this point only new extensions and new institutions for what we have traditionally called higher education have been considered. Although "post-secondary education" is often seen as synonymous with higher education, it is more properly used as a generic term for all institutions that facilitate youth and adult learning, whether or not degree credit is involved.

In an ignorant society, we can no longer afford to ignore all the institutions that facilitate serious learning. Stanley Moses, of the Educational Policy Research Center at Syracuse, has estimated that, in 1970, "The Learning Force" in the United States involved 124 million persons, including 64 million students in elementary, secondary, and higher education, and 60 million students in the educational periphery of corporate and military training programs, proprietary schools, anti-poverty programs, correspondence schools, and other adult education programs conducted by service organizations, unions, schools and colleges, etc. Although this estimate is probably high and the real total may only be 10 million or less when viewed in full-time equivalents, there are nevertheless many persons spending many non-credit hours in improving their skills and knowledge so that they may be better workers, citizens, parents, and human beings.

In addition to organized programs, many people engage in self-directed learning projects. Allen Tough, of the Ontario Institute for Studies in Education, has discovered that about 70% of all adult learning projects are planned by the learner himself, while less than 1% of this learning activity is motivated by credit. This independent learning will be particularly enhanced with the advent of the "multiscreen home information center." In the near future, many of us (starting, of course, with the most affluent) will not only have the television screen with an expanded variety of source options, but also a picturephone, a computer terminal, an ultramicrofiche reader, and/or some multipurpose screen. We may soon have instant access to the world's knowledge, although it is uncertain whether we desire this option and whether we are capable of utilizing it.

An ignorant society should promote all forms of constructive learning. And it is a matter of simple justice to bestow credit—if credit is desired—for what one knows regardless of where or how the knowledge is acquired. Thus we are beginning to see mechanisms for promoting academic equity, such as the New York External Degree. But there is a major question as to whether the new credit only programs will acknowledge transdisciplinary learning, or entirely new combinations of learning experiences, or other learning that is equivalent to—but different from—that offered by the traditional academic disciplines.

One approach to promoting equity might be through new degree-granting authority for research institutes and corporation training schools. Even if these activities are not directly legitimated by the authority to grant degrees, they will probably receive greater attention in forthcoming years. If better information becomes available concerning who actually learns what under differing circumstances, the public may well find good investments in non-credited formal education, or in independent learning efforts. The 1971 Newman report (cited earlier) has recommended establishing informal colleges or local learning clinics, with clients obtaining credit (if desired) from a regional examining university.

An ignorant society can no longer afford the mythology of credentials; learning assumes higher priority. This fact is only dimly recognized at present, but it will become more apparent to more people as we increasingly recognize our massive learning needs, and the extent to which our fetish for credentials has inhibited learning. To this end, the College Entrance Examination Board established in 1971 a Commission on Non-Traditional Study, chaired by Samuel Gould, former chancellor of the State University of New York. And the Graduate Record Examinations Board, allied with the Councel of Graduate Schools in the United States, established a Panel on Alternate Approaches to Graduate Education in late 1971.

New Shape of Education in 1980 Will Invalidate Forcasts

The wide variety of proposals and programs listed here are overlapping, complimentary, and competitive. Although the ultimate shape of any single program cannot be outlined, it seems virtually certain that some array of extended programs, electronic universities, and the new credentialing will be apparent to all of us by 1975. By 1980, the new architecture of higher learning will be dramatically different from that which we accept today.

In view of the changes in the structure of education, the traditional projections of staff and enrollments in campus-based institutions will prove totally inaccurate. There will be an entirely new framework of students in traditional and non-traditional programs, engaged in non-credited learning or receiving credit from a variety of sources that may or may not be related to these programs. More-over, the traditional basis of estimating demand for higher education —utilizing the "baby body count" of graduating high school seniors —will become totally obsolete in the era of post-secondary educa-tion. More high school graduates may decide to work first and study later, or try some alternative to the conventional age-graded lock-step. Indeed, the traditional projections of enrollments are not only a misleading estimate of the future, but they also serve to inhibit the necessary invention of new educational approaches (which is, nev-ertheless, taking place.)

The new institutions and new credentials will not necessarily alle-viate the problems of our ignorant society. We may very well find ourselves with a second-rate duplication of the obsolete higher edu-cation that presently exists. The electronic university may become a de-humanized technocratic monster, promoted by legislators as a cheap solution to the financial crisis of publicly-supported campus-es. There might be substantial unemployment of faculty, or a sub-stantial reduction of status for professors shifted from their small but autonomous ponds to become tutorial assistants in an oceanic enterprise where only the superstars can do their thing. Employers may sniff at the new degrees earned merely by examination or through non-campus programs. The new opportunities may give us a sense of overcoming ignorance when in fact we may only be recog-nizing new ways to give credit for fragments of knowledge. Such negative consequences—and many others—should be anticipated and guarded against.

On the other hand, the new institutions and procedures may create a free market for widespread and significant learning. The new learning would release the humanistic potential of many people throughout the world, greatly enhancing the prospects of the humane society that is advocated by so many futurists. Facing genu-ine competition, traditional institutions of higher learning would have to innovate or perish. New flexibility and openness at post-secondary levels would ultimately impact on secondary and elemen-tary levels of education, and would break the mandatory monopoly of public schooling, creating many paths for attaining a high school diploma, or acceptable equivalents. In turn, high schools would increasingly gear their programs to preparing students to utilize fully the entire range of post-secondary opportunities for entire lifetimes of learning.

There is only one negative consequence of a successful emergence of new institutions and crediting procedures. As the strength of these new options grows, we will increasingly face the painful question of what learning is to be valued in our society. But this is a necessary task if we are to cease being an ignorant society.

29. Youth and Jobs: Educational, Vocational, and Mental Health Aspects*

Milton F. Shore

Eric Erikson[1] has clearly formulated the task of adolescent development as that of the formation of psychological identity. It is during adolescence that cognitive development becomes fully mature. What is needed is the organization and integration of all aspects of experience that will aid the person in his adjustment to adult life. Erikson has also delineated the manner in which identity formation is dependent upon the historical, sociocultural, and value systems of a society at a given time. One aspect of identity formation noted by many students of adolescence is that of beginning to delineate a vocational direction.

Work plays an important role in the daily life of adults. However, it is during the adolescent period that major decisions are made with regard to work; its nature, its quality, and its relevance to the self-image of adults. It is during the adolescent phase that the young person is clearly exposed to the values inherent in the society with regard to occupations and vocations. These values in turn are dependent upon the current state of technological and historical development in a given culture. For example, in the early part of the century it was important for young people to be protected from exploitation. In order to protect them, child labor laws were passed. But these laws are currently being reevaluated for in some ways they have been found to prevent young people who should work from being employed. Over the last few decades, as technology has expanded and automation has increased, the meanings of many jobs have changed. Work is no longer within the family context but takes place in communities away from home. More and more young people are unaware of the details of their parents' occupation or what

---

*This paper was written for the Task Force on Work in America set up by the Secretary of the Department of Health, Education, and Welfare, Washington, D.C. and will also be published in the *Journal of Youth and Adolescence*.

various jobs require. More recently there has been an increase in both parents working, with a large campaign under way for the establishment of day care centers. Technological change has also resulted in large unemployment for young people, especially for youth from minority groups.

In light of all of these changes in the employment area, there has been a need to reevaluate the relevance of education to the work world in the United States. An in-depth study is currently being done on a grant from the National Institute of Mental Health on the meaning of work for young people, in an effort to determine the changing attitudes toward work. Newman,[2] in a report to the Federal Government, has suggested new directions for work-study programs in university settings. Coleman[3] has recommended that schools teach basic skills, but that more of the education beyond the basic skills be in the community and in work settings.

The research on the psychological aspects of employment has also been markedly influenced by social values. Most of the research has focused on how an individual chooses an occupational role and the motives related to these vocational choices. Much research has been reported on the entrance to the labor market and some of the ways by which one's employability is increased or decreased (i.e., manpower studies). Only rarely has the reverse problem been studied, that is, the importance of the work experience as a factor in the personality growth and development of the adolescent. One example highlights the difference in approach: Job changes are often viewed as an example of personal instability. However, Kohen and Parnes,[4] in a recent research study, have shown that job changes, on the contrary, are frequently associated with rising status and rising income. A job change may indeed be a necessary step in the personal development of an individual if he is highly motivated. It appears that what has happened is that often we are more interested in the relationship of the individual to the job and keeping the person on the job than we are in the relationship of the job to the individual and his personal growth.

The Adolescent and Work

General Issues

The Joint Commission on the Mental Health of Children[5] (set up by congressional mandate) recognized the mental health aspects of work for adolescents. In a chapter entitled "Employment Problems and Issues Related to the Mental Health of Children and Youth," they noted the dearth of material in the area, and recommended that more time and effort be put into exploring in detail the mental health aspects of employment in young people. Much of the work done up to now has been haphazard and uncoordinated. There have been some work programs for the disadvantaged, some vocational training programs in high schools (often for lower class youth only), a few work-study programs, and very few apprenticeship programs. Most of these work programs have been isolated, poorly planned, limited in number, and available to only certain groups. Only a few of these programs have been carefully and systematically evaluated.

Review of Studies

As stated above, there have been many studies on the effect of social class, race, and education on job career patterns in youth. Likewise, the psychological elements that go into job satisfaction, the personality factors that affect performance on the job, and the personality variables related to vocational choice have all been studied. These areas have been extensively reviewed in Borow.[6] But surprisingly little has been done on the influence of the work experience itself on personality development in young people. Those studies that have been done on the effect of employment on psychological development fall into two general areas: the naturalistic study and the therapeutic study.

In the naturalistic study no effort is made to bring about changes in behavior. Young people who are employed are observed and studied, formally or informally; this is usually done over a period of time in order to determine how their personalities change as a result of the work experience.

The second methodology systematically attempts to bring about change and alter the adjustment of individuals. In this therapeutic approach, the aim is not only to facilitate adjustment to work, but also to influence the individual's total life so as to affect his relationships to others outside his area of employment. Examples in this area include the efforts to assist disadvantaged youth in overcoming the deep personal scars left by the experience of poverty. One can also include the work programs for delinquent youth which aim to bring about behavioral changes in areas other than employment per se. The studies in the two areas, naturalisitic and therapeutic, will now be discussed.

Naturalistic Studies. Engel, *et al.*, in an exploratory study, used clinical interviewing techniques and personality tests to investigate some of the dimensions of a group of boys, 8 to 14 years of age, from different socioeconomic levels who were working at a variety of jobs in a suburb outside of Boston. Five areas, some of which were directly related to work, and some of which were not, were explored: (1) the nature and extent of commitment to work (work-mindedness) as related to a sense of identity; (2) the   activity-passivity dimension; (3) the interests and future vocational plans of these young people and how these plans were conceptualized in terms of the continuity between past and present (occupational orientation); (4) time dimension in the future (concept of life span); and (5) relationship with adults. The authors found that those elements least related to specific occupational choices were the ones that seemed more highly advanced in these youth. It should be remembered that these were preadolescent and early adolescent boys, a time when specific vocational directions would not be expected. The investigators were impressed by the maturity of these boys, and particularly by their way of handling adults. They felt that these boys were more active in their orientation than one would expect of boys their age. Unfortunately, there was no control group in this study. It is possible that the boys who were involved in work were a self-selected group, that is, the characteristics that were found were those that may have been the ones that led them to seek employment in the first place rather than the results of the work experience itself.

Kohen and Parnes, *op. cit.*, on contract to the United States Department of Labor, have undertaken a longitudinal study of 4300 young men of different racial and economic backgrounds, 14 to 24 years of age, to determine those factors that are most important in their choice of career direction, either with regard to school or within the labor market. Included in the interviews were two personality dimensions—aspiration level and internal-external control (whether the person feels himself a victim of fate, or able to bring about changes in the external world). The authors reported that those youths who had work experience had greater and more realistic aspiration levels than those who remained in school. The findings on internal-external control have not as yet been analyzed.

There have been a variety of situations where naturalistic studies would have been possible, but unfortunately were not systematically undertaken. However, observations, case studies, and anecdotal material reveal many changes in youth as a result of work experience. It is noted, for example, in the Newman Report, *op. cit.*, that interest and persistence appeared greater in those youth who participated in work-study programs in universities. Many educators reported that those GIs and Peace Corps members who returned to school after their work experience felt a greater sense of purpose, a greater enjoyment of studies, greater appreciation of the relevance of studying, improved ability to make a career choice, and much less fear of the larger society.

Currently, youth are involved in a variety of youth-initiated and youth-run projects. They are setting up their own health services. They are part of efforts to develop alternatives to public school education. They are active in new mental health service delivery systems such as Hot Lines and free clinics. They are doing their own research and evaluation. It would be valuable to study the effects of the involvement of these youth in these various work activities on their identity formation during adolescence.

Therapeutic Studies. The aim of a therapeutic program is to alter current adjustment patterns and develop ways for the individual to make a better social and personal adjustment. This has been observed in two types of therapeutic work programs, those that have consciously attempted to bring about specific changes in youth through employment and have evaluated to see whether these changes have indeed occurred, and those programs where the interventions were not related to employment, but had some other purpose such as research, and where changes in the adjustment patterns of youth were found to occur.

The most massive planned recent intervention program using employment as a tool to bring about change is the national effort to reverse the destructive effects of poverty, a condition which has generally been seen as a major cause of personal, social, and physical problems. Three large-scale Federally-funded programs related to employment have been developed for the poor: the New Careers Program, the National Job Corps, and the Neighborhood Youth Corps.

New Careers Programs are efforts to train paraprofessionals in many areas, especially as technicians, associates, aides, human service workers, etc. These programs, some of which are affiliated with junior colleges or community colleges, others of which have their own job training and career ladders, not only attempt to aid the person in his employment, but also help with the person's over-all adjustment.* One of the dangers in such programs is that they easily

---

* Not all New Careers Programs are for low socieconomic groups. Some have been developed from middle-class groups, especially for women who are returning to the job market.

can become self-selective, that is, those young people who are willing and able to profit from the employment opportunities offered with a minimum amount of ancillary services, such as remedial education or counseling, continue in the program, while the youths who do not want these services often drop out. Thus, there will remain a core group of "unreachable youth" who continue to be community problems.

There are some case studies of New Careers Programs. Grant and Grant[8] have noted "there have been increased feelings of competence and self-worth as a result of program participation, particularly as participants have shifted from welfare status to earning some money. Attention is also often given to more external manifestations of role changes, shifts in dress, speech, work habits and attitudes. These have not been systematically studied, nor the experiences on the job that lead to them nor the relation to actual job performance (p. 29)."

In contrast to the New Careers Program, the National Job Corps was aimed specifically toward high-risk disadvantaged young men and women ages 14 to 22, who were unemployed and out of school. Twenty-five percent of the 35,000 enrollees in the Job Corps had a past history of antisocial behavior. Counseling, education , and job training were integrated into the program. The mental health components of the Job Corps Program have been described by Scherl and Macht.[9] Although there is no hard data, general evidence suggests that the program was successful in about 35% of the cases, that is, in returning to his original community, a trainee deemed successful showed improvement in general adjustment, as well as in the ability to handle future employment. Considering the fact that this was a group of extremely high-risk individuals and that the programs varied greatly, such change appears significant.

The Neighborhood Youth Corps did not take children away from the local communities. Instead, youth were given opportunities for work experience and education aimed toward greater employability in their local areas. Youth in this program were 14 to 21 years of age, and the length of participation in the program was six months. Participation was entirely voluntary. The goal was, after the six-month period, for the individual to be able to successfully find employment on his own. Unlike the Job Corps, which was only informally evaluated, systematic efforts have been made to more carefully study the effect of employment on Neighborhood Youth Corps young people and their personality functioning. Scales have been developed both for evaluating areas relevant to work assessment and for areas related to general psychological functioning. For example, the social research group of George Washington University[10,11] has been interested in studying changes in impulse control, internal-external control, achievement motivation, and optimism and self-confidence. In addition, vocational orientation, skills in seeking and maintaining employment, changes in self-esteem, control of hostility, job motivation, and practical reasoning have also been assessed. On the basis of preliminary findings, efforts have been made to make the programs more individually oriented. Four subgroups of employees have been identified, each requiring different strategies—the disadvantaged graduate, the adverse-situation individual, the rebel, and the low-self-esteemed person. The program evaluations have led to recommendations for program changes that would more adequately integrate work experience, remedial education, and counseling over longer periods of time and in creative and innovative ways. One such recommendation, for example, was that the counselor should be knowledgeable not only about mental health, but also about educational training, remedial resources, and job opportunities.

Another area of therapeutic intervention through jobs are the efforts specifically to deal with antisocial young people. Although the data are primarily anecdoctal, in a community where a psychologist was employing young people as research assistants in a study of adolescents, the police reported significant reduction in antisocial behavior.[12] Since reported antisocial behavior is a function of police response to behaviors that might be provocative in nature, a change in the feelings of the police themselves may have brought about reduction in reported crimes.

The Mobilization for Youth Program in New York, oriented toward reducing delinquency through changing the opportunity structure within a community, found that employing some antisocial youth as tutors ("homework helpers") for younger children in academic subjects not only reduced the antisocial behavior of the tutor, but also resulted in improvement in the tutor's academic skills. This program has spread to many other settings.[13]

Massimo and Shore[14] developed a comprehensive vocationally-oriented psychotherapeutic program for suburban adolescent boys who had dropped out of school and who had long histories of antisocial behavior. Remedial education, counseling, and job placement were an integral part of the program which was totally administered and carried out by one person. Each part of the multidimensional program was set up to meet the boys' specific individual needs. Through using work as an entree for all the other services, the aim was to bring about significant changes in personality, especially those personality dimensions that seemed most closely associated with antisocial behavior. The program was very carefully evaluated. Significant changes were found in all personality dimensions (feelings about oneself, control of aggression, and attitude toward authority) after ten months of intensive work in the program. The personality changes were highly correlated with major improvement in academic achievement and overt behavior. Two to five years after treatment, the treated group continued to improve, showing significantly better marital adjustment and general social adjustment, as well as a significant better employment record.[15]

Psychological Effects of Work

The author, in a previous publication, [16] attempted to delineate those dimensions of personality functioning that might be affected by work experience in the adolescent in relation to his developing identity. These were: (1) success on the job can help build self-esteem; (2) money obtained on the job helps the adolescent to disengage himself from his parents and become independent and interact more with his peer group; (3) employment experience can help increase the adolescent's acquaintance with different types of work before he decides on a vocational choice; (4) work opportunities can offer a chance to deal with and identify with adults; (5) activity on the job may serve to drain off many of the excess energies of adolescents into constructive channels; (6) a job may help the formation of sexual identity and the resolution of many sexual concerns of the adolescent; (7) a job can help test out new skills against reality and permit the assumption of responsibility; and (8) a job can permit the adolescent to be in an active rather than a passive role.

Summary and Conclusions

Although much has been written about the personality factors in job choice, little has been done in systematically investigating the effect of work experience on adolescent development. Instead, the social climate has been aimed more toward keeping young people out of the job market and maintaining them in school, even though schools may offer them very little. The few studies that have been reported seem oriented primarily around high-risk groups (the culturally disadvantaged or the antisocial youth), rather than studying how employment relates to normal development. From those studies that have been reported, however, certain generalizations can be drawn: (1) Work experience can play an integral part in the personality development of the individual in areas other than those specifically related to employability and career choice. (There have been some suggestions that work experience could even be introduced as early as at the elementary school level.) (2) In adolescents the experiential level is a major one, so that work becomes meaningful not only in terms of anticipation of future employment, but in terms of everyday activities. Working at these everyday activities appears to be an important element in aiding identity formation. The fostering of adult role models and learning through identification is significant. (3) Employment of adolescents should be meaningful and challenging. There must be a direction, a purpose, and a goal to the work. Research has found that the closer the adolescent is to a real-life experience, the more effective the experience is in bringing about positive attitudinal changes.[17] (4) The work experience should as much as possible be relevant to the individual's own psychological development. Only when the adolescent is personally involved is he able to grow and work out his unique identity. (5) There should be a diversity of work choices. The adolescent should be able to shift jobs and experience a variety of employment opportunities without having to make a final choice early. A wide range of possible experiences would reflect the diverse interests of many young people. (6) The work must be compensated. The adolescent should not be forced into volunteer activities unless he chooses to participate in them. Greater opportunities for financial remuneration should be developed, since money in our society is so closely associated with self-worth. (7) Any work programs for adolescents must be multidimensional and include remedial education and opportunities for counseling, as well as job placement, all integrated and closely tied together in a well-planned, well-coordinated program.

References

1. Erikson, E. Growth and crises of the healthy personality on identity and the life cycle. *Psych. Issues,* # I, 1, 1959, pp. 50-101
2. Newman, F., *et al. Report on higher education.* March, 1971, U.S. Dept. of Health, Education, and Welfare, United States Government Printing Office.

3. Coleman, J. S. *How do the young become adults?* Center for Social Organization of Schools, Report #130, May, 1972, Baltimore, Maryland.
4. Kohen, A. I., and Parnes, H.S. *Career thresholds.* Center for Human Resource Research, Ohio State University, Columbus, Ohio, Vol. III, June, 1971.
5. Joint Commission on Mental Health of Children. *Crisis in child mental health: Challenge for the 1970's.* Harper and Row, New York, 1970.
6. Borow, H. Development of Occupational motives and roles. In: *Review of child development research.* L.S. Hoffman and M. C. Hoffman (Eds.). Russell Sage Foundation, New York, 1966, pp. 373-422.
7. Engel, M., Marsden, G., and Woodaman, S. Children who work and the concept of life style. Psychiatry, Vol. 30, 4, Nov. 1967, pp. 392-404.
8. Grant, D., and Grant, J. *Evaluation of new careers programs.* Unpublished paper, Social Action Research Center, Oakland, California.
9. Scherl, D. J., and Macht, L. B. An examination of the relevance for mental health of selected anti-poverty programs for children and youth. *Community Mental Health Journal,* in press.
10. Walther, R. H. *The measurement of work relevant attitudes.* Final report, U.S. Department of Labor Contract #41-7-004-09, October, 1970.
11. Walther, R. H., *et al. A proposed model for urban out-of-school Neighborhood Youth Corps Programs.* Manpower Research Projects, George Washington University, 1969.
12. Roemer, D. V. Adolescent peer group formation in two Negro neighborhoods. Unpublished Ph.D. dissertation, Harvard University, November, 1968.
13. Gartner, A., Kohler, M., and Riessman, F. *Children teach children. Harper and Row, 1971.*
14. Massimo, J. L., and Shore, M. F. A comprehensive, vocationally oriented psychotherapeutic program for delinquent boys. *Amer. Journal of Orthopsychiatry, Vol. XXXIII, No. 4, July, 1963.*
15. Shore, M. F., and Massimo, J. L. Five years later: A followup study of comprehensive vocationally oriented psychotherapy. *Amer. Journal of Orthopsychiatry,* Vol. 39, No. 5, October, 1969.
16. Shore, M. F., and Massimo, J. Employment as a therapeutic tool with adolescent delinquent boys. *Rehab. Counsel. Bul.*, 1965, 9, pp.1-5
17. Walther, R. H. *Strategies for helping disadvantaged groups.* Paper for International Conference on Trends in Industrial and Labor Relations, Tel Aviv, Israel, January, 1972.

30. Identity Group Psychotherapy with Adolescents*

Arnold W. Rachman

The aim of this article is to demonstrate the clinical efficacy of employing group psychotherapy in treating the adolescent identity crisis. The adolescent period of human development can be viewed as one of the most crucial psychological periods in the human life cycle. Developmentally, adolescence is the rallying point or bridge between childhood and adulthood. As childhood is the foundation upon which adolescence rests, adolescence is the foundation of adulthood. Erik H. Erikson's theory of human growth and development pays significant tribute to this crucial role of adolescence and provides a unifying concept of ego identity, which well serves as the basis for a theory of group therapy for dealing with the adolescent identity crisis (Erikson, 1950, 1959, 1968).

Historically, individual psychotherapy has been considered the treatment of choice with adolescents. This discussion challenges the traditional notion, by suggesting that group psychotherapy is the most meaningful therapy for adolescents in the midst of an identity crisis. Individual psychotherapy is considered an adjunct therapy to be used to supplement group sessions, as needed.

Although this article presents clinical material illustrating the actual conduct of adolescent group therapy dealing with the identity crisis, the beginning sections focus on a theoretical foundation for such clinical practice. A meaningful and relevant theory is indispensible to, and cannot be divorced from, meaningful and relevant clinical practice. In fact, without such an underpinning, clinical practice with adolescents can be a haphazard, disorganized, difficult, and confusing enterprise. The practitioner of adolescent psychotherapy has a particular mandate to be organized, consistent, and clear in his method, technique, and mode of therapeutic inter-

---

*This paper is an expanded and revised version of a previous publication, "Group Psychology in Treating the Adolescent Identity Crisis." *Int. J. Child Psychother.* Vol. 1, January, 1972.

vention. Adolescents need direction, organization, consistency, and clarity in their attempts at identity crisis resolution. The field of adolescent group psychotherapy also demands a comprehensive and meaningful theory that relates to the essential psychological conflict of adolescents, while providing a contemporary rationale for clinical practice. Much practice of group psychotherapy with adolescents has relied on a model of either child or adult group therapy for its concepts, practices, and process.

Concept of Ego Identity

The major theoretical construct in this frame of reference is the concept of ego identity as first described and elaborated by Erikson (1950, 1959, 1968). There are several basic rationales for relying on the concept of ego identity for adolescent psychotherapy:

1. The successful resolution of the identity crisis of adolescence (ego identity vs. identity confusion) is the major intrapsychic and interpersonal conflict of adolescent development.
2. The conceptualization of the identity crisis identifies a universal psychological phenomenon of adolescence which transcends culture, society, and historical era.
3. Ego identity is the major organizing principle of the ego's functioning. It is the mechanism by which the individual maintains a continuity in his personality and a continuity of relatedness to significant others.
4. A developing sense of ego identity in adolescence prepares the individual for adulthood and can provide him with the crucial capacity for an intimate relationship with a sex and love partner. The person who has not adequately solved his identity problem during adolescence will be faced with its recurrent ghost throughout his adult life. Resolution of the identity crisis can be postponed, but it cannot be denied.
5. Contemporary adolescents are going through a protracted identity crisis period, which has become a distinguishing feature of our age. Clinicians have been noting an increase in the psychological disorder known as "existential neurosis" or "borderline schizophrenic reaction." This disorder is a severe form of an identity crisis, with the negative stage of the crisis-identity-confusion predominating.
6. Contemporary society is characterized by certain negative psychosocial forces which are retarding ego identity development in our youth. Two such problems are adolescent drug

abuse and the identity crisis of the American family (Rachman, 1973).

The Adolescent Identity Crisis:
Ego Identity vs. Identity Confusion

Ego Identity. Ego identity has three distinct aspects: an intrapsychic or personal identity, and interpersonal or group identity, and an ideological or philosophical identity.

The intrapsychic aspect of ego identity refers to an adequate sense of oneself as a separate, functioning, positive, meaningful person with a sense of destiny and goal directedness. Colloquially speaking, ego identity is when:

> You know who you are and where it's at; where you want to go and how you're going to get there. And, inside, somewhere in the middle of you, you have a good feeling about yourself, and no one can take it away from you.

Identity formation is the process of discovering who one is as a person, what one's distinct, peculiar, idiosyncratic assets and liabilities are. This identity search can be exemplified in a creative period of self-discovery, as in George Bernard Shaw's young adult withdrawal from society (Erikson, 1959) or in a protracted, severe identity crisis exemplified by Martin Luther's agonizing young adulthood (Erikson, 1958).

The basic implication for psychotherapy as it concerns the sense of personal identity is the individual's need to have a period of creative retreat in the service of self-exploration. The social structures that reinforce withdrawal and introspection in our culture have been changing; for example, college campuses are no longer the retreats and ivory towers they once were. Opportunities for "retreats of self-actualization" are becoming scarcer for our youth. Perhaps this is why Eastern philosophy, with its focus on meditation and self-absorption, have much appeal to contemporary youth. Psychotherapy may also become a significant social structure, in which young people can have an opportunity for creative withdrawal in the service of personal identity formation.

Identity formation has the implicit notion of self-actualization, the individual's capacity and motivation for becoming what he is as a person. As such, Erikson's notion of ego identity is compatible with the contemporary humanistic and existential movement in psychology, psychiatry, and psychotherapy (Allport, 1954; Maslow, 1968; May, Angel, and Ellenberger [eds.], 1958; and Rogers, 1961).

Identity formation is also a process of discovering one's place in society, one's mission in life, and the specific meaning life offers one. Erikson (1968) describes this development as follows:

> The end point of this stage is a development of fidelity as a virtue. That is, a developing capacity to be faithful to some ideological view. Without the development of a capacity for fidelity the individual will either have what we call a weak ego, or look for a deviant group to be faithful to.

The fidelity which Erikson describes is basically related to the faithfulness to an ideological point of view. Without a philosophy of life—a cause for which we exist—to provide overall meaning to our existence, one feels an existential vacuum in his life. As such, Erikson's thinking once again has an existential flavor. Identity formation helps define the meaning of one's existence, creating new value and direction.

Fidelity can also refer to the value of valuing oneself. Fidelity is being secure in knowing who one is and being faithful to this sameness—that is, feeling that one will be the same person tomorrow that one is today, a kind of psychic balance and predictability. It does not refer to a rigid, inflexible, compulsively oriented intrapsychic and interpersonal stance. The sameness is experienced as a good feeling; one knows who he is and what he is becoming.

One can also be faithful to some meaningful group—social, political, or familial. Therapy group affiliation may be replacing the more traditional groups in our culture, such as family and church (Rachman, 1969-1970). The need for group affiliation continues because man is a social being; he wants to belong. But as society changes, the kinds of group affiliations change.

The implication for psychotherapy of an adolescent's need for a sense of philosophical identity relates to the relationship between adult authority and the adolescent. Adults need to provide adolescents with meaningful, positive ideologies with which to identify. A psychotherapist needs to have a meaningful, positive, consistent, personal and professional frame of reference with which adolescents can identify. A psychotherapist with adolescents must stand for something and make his stand known.

The process of identity formation is also an interpersonal one. It occurs not only within the individual but also between the individual and the group:

Identity expresses a mutual relation in that it connotes both a persistent sameness within oneself (self sameness) and a persistent sharing of some kind of essential character with others (Erikson, 1968).

Adolescence is highlighted by the psychosocial mandate to form positive, meaningful peer relationships. An individual's capacity throughout childhood for peer group affiliation will determine his capacity as an adolescent for group identity resolution. Identity formation is not complete without such an encounter.

At all stages of the life cycle, ego identity "transcends mere 'personal' identity; that is, the knowledge of who you are" (Evans, 1969). According to Erikson (1968), peer group affiliation is a psychosocial need of man:

> Personality, therefore, can be said to develop according to steps predetermined in the human organism's readiness to be driven toward, to be aware of, and to interact with a widening radius of significant individuals and institutions.

Such a view recognizes man's inherent social nature. An individual's growth and development is directly related to the interaction with significant others throughout the life cycle (Mead, 1934). The most pathologic identity problems occur when individuals have been seriously deprived of meaningful human contact; for example, feral children reared in isolation of human contact (Bettleheim, 1954).

An individual is always dependent upon some form of group affiliation for the basic ingredients of a sense of identity, self-esteem, ego strength, personal consistency, and a sense of mastery of the environment. How others evaluate and respond to us determines what we feel and think about ourselves. Adolescents have the opportunity to crystalize emotional separation from infantile dependence upon parental influence. If the crisis of group identity is successfully resolved, the adolescent heads toward adulthood with the capacity to hear and respond to *the voice of the group*. As an adult, one's peers should have significant influence upon one's thinking, feeling, and behaving. During adolescence one begins to break the potentially neurotic bind of hearing only *the voice of the parent*. Many clinicians are faced with patients in adulthood who are only cordial to the voice of a parent, usually the mother. The adult patient so neurotically bound is not free to hear and respond to a peer, ever searching for the surrogate parent to finally fulfill unresolved infantile needs.

Identity confusion. The psychological danger of the adolescent stage of development is identity confusion, the negative stage of the identity crisis. Erikson (1959) has defined identity confusion as:

> You are not sure, you are a man or a woman, that you will ever grow together again and be attractive, that you will be able to master your drives, that you really know who you are, that you know what you want to be, that you know what you look like to others, and that you will know how to make the right decisions without, once and for all, committing yourself to the wrong friend, sexual partner, leader or career.

Colloquially speaking, identity confusion is when:

> You're up for grabs. You don't know where it's at, or what's happening. You can't get a hold of anything. You don't feel together. You don't know where your head is at. You are always grabbing onto people for a piece of them. You are what they are. You feel what they feel. You don't know where the *you* is.

Identity confusion, although the negative stage of the identity crisis, can be a normative crisis. All adolescents pass through a period when feelings of confusion, disorganization, impulsiveness, lack of commitment, and inconsistency predominate their thinking and behaving. Therefore, adolescent confusion is not an affliction or disease, but "a normal phase of increased conflict characterized by a seeming fluctuation in ego strength as well as by a high growth potential" (Erikson, 1968).

It must be emphasized, however, that such a normative crisis has the inherent potential for psychopathology as well as for self-actualization. Which direction the adolescent takes depends upon his previous personality development (perhaps especially the development of ego strength) as well as his interaction with adults and society. Erikson speaks of adolescence as a period of psychosocial moratorium, a temporary delay of adult commitments. The adolescent, supported by his culture, should be given the opportunity, encouragement, and support for "free role experimentation" with a variety of psychosocial roles. This moratorium should be a period characterized by a "selective permissiveness" on the part of society and a "provocative playfulness" on the part of youth. It can lead to deep yet transitory commitment by the adolescent, and it ends in a more or less ceremonial confirmation of commitment on the part of society. Such moratoria show highly individual variations.

If society provides periods of psychosocial moratoria, it allows adolescents opportunity for free role experimentation, thereby enhancing the self-liquidating, transitory aspect of identity confusion. After a period of experimentation and withdrawal, the adolescent can move along toward positive identity formation. Identity confusion will be replaced by ego identity. When society does not support such periods, the individual's own ego strength becomes paramount. It is then necessary to create a personal psychosocial withdrawal—to withdraw by oneself, for oneself, to find oneself. Many of our young people can accomplish this developmental task; unfortunately, an increasing number of adolescents and young adults cannot and thus turn towards psychopathology. Besides personal pathology, social conditions can lead to identity confusion: a lack of positive and meaningful adult leadership, a lack of meaningful ideology with which to identify, and little or no opportunity for free role experimentation.

It is when identity confusion predominates that psychotherapeutic intervention is crucial and mandatory. However, group psychotherapy can also be meaningful for adolescents with adjustment reaction difficulties, because the problem of ego identity resolution often lies underneath the adjustment difficulties.

Group milieu and ego identity. The most basic implication of the concept of ego identity for group psychotherapy with adolescents, which follows from Erikson's theory, is that adolescents must develop peer group affiliation to gain a sense of ego identity. As a defense against identity confusion, adolescents (all of whom are threatened by this negative stage) are emotionally inclined towards peer group membership. Group membership, then, represents a "life saving device," or the necessary and sufficient conditions for identity formation in adolescence. Adolescents, according to this theory, can enhance their self-esteem only by their own action in the culture of a peer group that is positive, meaningful, and continuous.

In a group therapy setting, adolescents can perceive and support each other in their common struggle to discover who they are as individuals and to whom they belong. They can perceive the same ego struggle within each other, feeling more aware and comfortable with their own struggle. By identification with the significant others of a therapeutic peer group, the prototypical defensiveness and psychological myopia ascribed to adolescents can be converted into psychological awareness and insight.

Ego identity is an integration of intrapsychic and interpersonal functioning. The person and the group are interwoven in a social, cultural, and historical matrix. The relationship is mutual and reciprocal. An individual gives meaning, significance, direction, and support to a group. The group serves similar functions for the individual. We are then led to reorient our thinking regarding anxiety in the interaction between personal and group identity. We can conclude there is no individual anxiety (intrapsychic anxiety) which does not reflect a latent concern common to an immediate and extended group. Individual anxiety—for example, neurosis—is of concern to and affects others in a given social group. Group therapy and family therapy acknowledge this concept as an essential ingredient for the diagnosis of pathologic interaction. The emphasis on the psychosocial context for identity formation also acknowledges the social imperative of man and his human nature.

Erikson's theory offers one of the most meaningful and basic rationales for including a patient in a group therapy experience. A primary contribution of group psychotherapy is to foster separateness and independence from infantile dependence upon parental figures, while fostering relatedness to peers (Wolf and Schwartz, 1962). Erikson's theory emphasizes adolescence as the period in which relationship to peers is paramount for the successful resolution of the identity crises. The group therapist and the group can become the surrogate family, providing a corrective emotional experience that can lead to new meaning and new ways-of-being for the adolescent. Children and adolescents can cope with their negative experiences within their original family milieu by creating in fantasy imaginary siblings and parents (Bender and Vogel, 1941; Burlingham, 1945; Rachman, 1967; Rapaport, 1944; Epstein, 1967).

Adolescents need to confront a meaningful authority figure in a therapeutic or corrective emotional climate to provide the bridge for separation from infantile ties with parents while moving towards peer relationships. They gain a greater sense of independence, a feeling of ego strength, and a sense of mastery by such meaningful confrontation. A therapy group of peers provides the adolescents with the necessary emotional support and courage to confront an adult authority figure. There is greater risk of losing the favor of the parental figure in individual therapy: "The therapist will not like me if I tell him off; I have to be a good guy with him." A fellow group member, confronting the therapist, can introduce a new way-of-being to an adolescent. Initially, the adolescent merely observes, risking nothing. Gradually, silent confrontation occurs in the intrapsychic sphere. With the encouragement of the group therapist and the group, the adolescent risks a direct confrontation, opening up a new way-of-being in the group.

In an adolescent group therapy setting, authority is vested in the group, which can explore, interpret, and develop insight into a member's identity problem. An adolescent does not have to listen only to the voice of the adult authority, the therapist; he can listen to and respond to the voice of the group.

Contemporary Group Techniques in Treating the Adolescent Identity Crisis

The basic aim in the technique of group psychotherapy with adolescents is to establish and maintain structures and functions within the group process which foster identity crisis resolution. A fuller explication of the structures and functions involved in beginning and maintaining adolescent psychotherapy groups can be found elsewhere (Rachman, 1973).

The present orientation for the clinical practice of group psychotherapy with adolescents incorporates contemporary developments in encounter and marathon group psychotherapy, within a humanistic psychoanalytic frame of reference (Rachman, 1969-1970, 1971). Encounter and marathon techniques provide the opportunity to foster the crucial activities of free role experimentation, psychosocial play, and free elaboration of fantasy and dream material, which are necessary for the *identity search*.

The identity search aimed toward resolving the identity crisis occurs in the following process:

1. The group therapist brings the identity crisis into the group's conscious awareness. The three spheres of identity formation are considered for ego examination by asking the basic identity questions: Who am I? With whom do I identify? What do I believe in? Where am I going?

2. Individual identity problems are identified by focusing on identity conflict areas particular to group members. Group members are asked to describe their identity conflicts and feelings. Feelings are sorted out. By sorting and identifying feelings as one's own, one deals with identity confusion and disorganization.

3. The group therapist provides the encouragement and impetus for the identity search. Through free role experimentation,

psychosocial play, exploration of fantasies, dreams, early recollections, and transference reactions, and group interaction,
the adolescents are encouraged to experiment with a variety of
different roles, to become aware of alternate ways-of-being in
the world, and to become cordial to the alienated portions of
their identity.
4. The therapist encourages group members to make decisions,
develop choices, and take a stand in their developing identity.
He helps them to translate their identity stance into overt
behavior, functioning both within the group and outside it.

The following clinical illustrations by no means exhaust the possible significant variables or crucial interactions of adolescent group
psychotherapy in identity crisis resolution. A forthcoming publication should be consulted for a fuller treatment of this topic (Rachman, 1973). These cases demonstrate the applicability of group psychotherapy in various settings with diverse patient populations.

Treatment of Neurotic and Borderline Symptoms

The first clinical example illustrates the use of encounter techniques in analyzing a dream presented to an adolescent group with
neurotic and borderline problems.

The basic aim in the exploration of the dream is: to encourage the
adolescents' full exploration of the dream material; to reduce their
superego feelings of guilt and shame toward id impulses reflected in
the dream; to side with the developing ego identity elements in the
dream (those aspects of the dream material that show a source of
positive direction, self-esteem, sense of mastery); to encourage
identification of one's own feelings; and to develop insight and
understanding of identity conflict areas. Early in therapy, dreams
are prognostic and diagnostic indicators of identity crisis areas. During the working-through and termination phase of therapy, they can
become indicators of the dreamer's rehearsal for new ways-of-being
in the world as he experiments with new roles and identity alternatives. The therapist, during this later period of therapy, interprets
the "rehearsal for change" and "the outcome of change" reflected
in the dream.

Dave, the most passive and isolated group member, says he feels
he is changing, "I feel more sure of myself." He tells the following
dream, which he says reflects a growing sense of identity in terms of
standing up for himself and wanting to be part of a group:

All of the group is there. All having a good time. Trying to force myself to get in there. Felt very rejected. All saying a lot of things. I was saying least of all. Felt I was going to scream, yell.

The group then begins to deal with the dream material. Robert, in a somewhat angry, challenging manner, chooses to deal with the rejection theme in the dream. He asks Dave why he doesn't tell the group how he feels, so that the group can help him.

Dave: Feel more part of the group now. Want to say things. That's why I had the dream. I want help to say things.

Therapist: Dave, you're right that you're dream shows you are trying to reach out to the group and become more open, emotional, and close to the people here. Robert is also right when he tells you there are things you do, which keep you and the group apart. Remember, when you and Stan had the telephone encounter about being lonely and without friends? (This encounter has been published in full [Rachman, 1971].) We all became aware then how you keep people from getting close to you.

Dave: Yeah, I think I had the dream because of something like that. I asked Charlie for his telephone number, than I lost the paper with the telephone number on it.

Robert: Your subconscious is copping out on you again, just like that time Dr. Rachman asked you to call Stan up for a meeting and you said you couldn't make the meeting. (Robert begins to intensify an angry interchange, using Dave as a transferential object, out of his need to break open his own defensiveness and emotional distance.)

Therapist: Bob, you're getting angry at Dave because you want to break open your own problem in getting close to people.

Robert: Yeah, you're right. I was beginning to feel that, like I was getting angry at Dave, instead of listening to what he was saying.

Therapist: Let's set up an encounter situation, so we can help Dave break through to his wanting to get closer to the group. Dave, let's use the situation you mentioned with Charlie. (Therapist sets up split-ego technique [Rachman, 1971].) Dave, I want you to talk to the two sides of you—the part of you (1) that asked for Charlie's number and wants to call him up to meet him and the part of you (2) that lost the telephone number and is frightened to meet him or is not interested in getting to know him. When you are sitting on the couch, you'll be the part of you that's trying to meet Charlie; when you sit on the empty chair opposite you, you'll be the part of you that doesn't want to contact Charlie. I want you to keep talking to both parts of you, moving back and forth between the couch and the chair.

Dave (1): I think I'll call Charlie tonight.

Dave (2): No, I really don't want to.

Dave (1): Well, I really should call him.

Dave (2): I can't do it. I can't call him. It's no use.

Robert: Dr. Rachman, can I talk to the part of Dave that doesn't want to do it?

Therapist: Great, do it!

Robert then goes on to interpret what he witnessed, as Dave attempted to encounter the portion of his ego that reinforces distance and isolation from others. He plays Dave (2), while Dave is the part of himself that wishes to move towards peer relations. Robert's responses focus on Dave's fear, because of his attachment to his mother, to be responsible to a peer. Robert's own poor self-esteem (he has limited intellectual and emotional resources, further limited by his resignation to inactivity and failure, self-pity, and masochistic maneuvers) prompts his focusing on Dave's similar deficiency. Dave appears to need a rest from the intense emotional experience and some time to incubate about the dynamic material offered by the group.

The group interaction moves to another member, Stan, when the therapist observes his inactivity in analyzing the dream material or the encounter situation—especially since he was the original member involved in the aforementioned telephone encounter. Stan says he is preoccupied with a problem of his own. He is having continued difficulty with his physical education course and its teacher.

Robert, once again attempting to encounter his own defenses vicariously, challenges Stan to participate in an encounter with him. Robert focuses on Stan's inability to follow through on the group's previous encouragement to develop some positive attitudes and behaviors towards physical activity, in order to cope more adequately with his problem. Stan remains solidified in his contention that he disdains physical activity and is totally incapable of it. He resists changing this defensive stance in spite of demonstrated physical ability, volunteer help with athletics from group members, and creative suggestions for improving his physical ability.

Stan reluctantly enters the "cop-out encounter" with Robert, playing his negative self who can't perform athletically. Robert responds to each negative statement by Stan with "That's a cop-out." This confrontation is continued until Stan finally admits that to overcome his resistance he must change his negative identity.

At one point in this confrontation Dave, the subject of the dream discussion, interrupts the interaction by yelling at Stan, "You're copping out, just like me. Why don't you try, just once, to say I can do it, I can succeed?" Apparently, Dave had incorporated the interaction surrounding his dream and its exploration and had begun to work on his identity problem of becoming connected to a meaningful peer group (his psychotherapy group).

In the group sessions that followed Dave became increasingly more active, assertive, and challenging with the group. He also began to develop friendships with group members outside the sessions. The years of childhood spent in almost total isolation from meaningful relatedness to peers came to an end.

Identity Crisis Resolution in a Male Delinquent Adolescent

Identity confusion can lead to serious psychopathology: "When such a dilemma is based on a strong previous doubt of one's ethnic and sexual identity, delinquent and outright psychotic incidents are not uncommon" (Erickson, 1968). The following case highlights the resolution, by means of group therapy intervention, of a severe identity crisis in a delinquent adolescent male. An abbreviated version has been previously reported (Rachman, 1969).

Johnny, age fourteen, was referred to the author's delinquent adolescent group by the courts. The group was conducted in an outpatient psychiatric clinic whose population was drawn from disadvantaged families. Johnny had a history of aggressive and sexual acting out since childhood. His areas of identity confusion are listed in an "ego identity profile," which the author develops for each adolescent. The profile involves personality functioning in the three spheres of identity formation: personal identity; group identity; philosophical identity.

Johnny's intrapsychic or personal sphere of identity showed marked areas of confusion. A borderline adaption was in development. Almost all ego areas of functioning were in conflict and crises. Johnny's thinking was confused and loosely associated. It was sometimes difficult to follow him in conversation; one had the feeling that he didn't know where he was going in a conversation. Johnny's social judgment was poorly developed. His capacity to discriminate socially acceptable ways of thinking and behaving was impaired, with id impulsivity predominating. He could respond more readily on the basis of his own inner distorted needs. Weak ego development exhibited itself in his capacity to be easily led into delinquent acts by his peers. Sexual confusion was a marked aspect of Johnny's identity problems. He had had homosexual experiences as early as his tenth year, when he was first arrested. He was not, however, committed to homosexuality, nor was he actively engaged in homosexual experiences when he entered group psychotherapy. At this time homosexuality was primarily at a latent level, confined to a friendship with a homosexual. Johnny was actively interested in heterosexuality. Although he had no meaningful, sustained loving relationship with a girl, one felt he longed for such a positive involvement.

Johnny's family and its social milieu offered him limited and negative opportunities for identity formation. His biological family and its functioning revealed a psychosocial theme of individual and group alientation. Each member of the family suffered from personality disturbance and was negatively related to one another. Johnny's description of his family's relatedness to one another speaks for itself as a model of familial alienation:

> My father is a mean son-of-a-bitch; he used to beat me silly. Once when I was a kid, he pushed my face into a corner of our room and split my head open. He doesn't give a shit about any of us. He goes his way; we go our way.
>
> My brother doesn't have anything to do with the family. He lives by himself. My older sister is divorced, with a kid; lives with my grandmother. My younger sister lives at home; she works, goes out, I never see her.
>
> My mother is the only one who talks to everyone, even though no one is interested in talking to her. She and my father don't get along. She's always complaining about him; he doesn't give her enough money for the house, he gets drunk, comes home mean and angry.

Johnny's relationship with peers was predicated on being a member of a neighborhood gang, whose main activities were various feats of physical aggression within the group and with rival gangs as well as destruction of property. Johnny followed no one, although he was susceptible to influence by fellow gang members. His ego-ideal was the strongest and the most sadistic gang member. He had found a negative identity as a delinquent. Johnny had two inadequate parents who did not provide him with appropriate models of identification—a mother who was emotionally, mentally, and socially immature and weak; and a father who rejected him. His membership in a delinquent gang was a complex phenomenon. On the one hand, it was an opportunity for sadism and aggression. But it was also an attempt to gain a sense of ego identity, a sense of belonging to a meaningful group.

Johnny's third sphere of identity confusion was the intellecutal and ideological sphere. His school achievement was poor. Johnny was placed in a special class for behavior problems in junior high school. Thus school became a custodial situation, to keep him either until he was ready to drop out voluntarily or until he was of legal age for dismissal. The educational system, his family, his social milieu, and his personal problems had formed an unwitting alliance to divest Johnny of any positive meaning in or relatedness to formal education. He was, however, a young man educated in the streets, who still valued learning. He wanted to learn some kind of trade. He wanted to learn more about himself and his problems; he longed for a goal in life.

Johnny had no meaningful ideological viewpoint, but he generally believed in people and had positive feelings towards some. His conception of life and its meaning—in actuality, his differentiation between life and death—was seriously confused. Johnny began group psychotherapy with a developing belief in reincarnation. He questioned whether he had had a previous life. Perhaps this was a "life saving fantasy" (Rachman, 1967)—his unique way of communicating dissatisfaction with his present negative life and wishing for another, more positive life. This belief helped him to maintain ego integrity, to sustain a desire to continue his present life, and to hope for a better existence. This interpretation does not disavow the pathologic thinking process and depersonalization potential in such a fantasy.

Johnny was one of the most active participants in the group sessions during his two-year period. Initially, his participation revealed unusual modes of thinking and feeling. One of his first therapeutic interactions regarded his thoughts about reincarnation. Johnny asked the group and its leader, "Do you guys believe in life after death? Lately, I have been thinking that maybe I died once before, and now I came back as a different person."

Apparently, Johnny had brought this subject up before to his gang member friends, who laughed off his ideas. They appeared to regard him as a "likable nut," who had peculiar ideas, but essentially was harmless. In essence, then, they reinforced these unusual ideas, helping Johnny to solidify an identity as a "likable nut." Johnny knew, however, that these ideas were serious and needed attention. He also wanted to experiment with a new identity.

The therapy group, with its reaction to the revelation and exploration of his reincarnation fantasies, provided Johnny with a new opportunity in identity formation. Their first reaction was to ridicule the fantasy:

Joe: Man, you're nuts.

Danny: You probably were a monkey in your first life, man.

Johnny: Fuck you guys.

Walter: I think I know someone who believes in that stuff.

Johnny had previously made an ego-syntonic adaptation to these fantasies (reinforced by his participation with and feedback from his friends). He was shocked, as well as angry, resentful, and hurt, by the group's challenge of his fantasies.

With the help of the group therapist, the group began to therapeutically explore the meaning of Johnny's life-after-death fantasies:

Therapist: You guys are dumping on Johnny because he is making you uptight about talking about a spooky subject like life after death. Let's see if we can help him and learn something about him and each other from this. I'm sure all you guys have had some weird thoughts or feelings at one time or another.

Johnny: Wow, that makes me feel better. Doc, what do you think about this stuff? Do you think I'm nuts?

Therapist: I think you're trying to tell us that you are very uptight about your present life. Like, you're unhappy about what's happening to you; maybe in your family, in school, and so on.

Johnny: Yeah, I sure am. My family life is all fucked up. My old man is either beating up on me, or he tells me to quit school and go to work so I can bring money home.

In this session and many more sessions to follow, the group focused on the message and themes contained in these fantasies. Johnny was telling the group he was so unhappy about his past state of being that he wanted to make some drastic change. He was telling them that he was very confused about his identity—who he is, where he came from, and where he is going. He was saying that he had to resort to magical (primitive) modes of thinking and feeling, in order to resolve his conflicts and problems. He was wondering out loud whether he was really crazy—a "likable nut."

The group's therapeutic exploration of his underlying feelings, with the direction and support of the group therapist, made a significant positive impact on Johnny's thinking and behaving. He began to explore the meaning of his personal identity and its relationship to significant others. He began to perceive his identity crisis; the lack of positive meaning in his past life; his negative relationship with his father; his confused self-image; the negative identity he had formed as a delinquent gang member; and his need to create new meaning and positive direction in life. The group provided Johnny with: first, the awareness of his identity problems; second, an opportunity to experiment with new identities, new roles, and new ways of being; and third, the opportunity to solidify a new identity, an alternate to being a juvenile delinquent.

By challenging his reincarnation fantasies and helping him explore their underlying meaning, the group provided Johnny with an alternative mode of being in the group. Johnny no longer had to appear a "likable nut" to gain group support or status. The group was telling him: "You don't have to be crazy and confused for us to like you. We'll like you, support you, pay attention to you, if you work on your head—find out who you are and where you're going!" As group therapy progressed, Johnny's bizzare thinking and its accompanying anxiety and disorganization diminished.

Another significant problem area for Johnny was his negative identity as a delinquent and the related difficulty in controlling hostile and aggressive impulses. In the social milieu of a delinquent gang, an adolescent with severe identity problems is faced with a serious dilemma. On the manifest level such a group offers a sense of identity: there is a group name; there are group activities; there are group goals; and there is a status position within the group for each member (even if it reinforces a negative identity). In many important spheres of intrapsychic and interpersonal functioning, delinquent gang affiliation provided Johnny with an identity. One must keep in mind that having any identity—whether as a delinquent, hippie, faggot, junkie—is preferable for an adolescent in the midst of severe identity confusion to feeling that he has no identity at all.

Initially, Johnny's participation in the therapy group was a report of aggressive and sexual acting-out behavior by himself and the members of his delinquent gang. He told tales of individual and gang-related activities of sadism, fighting, stealing, destruction of property, and molesting of girls. Reports of gang wars by Johnny and other group members were dramatic and vivid examples of aggression, hostility, and sadism.

The therapist introduced an encounter situation, in the framework of a "fantasy gang war," in which the group's role was to imagine a gang war taking place in the here and now of the group therapy session. Group members were encouraged to fully delineate their plans of aggression. The emotional climate of such an encounter was heightened by stimulating intense verbalization of affect. The group therapist took the lead, freely expressing verbal aggression and hostility to the fantasied rival gang. Gradually the group echoed the feelings, and a chorus of anger, hostility, and aggression emerged.

Although fantasied aggressive interactions were developed in the role-playing encounter, physical contact between members was discouraged as before (Rachman, 1969). The strong verbal interaction served as a discharge of impulses.

After the heightened feelings during the simulated gang war situation, the group therapist led a therapeutic exploration of the meaning of the experience for each group member (Rachman, 1971). The encounter situation attempted to enhance certain ego-syntonic feelings that delinquent adolescents have suppressed from their awareness. In the analytic exploration of the encounter situation, they can become aware of anxiety, fearfulness, vulnerability, and danger. The emotional climate of a therapy group allows these adolescents to drop their facades of hyper-aggressivity and to share with each other significant feelings of anxiety and vulnerability; for example, "one can get killed in a gang war." When this begins to occur, the group therapist is able to introduce alternative ways-of-being to the group, which focus on verbal means of settling disputes.

Johnny was involved in a dramatic illustration of this therapeutic approach, which proved to be a turning point in his attempt at identity crisis resolution. The group had been meeting weekly for about eight months, when Johnny brought in his plan to settle a personal dispute. He had been unjustly accused of demeaning a former girlfriend by calling her a whore. The girl's present boyfriend and Johnny were prepared to mobilize their gangs and fight it out. At the beginning of the session Johnny was convinced of the efficacy of his plan. When he presented his gang war plan to the group, the group challenged it immediately. He was noticeably shaken. Angrily he asked the group to "come up with something better." He was apparently intensely anxious about the upcoming fight, and the group's reaction had intensified his anxiety. He said that he didn't sleep the previous night because of the fear he would be killed in the fight.

Once again, the group challenged Johnny's identity—this time his negative identity as a delinquent. The group first questioned and ridiculed his ideas and plans, then began to explore the entire dispute. They suggested that Johnny did not do enough to prove his innocence, that his going along with the gang war could be interpreted as an admission of guilt. They pointed out that violence and acting out were his prime vehicles for settling any dispute, whether large or small. Past reports of such behavior and their negative consequences emerged. Peaceful, non-violent means of handling the situation were discussed. The group, in collaboration with the therapist, formulated a plan to settle the dispute by "talking it out" in a small group situation; the girl, the girl's parents, the boyfriend, Johnny, and his friend (for support) would peacefully settle the dispute, averting the upcoming gang war.

By the end of the session Johnny had reformulated his plans in a constructive way and decided to put these ideas into action the same night. The session ended with the group wishing him luck.

The follow-up to this incident revealed that the social crisis of a gang war was averted due to Johnny's peaceful efforts. This incident had social significance for Johnny's friends outside the group sessions, because it demonstrated to them a new, workable way to handle conflict. The incident and Johnny became famous in the group sessions to follow. It was used by the therapist and the group members to reinforce the value of "talking it out" rather than "fighting it out" in changing one's aggressive behavior and in avoiding a social crisis.

Highlighting Johnny's struggle has, by necessity, excluded a fuller discussion of the group. But Johnny's struggle for identity was also their struggle for a positive, meaningful sense of themselves and of others. His struggle gave them all hope and faith in their capacity to change and become themselves more fully. After several years in group therapy, Johnny and the group therapist terminated their relationship by mutual consent. Johnny felt he had found a sense of himself, "I feel I know where I am trying to go now."

Adolescent Drug Abuse: The Search for Identity

The psychosocial context is crucial for ego identity formation. One of the most serious social problems of our time, adolescent drug abuse, presents a negative psychosocial context for identity formation. I have previously attempted to explain adolescent drug abuse as a "search for identity" (Rachman, 1972).

1. Contemporary adolescents feel alienated, confused, and disoriented. They don't really know where they are going, what to believe in, or whom to follow. They are suffering from an *identity crisis*.

2. There are psychosocial forces in our culture which have contributed to the alienation and confusion of our youth. Specifically, there is a pervading sense of alienation and loneliness fostered by our growing technocratic society.

3. Therefore, our adolescents and young adults are showing us the results of identity confusion. In an "age of identity confusion," pathologic adaptations are most likely to develop in

order to deal with the underlying anxiety about one's existence.

4. Drug abuse is one such pathologic adaptation. Drug abuse among ghetto youth has demonstrated that an artificial, euphoric, semiconscious fantasy state is preferable to the dehumanizing reality of the ghetto. Now we are astonished to see that middle-class youngsters share a similar negative view of their families and their environment, even though they have material comfort and luxury.

Adolescent group therapy can provide an alternative to drug use by creating a positive psychosocial context in which adolescents can find meaning, direction, and position in group affiliation, as demonstrated in the following incident in a psychotherapy group.

Hal (waiting for a lull in a group session): I have something very heavy I want to talk about. I have been thinking about taking acid (LSD) and I want to talk about it first. I want to know if anyone here has taken it and what they think about it, and I want to know what Dr. Rachman thinks too.

Alan (a "pot head," on probation for selling marijuana when he joined the group): Man, are you kidding? That's crazy to take acid. It will mess up your mind.

Stan (a nondrug-user): I don't understand why you want to take any drugs that could hurt you. Why do you need drugs?

Karl: Wait a minute, acid can bring you insights. I took it several times, and it can really open up your head.

Therapist: Yes, that's true for you, Karl. Some important feelings about your mother came out under acid. But you also got fucked up under acid. You had bad trips.

Alan: Yeah, man, don't you remember when you told us about going up to the Empire State Building under acid and thinking about jumping off?

Karl: I guess so, but I didn't jump. I was only thinking about it.

Hal: I feel I need something to open up my head. There are things I want to get to. Like, I want to really understand myself, get deep insights into myself. I want to find out why I have trouble getting along with my father. I want to know why I can't express my feelings, especially when I get angry.

Alan: Look man, I took acid a couple of times, and it didn't do any of that for me. It made me sick and scared. I had the shakes; I got paranoid.

Karl: Hal, my advice is, like you want to learn something about yourself, but you're thinking about the wrong teacher.

Hal: Maybe, but I want to change now. Man, like I was thinking about heroin; it would be so cool to feel calm with no hassles.

Marv: Heroin, are you kidding?

Therapist: The more you talk, the more worried I get about you. I've worked with a lot of kids who take all kinds of drugs, but you are the first one who's told me they want to take heroin because it will be good therapy for them. People who take heroin usually figure their life is fucked up; they don't care what they take to get away from it all. I've never seen anyone talk about taking heroin in such a positive, enthusiastic way, with no sign of being uptight about how it can fuck your mind, your body, your whole life.

Karl: Listen, if you gotta take something powerful, take acid rather than heroin. Take mescaline.

Marv: Bullshit, don't take any of that. Why don't you take therapy, man? You've only been in the group a month, right? So give the group a chance. Turn on to us and Dr. Rachman. Like, I feel therapy is the greatest thing that ever happened to me in my life. I'm doing so much better in school, I will be able to go to college; I'm getting along better with my folks; learning to make it with chicks; feel better about myself as a person. It's out of sight. It could happen to you, too. Dig it.

Karl: I've changed my mind. My advice to you is, although acid can bring insights, it's not worth the price. I thought I would take it again, but I'm not sure now. I seem to be doing better without it. I've met this girl who is real cute; I'm doing good in school now.

Dave: You also changed in the group. You're less uptight, smiling more, getting along better with us.

Therapist: You sure are, and you and I don't have the hassles we used to have. I really feel good about that, Karl.

Hal: Dr. Rachman, I'd like to hear what you think about drugs.

Marv: He's against all drugs. He doesn't even think you should smoke grass.

Therapist: I'm glad you asked; but if you didn't ask, I was going to tell you anyway (group laughs). First, I'd like to pull together some of the things I've heard you tell us today about your head. Then I'll go into my "drug rap," since you haven't heard it before. I like to give everyone a full dose of my rap, so there will be no question about where I stand on drugs.

I think you've made a very positive step forward towards us today, by admitting to us how troubled and fucked up you feel sometimes. Before today, you weren't willing to let us into your head. So, welcome to the club and congratulations for joining us. The group and I invite you to get high here. We will help you get as deep into your head as we can and you will let us.

Following is a composite of the "drug rap" I usually offer. At this session it was not necessary to go into all the material, since much of it had been covered in the interaction.

I guess it is time for my lecture on drugs. Here's where I stand on drugs. I am basically a puritan when it comes to drug use. I firmly believe that any introduction of any chemical substance into my body is undesirable, and I try to avoid it whenever I can. I see all chemical substances introduced into my body as potential poisons. Any chemical or drug can become a body poison, if it is abused. By chemicals or drugs I mean all drugs, everything—aspirin, Alka-Seltzer, sleeping pills, tranquilizers, penicillin, Allerest, nicotine, alcohol, grass, acid, speed, goof balls, dope. Of course, there are some drugs that I take at some time or other; for example, aspirin, Excedrin, Allerest, alcohol, nicotine. So, I am also a drug user. But I try not to cop-out. I try to be honest with myself. When I have a headache, nine times out of ten it's because of tension anxiety. I'm probably pissed off about something I don't want to admit to. I should really sit down and have a talk with myself and find out what and at whom I am angry. Sometimes it works; sometimes it doesn't. I have to live with it not working all the time.

It's important to admit to yourself that taking drugs is a kind of cop-out—a magical, chemical, fairy-tale way of not dealing with the real thing that is bothering you. Take a look at TV any night and see how much of America and the Adult Population cops out and is into drugs. Aspirin, antacid, sleeping pill, tension-relieving pill commercials are all examples of how uptight many adults are, how much anxiety they have, and how much they turn to pills and drugs to get relief.

Now, my thing about the new drugs—grass, acid, speed, dope, and so on. I put grass in a bag separate from all other mind-expanding drugs. This is what I think about grass. If you feel you have to have some drug, you should first ask yourself why. Grass, as far as we know right now, does not seem to be as dangerous as the other stuff. The other stuff, all the rest, is deadly poison.

I am not for smoking grass. I will admit I've thought about trying it, out of curiosity, several times. Perhaps someday I will. I guess I haven't because I haven't been moved to do so; I don't feel the need. All the rest of the mind-expanding drugs are deadly poison. You really shouldn't try them, even once. They can fuck up your genes, your head, and your body. If you take them, you can freak out, maybe die.

I would like you not to take any of that shit. If you feel you need to take something, come in and let's talk about it. I'll try to turn you on to something that will give you a natural high (therapy and life) and is good for you.

The group session ended with Hal deciding not to experiment with LSD. He also made it clear to the group and the therapist that he was glad to be dissuaded from taking the drugs he mentioned, and he was grateful to be able to turn to us for help with the problems.

Role of the Adolescent Group Therapist

The present orientation signals a re-evaluation of the traditional role of the group therapist. The traditional conceptualization of the therapist's functioning as a neutral, objective, and passive figure is rejected. In fact, the blank screen or "tabula rosa" approach for the adolescent therapist is considered antitherapeutic behavior.

Adolescents need compassionate, demonstrative, active involvement by the therapist. Neutrality, passivity, "strict objectivity" and a rigidly defined therapeutic role encourages emotional distance, negative transference, and a pseudo-therapeutic relationship.

The group therapist's capacity to enter into a humanistic active relationship with adolescents enhances the therapeutic exploration of identity conflicts. Adolescents will not unfold themselves to a passive, indirect, neutral, inhibited authority figure.

It is only through an emotional encounter in the here-and-now, where the adolescent is invited to participate in an open, direct, honest, lusty dialogue, that "true meeting" can take place.

Identity Group Psychotherapy, therefore, also focuses on the concept of ego identity in regard to the functioning of the group therapist. In order to aid in an adolescent's ego identity formation, the group therapist needs to emphasize several aspects of his functioning:

    1) The identity search of the therapist
    2) Identity role modeling
    3) Identity countertransference
    4) Self-actualization of the therapist

The adolescent group therapist needs to establish his own identity search in the areas of personality functioning relevant to an emotional encounter with adolescents. The analysis of unresolved identity conflicts, in the therapist, becomes an integral part of the therapeutic work. The therapist needs to maintain a therapeutic attitude toward exploring his own resolved indentity conflicts in the areas of authority, dependency, aggression, sexuality, and affection. The more aware and related the group therapist is to his own identity conflicts, the more understanding, empathetic, and hopeful will he be in helping adolescents find their identity. The therapist's ongoing identity search will also enhance his capacity to offer himself as an "ego identity role model" to the adolescent group.

Identity Group Psychotherapy relies heavily on the capacity of the group therapist to offer himself as a model with whom adolescents can identify. Identity role modeling is the adolescent's temporary borrowing of a portion of the therapist's ego to aid in the identity search. By emulating and patterning themselves after significant adults in their life, they hope to gain a sense of ego mastery and organization and temporary relief from identity confusion. Drug rehabilitation programs have intuitively sensed the dynamic significance of identity role modleing, and rely on it to help adolescent drug abusers (Rachman and Heller, 1973).

Inherent in the identity role modeling functioning of the group therapist is a democratic and humanistic philosophy of man and psychotherapy which aims toward enhancing personality growth, individuation, self-determinism, and self-actualization.

Several components in the relationship attempt to synthesize this concept:

1. The therapist is an adult authority with a positive sense of himself and the direction in which he is going. He is someone who is working on his own identity.
2. The therapist is caring, warm, understanding, and passionate—yet firm, assertive, and direct in his interaction with the group.
3. The therapist is willing to risk himself in the relationship and to share his own feelings, thoughts, and behaviors. He develops a humanisitic, person-to-person relationship. Yet the therapist is always an authority in the group.
4. The therapist takes definite stands in the relationship, expressing and sharing his values, ideas, and beliefs in a compassionate, humanistic way. He offers these as hypotheses for the group to accept or reject; he allows them "psychological room to breathe."
5. The therapist encourages the adolescent to have a meaningful dialogue with him and the group members, emphasizing empathetic understanding and creating meaning, rather than judging or prohibiting feelings, thoughts, or behavior. Since we are all brothers in the human community, there are no alien feelings, thoughts, or behaviors.

Identity countertransference is the crucial sphere which helps the group therapist to become aware of, to own, and to resolve his identity conflicts. Adolescents when formed into therapy groups stimulate the greatest variety and intensity of countertransference reactions in the group therapist.

An ongoing program of analyzing the group therapist's counter-transference, therefore, contributes toward the necessary and sufficient conditions for adolescent group psychotherapy. It:

1) Enhances the therapist as an ego identity model
2) Provides the group with a heightened sense of emotional encounter with the group therapist and with each other.
3) Allows the group therapist to develop a humanistic rather than a defensive stance.
4) Enhances the group therapist's sense of "being alive" in the relationship; provides new vistas for emotional experiencing and understanding.
5. Provides the therapist with opportunities for self-actualization and ensures a sense of flexibility in personality functioning.
6. Reduces the therapist's need for acting out identity conflicts with the group.

Adolescent group psychotherapy is one form of psychotherapy that has inherent opportunities for personal growth and personality change. The most basic non-defensive stance for the group therapist when confronted with identity feelings and conflicts stimulated by group interaction is a direct encounter with them, aimed toward personal growth and identity development. The act of giving or sharing oneself with a group is a significant opportunity to understand oneself more fully. The therapist can analyze what he has given to others (or has not been capable of giving).

Since adolescent groups stimulate intense feelings in a therapist, that is, expose "weak points," one must be willing to deal effectively in this area. This would mean a willingness to sustain a certain amount of personal vulnerability, to have "personal wounds" opened up from time to time. If a group therapist isn't open to experiencing and dealing with intense feelings, one could expect limited success with adolescent groups. If, however, one is open to an ongoing program of becoming aware, experiencing, and analyzing identity conflicts, eventually "the sweat" is taken out of working with adolescent groups. Then, working with adolescents in groups becomes a joyful, easy, exhilarating, lusty experience.

References

1. Allport, G. W. (1954), *Becoming: Basic Considerations for a Psychology of Personality*. New Haven: Yale University Press.
2. Bender, L. and Vogel, F. (1941), Imaginary companions of children. *Amer. J. Orthopsych.*, 11:56-66.

3. Bettleheim, B. (1954), Feral children and autistic children. *Amer. J. Soc.*, 64:455-467.

4. Burlingham, D. T. (1945), The fantasy of having a twin. *Psychoanal. Study of the Child*, 1:205-210.

5. Epstein, N. (1967), A comparison in observation and techniques utilized in group therapy with male adolescent character disorders from varying socio-economic backgrounds. *Amer. Group Psychotherapy Assoc. Convention*, Chicago, Ill.

6. Erikson, E. H. (1950), *Childhood and Society*. New York: W. W. Norton & Co., Inc.

7. ———(1958), *Young Man Luther: A Study in Psychoanalysis and History*. New York: W. W. Norton & Co., Inc.

8. ———(1959), Identity and the life cycle. *Psychol. Issues*, Vol. I, No. 1.

9. ———(1968), *Identity: Youth and Crisis*. New York: W. W. Norton & Co., Inc.

10. Evans, R. I. (1969), *Diaglogue with Erik Erikson*. New York: E. P. Dutton & Co., Inc.

11. Maslow, A. H. (1968), *Toward a Psychology of Being*. New York: Van Nostrand Rineholt.

12. May, R., Angel, E., and Ellenberger, H. F. eds. (1958), *Existence: A New Dimension in Psychiatry and Psychology*. New York: Basic Books, Inc.

13. Mead, G. H. (1934), *Mind, Self and Society*. Ed. C. W. Morris. Chicago: University of Chicago Press.

14. Rachman, A. W. (1967), A life saving fantasy. Lecture at *Postgraduate Center for Mental Health*, New York City.

15. ———(1969), Talking it out rather than fighting it out: prevention of a delinquent gang war by group therapy intervention. *Int. J. Group Psychotherapy*, Vol. XIX, No. 4.

16. ———(1969-1970), Marathon group psychotheraphy: its originals, its meaning, its direction. *J. Group Psychoanal. Process*. Vol. 2, No. 2, Winter.

17. ———(1971), Encounter techniques in analytic group psychotherapy with adolescents. *Int. J. Group Psychotherapy, Vo. XXI, No. 3:319—329*.

18. 6—(1973), *Identity Group Psychotherapy with Adolescents*. Springfield: Charles C. Thomas (In press).

19. Rachman, A. W. and Heller, Margaret E. Peer, "Group Psychotherapy with Adolescent Drug Abusers," American Group Psychotherapy Assn. Convention Detroit, Mich., February 1973.

20. Rapaport, J. (1944), Fantasy objects in children. *Psychoanal. Review*, 31:316-321.

21. Rogers, C. R. (1961), *On Becoming a Person*. Boston: Houghton Mifflin Co.

22. Wolf, A. and Schwartz, E. K. (1962), *Psychoanalysis in Groups*. New York: Grune & Stratton.

Part Seven

SEX, SEXISM, AND SEXUAL STEREOTYPES

Flaunted, flouted, and falsified; maligned, celebrated, and suppressed—sex, that most intriguing of subjects—is the major topic of this section. Gadflies all, the authors prick the bubbles of superstition, hypocrisy, and obsoleteness that continue to pollute the realm of human sexuality.

31. Gadflying the Sex Thing*

Gertrude J. Williams

. . . your academic copier of fossils offers them to you as the latest outpouring of the human spirit, and what is worst of all, kidnaps young people as pupils and persuades them that his limitations are rules, his observances dexterities, his timidities good taste, and his emptinesses purities.

—George Bernard Shaw

Reflecting on current sex ideologies, including those expounded by many self-styled enlightened professionals, is often a *déjà vu* experience that smacks of Calvinism and Victorianism. A number of unquestioned, fossilized pronouncements are being foisted on young and old in schools, clinics, lecture halls, community centers —wherever the masses gather to mine the jewels of the so-called intelligentsia. Despite the quasi-liberal tone, much of what is being asserted by professionals is frequently just as subjective, moralistic and anachronistic as the lay versions of sex. Three major passé truisms related to traditional marriage, virginity in youth and the concept of perversion need to be defossilized.

Fossil I

It is Better to Marry Than to Spurn. One of the most crazed notions in this day and age is the assumption that the only fulfilling life style is traditional marriage. A hangover from the hunt and the hut, this old saw still permeates today's classrooms and clinics. Yet bearing numerous offspring is now considered antithetical to survival, and the sex role gap is rapidly diminishing. The very bases of the institution of traditional marriage, reproduction and division of labor

---

*This essay is a slight revision of an editorial published in the *Clinical Child Psychology Newsletter*, 1971, X, #2 and 3, 2-3.

by sex, no longer have their earlier survival value, and other interpersonal life styles are developing. Chosen singlehood, multilateral, group, trial and paramarriage as well as other individually drawn contracts and commitments are not rare arrangements to be righteously dismissed as withering on the vine, swapping, swinging or psychopathology. They may be the wave of an increasingly pluralistic future in which the institution of marriage, like other social institutions, contains a variety of options. A bill to legalize a three year marriage contract, to be renewed or dissolved without divorce, has already been introduced in the Maryland legislature.

Many young people, turned off by dating and courtship rituals and disenchanted by their parents' traditional marriage, are selecting new relational alternatives. The inevitable happy ending to the Goldwyn movies of the Forties, the strains of Lohengrin as the only option, is not appropriate to youth in the Seventies. Traditional marriage is becoming one of many possibilities for personal fulfillment. To continue to exert explicit or covert social pressure on youths to marry because this life style had survival value for their parents and grandparents widens the generation gap and is emotionally harmful to youth.

Fossil II

Better Dead Than Unwed in Bed. Ho hum. Virginity is still being touted for youth. The same old pastoral is being played by current sex educators as they glorify chastity in a quasi-scientific, humanistic guise. Adolescent sex relations are emotionally harmful, interfere with later appreciation of the beauty of sex in marriage, are too stimulating to assimilate at such a tender age, etc., etc. These mouthings, like those of the occasional pseudo-sophisticate who categorically recommends sex relations for all youth, are purely subjective fluff. The fact is we do not know whether celibate youths are more (or less) emotionally healthy than sexually active youths. We have little if any objective evidence about the emotional impact of sexual intercourse on adolescents. In fact, we do not know whether the presence or absence of adolescent sex relations makes any difference at all. Yet dogmatic opinion, passed off as fact, celebrates celibacy for all youth. In *Illegitimacy: Myths, Causes and Cures*, Phillips Cutright states: "The supposed ill effects of premarital sex on marital adjustment, marital stability and marital fidelity have never been documented, so long as premarital sex did not lead to an illicit pregnancy that was carried to term. It is the control of these unwanted pregnancies—not the control of premarital sex—that is the problem." (*Family Planning Perspectives*, Jan. 1971, Vol. 3, No. 1, Page 47.)

What are some of the ramifications of the chastity-for-youth admonition? For one thing, it further alienates youth because while the elders preach against sex relations, a number of youths are practicing it. Some are indifferent to these preachings. For others, needless irrational guilt is created. It is the male youth who is likely to be indifferent and the young female who is likely to feel quilty in response to unilateral expectations of celibacy. The old double standard is once again enthroned; male sexual activity is taken in stride and implicitly encouraged while it is the female who is exhorted to remain celibate.

In addition to widening the generation gap and perpetuating sexism, the better-dead-than-unwed-in-bed ideology may, by provoking guilt, ironically encourage a reluctance to use contraception among youths who violate the dictum. Cutright (*ibid*, page 43) refers to the finding that many young, unmarried women refuse to use contraceptives because of their "moral objections." He describes the condition as "a pseudo-moral barrier inhibiting both male and female contraceptive use. The term *pseudo*-moral seems appropriate because, if one wishes to take a moral stance on nonmarital coitus, then actual behavior indicates that traditional morality has already been abandoned."

Finally, certain subtle, age-ist prejudices are associated with categorical pro-chastity warnings. Youthful virginity is extolled, yet adult virginity is usually scorned, ridiculed and at best, pitied. In the clinical situation, the older virgin is helped to lift repressions and suppressions of sexuality so that sexual expression may occur, whereas the youthful virgin is usually helped to redirect his or her more intense sexual desires away from coitus. What is the scientific validity of these differential expectations? None! Another unfounded recommendation, passed off as sexual enlightenment, is the advice to youth to masturbate as an alternative to coitus, the implication being that masturbation is better for youth than sexual intercourse. *Mutual* masturbation is discouraged; young people are advised to play with their privates in private. Now an adult virgin whose exclusive sexual outlet is solitary masturbation tends to be viewed as in need of professional attention. At what age do virginity and solitary masturbation change from mental health promoters to expressions of emotional problems? It is becoming increasingly clear that specific sexual behaviors for youth are being advocated and repudiated by those who do not know what they are talking about.

The expectation of premarital virginity did have survival value in earlier times when a child born out of wedlock could not be cared for solely by the mother. The unwanted offspring of a nonmarital liaison became a severe burden to the woman's family and the community or else was abandoned. It is understandable that intense social pressures for premarital chastity were exerted. Now that contraceptives are available, what was once a necessity has become an outmoded ethos. We must quit our vacuous pretense of knowing the most desirable sexual outlets for young people and admit honestly that we do not know whether it is better for youth to remain celibate or to become sexually active. Our advice is based on opinion not on facts. Categorical encouragement (or discouragement) of youthful celibacy in this primitive state of our knowledge is an unwarranted imposition of one's own purely personal values on another and as such, borders on unethical behavior. We can best contribute to youth by helping them to examine the consequences of both celibacy and sexual activity; in the context of individual differences and the values, mores and styles appropriate to their unique environments, they can be helped to evolve their own choices of sexual behavior.

Fossil III

Perversions Are Crimes Against Nature. This stale, savage, mindlessly moralistic preaching continues to clutter the sex landscape. On what objective basis do laws and customs dare to dictate who should do what to whom? We express ardent concern about invasion of privacy by wiretapping, unethical psychological testing and research as well as other violations of human rights. Will we remain silent while archaic laws intrude on the sexual relationship, the most intimate, private and personal of all human transactions? Will we remain silent while human beings continue to be brutalized by irrational laws which punish non-injurious "crimes"? In most states, homosexuality between consenting adults is a crime. In addition to receiving unjust punishment, homosexuals may bear the stigma of having a criminal record and frequently, the humiliation of publicity and social vilification. Clearly, homosexual individuals are victims of the law. Heterosexual oral-genital contacts, including those between marriage partners, are also crimes; and some women have been able to obtain divorces on the grounds of fellatio. The most enlightened judge has no alternative but to sentence individuals "guilty of crimes" in which the consenting parties were not only not injured but in which the alleged criminal act was willingly accepted and enjoyed. One person's poison is another's meat. The law violates human rights when it intrudes on the expression of non-injurious personal preferences in sexuality.

What is a perversion? Who dares to decide in the Age of Aquarius what constitutes deviant sex behavior? In these days of environmental destruction by war and pollution, what clown in cap and bells dares to declare that non-coital sex activities are crimes against nature? In a statement bearing a disconcerting resemblance to a pronouncement by Moses from Mount Sinai, the American Psychoanalytic Association defined perversion as "a variety of sexual practices that deviate in aim or object choice from the accepted norm of heterosexual genital union" (*Glossary of Psychoanlytic Terms and Concepts*, 1967, page 67.) This statement is fairly representative of the views of the mental health professions. On what rational basis does heterosexual genital union constitute normality and acceptability? When survival of the race was dependent on replenishing the earth, it is understandable that the only socially sanctioned sexuality was coitus because it resulted in procreation. It is also understandable that non-coital acts, being antithetical to group survival because they did not result in procreation, were defined as crimes against nature and were unacceptable. These ideas are hardly applicable now when replenishing the earth is certainly not a goal, when unlimited childbearing is a crime against nature (and in that sense, a perversion), when prevention of childbearing is being strongly advocated, when non-coital acts being non-reproductive can be considered to have survival value for these times.

The vagueness, subjectivity and implicit moralizing inherent in the American Psychoanalytic Association's view of perversion are further revealed in the following mind-boggling afterthought: "True perversions should be distinguished from the occasional type of sexual act performed by people, usually during foreplay, whose conduct otherwise falls within the accepted norm." Variety-seeking persons are thus spared the onus of being labelled perverted providing they are straight most of the time and their so-called perversion is a means justified by a coital end.

What is a perversion? Who shall presume to decide for another what is acceptable sexual behaivor and what is not? Let us hope that psychologists will repudiate the spewing forth of empty moralisms in the guise of science, pronouncements that injure, frighten and stigmatize innocent human beings. Many homosexual individuals are forced by cruel social pressures into unfulfilling, unbearable marriages, and mental health professions may be a party to a truly injurious crime. Honesty impels us to admit that when partners consent, the notions of normal and deviate sexuality have little relevance in the world of today.

Gadflying Action

Let us bury the fossils that are polluting the sex scene of the Seventies. Let us actively endorse the repeal of all sexually repressive laws relating to "perversion", homosexuality, pornography, contraception and abortion. Let us work for the repeal of laws that bar physicians from prescribing contraceptives or treatment for veneral disease to minors without the consent of their parents; child advocates must vehemently counter such laws which are injurious to the physical and emotional health of youth. All of these laws are throwbacks to the long gone days when replenishing the earth had survival value and received the greatest social sanction, to the long gone days when non-coital acts and attempts to reduce the potential supply of people were therefore vehemently condemned, to the long gone days when social and economic arrangements made premarital sexuality tabu. The needs of people have changed, yet the world has not.

George Bernard Shaw commented : "The reasonable man adapts himself to the world; the unreasonable one persists in trying to adapt the world to himself. Therefore, all progress depends on the unreasonable man." Let us awaken society from its archaic slumbers! Let us persistently prod and poke and change the harsh sex dogmas that wound and scar! Come, let us be unreasonable. Let us change the outmoded world and make progress through action in behalf of authentic sexual enlightenment.

32. Liberated Women = Liberated Children

Margaret M. Horton

Historically, and into the present, the status of children and the status of women have been inextricably linked. Attitudes which oppress women also oppress children. Woman and children have been devalued, exploited, and subordinated together.

Aside from the biological ties, many cultural influences such as religion, education and political orientation have affected their positions. However, the type and effectiveness of the economic system has been and continues to be the single most important determinant, both for its own sake, and for its effect on values. Ethics will be sacrificed before eating. A look merely at our contemporary system by itself would be puzzling, for many of the values we hold dear were developed in response to needs which are no longer present. But the general development of economic systems explains a great deal about the manner in which women and children along with them came to be oppressed and why they have never been able to effectively change their status.

A gathering economy is considered to be the most primitive and was the first practiced by the human race. Food was obtained by foraging and by trapping small animals. Contemporary analogues indicate that there was probably very little division of labor along sexual lines. The position of women was nearly equal to men. Since paternity was unknown, children were identified primarily with the mother, but responsibilitiy for them was probably shared by the whole community to some extent. The status of children depended very much on the quantity of food available. When food was plentiful, children were accepted as they came. They may or may not have been ecstatically welcomed, but neither were they exploited for their economic value. When food was scarce, however, infanticide was frequently practiced, and women, as producers of such undesirable competition for resources, were denigrated accordingly.

With the development of more sophisticated weaponry, hunting began to take a more important role in economic life. In hunting economies, division of labor along sexual lines is generally quite pronounced. Furthermore, the status of women varies in inverse proportion to the dependence on hunting as a source of food; where hunting is the primary source of food, women are seen as quite lowly. Women's frequent pregnancies and nursing obligations precluded their going along on extended hunting trips, so women did not develop that skill. On the other hand, the camp had to function without the presence of men, so that when they did come home, their presence was largely superflous. Among nomadic tribes like, for example, many American Indians, women were indispensible but treated quite poorly. They did everything but hunt, even acting as the principal beast of burden. It is reported that when the natives along the lower Murray in Australia first saw pack oxen, they thought these were the wives of white men. Male children were desired because mortality among males was high, but females were seen as being easily replaced, and female infanticide was common.

While the men were out polishing their spears, women were busy inventing agriculture, and in so doing, signed themselves into bondage for the next 5000 years. This aspect of cultural development has always fascinated me because of the fact that the discovery of the wheel, which is usually attributed to a male, has received a great deal of emphasis and publicity. (Actually, since women were responsible for transportation it would make more sense to assign that credit to women. However, the development of agriculture, which is almost universally credited to women, has never received the emphasis it deserves even though its cultural implications were more profound and far-reaching. Obviously, the wheel is a symbol that has a great deal of appeal for our technological age, but it is equally obvious that there are other prejudicial factors at work here. The domestication of animals and plants was so successful that it made hunting obsolete, and men began to take over agricultural functions. Women could not successfully compete with men for the right to practice agriculture because they still had continual pregnancies and nursing to contend with. The ability to assure a continuous food supply allowed the establishment of permanent camps, and with a permanent location came the development of the concept of property and true patriarchy. When mobility has a high survival value, possessions are a hindrance. When stability exists, property represents a means of extending dominance over the environment. As men accumulated property, they desired to have children who would inherit it. The need to know that children were *theirs* led to monogamy and the imposition of strict sexual constraints on the female. Since males were growing the food, they were the property holders and began to consider women and children property to dispose of as they saw fit. Buying and selling wives began about this time and expanded to the practice of slavery in many parts of the world. Children were desired, particularly male children, because of their value as field hands, and they were exploited. The desirability of female children depended primarily on the relative worth of the bride price and the dowry.

This state of affairs persisted until the industrial revolution. Previously, women had functioned as the slaves of individual men, and those men had been relatively autonomous. Now great masses of men became subordinate to other men. Before, their work had been meaningful and integrated into their daily lives. Now their work was transformed into "jobs" which were boring, repetitious, and alienating. However, the fact that the jobs required few skills also meant that women were equally eligible to perform this labor. The same phenomenon that represented a step toward subservience for men was a step toward liberation for women. Initially, children were ruthlessly exploited as sources of labor, although they no longer had the value to the individual family that they had under agriculture. With the advent of child labor laws the economic value of children declined markedly, and the pressure on women to have many children lessened. Adequate birth control procedures were the final requisite to make the subjugation of women obsolete and unnecessary.

As the means of making a contribution to society shifted from making babies to making products, women began to demand access to the means by which they could make a contribution. They demanded the right to work, to vote, and to a decent education. However, the subservience of women had long since become functionally autonomous. That is to say, men liked having women wait on them hand and foot. If the economic dependence of women was to be the price, they were willing to pay it. Women had to fight for whatever gains they made. The eighty-year struggle for the vote stands as a reminder of the enormous resistance encountered in some of those battles. Women won many rights, but pressures from society and individual men prevented women from exercising their skills. The principal role open to women was that of wife and mother.

This was essentially the situation that Betty Friedan described in

1963 in *The Feminine Mystique*. Women were being disenfranchised by social norms.* There was great pressure on them to marry, have several children, and devote themselves thereafter to the joys of housework, cooking and to sacrificing themselves to their husbands and children. The alternative was to become a "career woman" which effectively cut them off from a meaningful family life. Everyone "knew" that career women were bitchy and domineering, and certainly no one would want to marry one. A lot of them probably were strong and aggressive because it always takes courage and determination to swim against the mainstream of social thought.

Actually, there was another, equally dismaying alternative: to attempt to combine a family with a career, which in effect meant holding down two full-time jobs. Working 40 hours a week did not release them from the obligations of housework. The Chase Manhattan Bank estimates that the average housewife works 99.6 hours per week, so even if she were an efficient organizer and had domestic help, she usually came home from a full day's work to cook supper, put the children to bed, and then attempt to appear sexually desirable to her husband.

During the Fifties, America was known as a child-oriented society for good reason. The average woman was denied a meaningful role in life except to live vicariously through her husband and children. Since so much of her self-esteem depended on her children, she was afraid to discipline them for fear they would not love her; that would mean she was a bad mother and, therefore, no good as a person. Of course, it was impossible for them to respect her under these circumstances, but she could still control them through guilt.** Inordinate demands were frequently placed on children to grow up in their parents' image because the parents had no life of their own: they were sacrificing everything for their children; surely they had the right to expect *something*. But that

---

*N.B. the way these social norms came about: The country and the economy had functioned beautifully during World War II with millions of men in the armed services and essentially contributing nothing to the productive processes. When they were demobilized, they had to make another place for themselves in the economy. It was time for Rosie the Riveter to move out and give them a chance, but she didn't want to. The great back-to-the-home-and-family-and-children ethic was created by men to induce women to leave the labor market so that positions would be opened for men.

**In *How to Be A Jewish Mother*, (Los Angeles: Price, Stern & Sloan, 1964), Dan Greenburg beautifully demonstrated the rules for controlling behavior through guilt. This book systematically treated a profoundly serious topic in a humorous manner, and thus, perhaps, made it easier to assimilate the truth.

something was sometimes more than the child could give. A mother would be afraid to have her children grow up, because if they did, she would not longer have an identity. So she artificially prolonged dependency needs into adulthood. The worst tragedy was that many women were pressured into having children they did not want. The mothers may not have been able to admit it to themselves, but the children certainly knew it. They were stuck in the classical double bind. It seems impossible to say enough negative things about this system; the data are certainly plentiful.

The Sixties was a period of awakening for many women and we now have that full-blown phenomenon that terrifies some, angers others, puzzles many, and inspires women everywhere: the Women's Movement. Men find themselves paraphrasing Freud's famous question, "What is it you women want, anyway?"

Let's get one thing straight right away. Women do *not* want to be men. They think they have something better going for them. The concept of penis envy as a motivating force is ludicrous and deserves an angry response only when it is spoken in pompous tones with the weight of authority behind it. Women think that, in general, men and "masculine" attitudes have made a mess of a world that is polluted with industrial wastes from dehumanizing factories that produce goods nobody really wants for the benefit of some fat capitalist who robs the poor and gives to the rich (himself), thus supporting a tax system which enables the perpetuation of an unjust war. So women are really more interested in changing the system than in making it in the present one.

What women do want is:

Equal training and educational opportunities

Equal opportunity to exercise those skills once they have been acquired

Equal rewards for work done

24-hour public child care centers

The right to control the reproductive resources of their own bodies

Equal responsibility for household and childcare tasks

Freedom from domination

Freedom from discrimination

Freedom from sex-role stereotypes

To obtain these changes, they are willing to: assume equal economic responsibility for themselves and their families; assume equal responsibility for the defense of the country; assume equal responsibility for decisions; give up protective discrimination; share equally the rewards of home and family life; and grant freedom from sexrole stereotypes.

Although critics find the social changes most anxiety-arousing because they have difficulty creating reasonable-sounding arguments for keeping women down, they usually attack the political and legal changes.*

The right to equal training and job opportunities are demands that few would dispute. Nevertheless, innumerable obstacles greet every woman who attempts to make something of her life. The list is painfully long. Many colleges and professional schools impose a quota on the number of women admitted. For example, Stanford maintains a 3:2 male-female ratio; at Princeton, the figure is 3:1; at Yale, 5:1. A larger number of educational institutions control admission ratios by demanding higher grades from women. Others refuse to admit women at all on the grounds either that women will distract men from their serious work or that women will drop their professional interests upon marriage, in spite of the fact that both these fears have been consistently proven groundless. Discrimination along sex lines is even more rigid in the trades than in the professions. Entrance into the most profitable trades is closed at each successive level beginning with the refusal to allow girls to take industrial arts in high school. Most trade schools will not accept women at all. Unions are extremely difficult for women to join. On-the-job training for technical skills is nearly nonexistent due to sex-role prejudice and a reluctance to promote women.

Similar difficulties restrict job opportunities and promotions, particularly in fields traditionally assigned to men. As a result, women occupy a disproportionate number of underpaid and menial jobs. According to the Bureau of Labor (1970), women are 97% of household workers, 60% of all other service workers, 75% of all clerical workers, and 31% of all factory workers. 51.6% of women workers occupy clerical or service positions as opposed to 13.8% of men. Many of these restrictions are even sanctioned by laws which forbid women working in specific occupations, restrict the number of hours they may work (which eliminates overtime pay), or restrict the activities they may engage in on the job. These are only a few of the external problems women encounter, and the social and psychological pressures have not even been mentioned. This pattern of discrimination against women affects children indirectly in numerous ways such as the perpetuation of sex-role stereotypes; however, it affects them directly and materially by confining women to poorly paid and marginal jobs.

---

*It *is* a step aove the *ad hominem* argument frequently heard: "Those women are just a bunch of frustrated, ugly neurotics who can't catch (or hold) a husband."

Some conservatives still frowningly declaim that women belong at home. They blithely ignore that women constitute 38% of the labor force, that 44% of all women over age sixteen work, that 63.4% of them are married, and that 55% of the married working women have children under eighteen. The idea that women have a "place" is obviously nonsense, as any reasonably open-minded look at women will demonstrate. Nevertheless, these myths persist. One of the most persistent, vicious, and difficult to deal with is the notion that working mothers are somehow doing irreparable damage to their children.

A recent poll[2] of *Psychology Today* readers, who are presumably better informed than the general public, revealed that 41% of male respondents and 24% of female respondents agreed with the statement "Children of working mothers are less well adjusted." In contrast, a review of the literature on maternal employment[3] from 1960-1970 revealed that children of working mothers were more assertive, more independent, less conforming, and higher school achievers where stable day care was available. Where problems did appear among children, family instability, unstable alternate care, and attitudes toward the morther working were more important factors than the simple fact that the mother worked. It is incredible that any ill effects of *parental* deprivation should be blamed solely on the mother with the father assuming no responsibility. However, since that is the case, unfair as it is, perhaps the research into maternal employment will lessen the burden of guilt that is forced onto working mothers. Other critics, under a humanistic guise, say that all work is dehumanizing and both men and women should go home. This attitude blatantly disregards the fact that ours is a complex society in which we are inextricably interdependent. Furthermore, work is often exalting; it is jobs that are dehumanizing. A return to the Fifties, with both parents in on the home glorification act this time, is not as satisfying a solution as is changing the rigidity of job structures.

It still remains that in the United States, women receive an average of 59% of the pay of men in the same occupation.* No rationalization can disguise the basic injustice in this fact. Equal opportunity and pay for women would have a profound effect on the lives of

---

Time Magazine (3-20-72) estimated that it would cost $109 billion, more than the total pretax corporate profits in 1971, to equalize pay scales. That figure does not even include the unpaid labor of volunteers or women who contribute significantly to their husbands' business. If you add in the $13,391.56 a year that the Chase Manhattan Bank figures as the value of the average housewife's labor, the figure becomes staggering.

many children. Children of divorced parents almost always go with the woman who must depend on the good will of her ex-husband for child support. One study in Wisconsin[4] found that within a year after divorce, 60% of husbands had stopped making full child support payments. If he decides to stop paying, court procedures seldom help, and she must then find a way to support the children in spite of multiple handicaps in the labor market. Thus, 38% of families headed by women (10.5 million) were classified as below poverty level in 1969, as opposed to 8% of families headed by men (13.5 million). Women head 43% of the poverty level families.

Arguments about public child care centers tend to be heavy on emotion and light on logic. Surely no one can deny that such facilities are sorely needed. Statistics released from the Department of Labor in March, 1970, show that half the mothers of school-age children, a third of the mothers of preschool children, and a fourth of the mothers of children under three are working. In fact, about half the women who work are married and have children, and most of them are working out of economic necessity. Eight million of them are raising children alone. And, as previously mentioned, stable day care is more important to children than the fact that their mothers work. But the cost and time involved in arranging for child care frequently almost nullifies a mother's salary.

There are a number of people genuinely concerned about the effects of day care on children and their concerns are legitimate. There is no doubt that facilities would have to be strictly licensed and inspected. A more enlightened philosophy than just taking care of bodies is also necessary. But the public schools have been functioning in a day care capacity for years. There is no evidence that children sent to our present day care centers are harmed in any way. On the contrary, the evidence indicates that children benefit from having their mothers work. In the first place, the mothers have lives of their own, and do not demand that their children live for them. They are free to live their own lives. When children are with their parents, their parents are happy to see them and not resentful that their entire adult lives are being sacrificed. It seems strange, considering that most mothers have little training or preparation, that their role in the child's life should be looked upon with such sanctity. There is nothing about bearing a child that mystically endows a woman with the ability to fulfill all the child's needs from parturition on. It is lack of love that harms children, but there is no evidence that love must come from one particular person or be administered all day every day. The reasons that America is the only industrialized nation in the world that does not provide public day care centers are that it would be expensive (yet 40% of the federal budget, or 78.3 billion dollars in 1970, is spent on the military) and, ironically, because we are an affluent nation that thinks it can afford to treat women as a reserve labor force to be called upon in times of need and disposed of when the crisis passes.

The right of women to control the reproductive resources of their own bodies is an issue with ethical overtones that frequently mask calculating policies. In general, the ethic that calls upon people to produce large number of children for society and the state is a holdover from the times when a large population represented military security or ascendency, and secondarily, when children were valuable labor resources. The Catholic Church, for example, which cites humanitarian values as the reason for its ban on birth control, is actually prescribing a morality which will ensure its own dominance by sheer number of the faithful. In a similar way, abortion reform in the U.S. is blocked because men, who are the legislators, would prefer to retain control over the child-bearing capacities of women. Only 11 states as of this writing (1972) have laws which result in abortion on demand. Polls consistently indicate that 60% of the population and 75% of women want abortion reform. It is sometimes argued that men should have a voice in the decision because a man might want the child though the women does not. If he wants the child and is willing to care for it, then he should have a voice, and the decision should be a private matter between the two of them. But no man should have the power to force a woman to carry his future child for nine months against her will; if he wants a child he should find a willing partner.

Prior to 1967, estimates of the number of illegal abortions in the U. S. ranged from 200,000 to 1,200,000 according to the Federal Commission on Population Growth. It is estimated that one-fourth of American women have had an abortion. Yet in New York, where abortion is legal, it is one-fourth as dangerous as a tonsillectomy in the U.S.* An unexpected benefit from the liberalized New York abortion law is that the maternal death rate fell from 5.2/10,000 live births to 2.9. The illegitimacy rate has dropped 14% and the birthrate is down 7%. True humanitarianism would dictate that no woman should be forced to have a child that she does not truly want,

---

*The death rate in New York from abortion is 4.3 per 100,000. In the U.S. deaths from tonsillectomy and adenoidectomy is 17 per 100,000. Childbirth is four times as dangerous as legal abortion.

and that every child brought into the world will be wanted and loved.

Of the desired social changes, probably the easiest to explain is sharing of houshold and child-care responsibilities. Even in the most liberal marriages today it is still the husband helping her with "her" housework. Pat Mainardi's classic paper, *The Politics of Housework*, delineates some of the difficulties in changing this situation even if both parties are reasonably committed to change. With respect to child care, much the same situation exists. The first week the thrilled father dutifully wakes up and "helps" with the two o'clock feeding. Maybe he'll even change a couple of diapers (as long as they're only wet). After the second week, his participation decreases, and the frequency of mumbled statements like "I'm really no good at this sort of thing" increases drastically. Children of both sexes should be taught that having a child is a joint decision which entails joint responsibilities for the development of that child; paying the bills doesn't make a father. There is nothing about the relationship between a mother and child that precludes other people. A child cannot help but benefit from having two people love and care for him/her instead of just one.

Domination means that any man has the right to tell any woman what to do, regardless. It is a by-product of the patriarchal system in which women and children are treated as property. It sounds archaic but it exists around us in ways that people do not even notice because it is an integral part of the system. The idea that a husband can forbid his wife to go to work, for example, and her acceptance of the fact that she must have his consent, if not his blessing, before undertaking such enterprises is domination because it is not reciprocal. Verbal assaults on the street are another example, ranging from cool appraisals of her probable ability in bed to obscene suggestions for making an empirical test of her abilties. Many men claim this is good clean fun, and that they are just being appreciative. Well, sometimes that is true, but usually not. Every woman knows the difference and knows that 95% of them are colossal put-downs. Physical assaults from rape to an unwanted pat on the fanny occur constantly. Americans are very sensitive about physical contact and consider if offensive to be touched without permission. Yet American men are able to violate this taboo with impunity every day. This teaches children that there is a hierarchy in which some people are allowed to do what most people are not supposed to do. They also learn that women must be inferior, or else these things would not happen to them, and that mothers must be helpless or they would not submit so meekly. Furthermore, any social hierarchy which rates women as inferior will be even more oppressive to children and will regard them as somehow less than human.

Discrimination comes in many forms. Anyone can recognize the discrimination involved in not hiring some individuals, not promoting them, or underpaying them. But what about the fact that women's work is undervalued relative to that of their male colleagues? Identical articles are consistently rated higher on profundity and writing style when the fictitious author is a man.[5] What about the fact that our language excludes women when speaking in generic terms? "Man, " "mankind," even *"humanity"* all exclude women to some extent. If you don't think that's so, ask yourself if you think the term "womankind" includes any men. When speaking of a person of unknown gender, the pronoun "he" is always used. What about the fact that there is only one woman U.S. Senator? How would you feel if there were 99 women Senators and one man? All this teaches children that women are inferior, not fully human, and not deserving of equal consideration.

Sex-role stereotypes are well documented[6] and would not be too much to complain about had not men appropriated for themselves most of the socially desirable traits like aggressive, independent, objective, active, logical, and self-confident. Women are left with a few good ones such as gentle, sensitive to others' feelings, and capable of expressing tender emotions.[7] Children as young as four and five are able to differentiate male traits from female traits and behave consistent with some stereotypes as early as 13 months. (Think about pink and blue blankets for a minute.) Boys learn early that it is unacceptable for them to cry. Girls learn equally early that they are somehow inferior to boys and develop a negative self-concept that lasts for life. If logic is a desirable human trait, then it is desirable for girls as well as boys. If gentleness is good, then it is good for boys, too.

One study[8] on the children of women who identified with the Women's Movement indicated that they were less sterotyped in their choice of toys and in their description of sex-roles than those with mothers not known to be active in The Movement. However, the study concluded "The family has some effect in eliminating sex-role stereotypes, but it alone cannot obliterate sex-typing, because of the pervasive influences of the rest of society."

Thus, children have invariably followed the fate of women. For too many centuries women and children have listed as subservient, inferior persons. If women are liberated from subservience, they can help children achieve inner freedom. If women are no longer viewed as property of men, they can give children a sense of self-ownership and integrity. If women no longer have children they do not want, they will be able to give love to children they do want. If women have lives of their own, they can permit children to have lives of their own. If women have control over themselves and their existence, they can help children develop self-control.

The liberation of women guarantees that each child will be wanted, not an accident; that every child will be cared for by two parents that love him/her, not by one in absentia and the other full of resentment; that every child can grow up to his/her fullest potential, not artificially stunted by inappropriate expectations; and that every child will have the chance to become a unique individual, and to be appreciated for what is, not what "should" be. When women are liberated, children can be liberated too.

References

1. Lubbock, Sir John, *Origin of Civilization*, p. 53.
2. Tauris, Carol. Woman and man. *Psychology Today* March 1972, *5* (10), 57-64.
3. Poenanski, E., Maxey, A., and Marsden, G. Clinical implications of maternal employment: A review of research. *Journal of the American Academy of Child Psychiatry*, 1970, *9*, 741-761.
4. *Time*, The Law, March 20, 1972, p. 67.
5. Goldberg, Phillip. Are women prejudiced against women? *Transaction*, 1968, *5*, 28-30.
6. See, for example, McKee, J. P., and Sherriffs, D. C. The differential evaluation of males and females. *Journal of Personality*, 1957, *25*, 356-371.
7. Rosenkrant, P., Vogel, S., Bee, H., Broverman, I., and Broverman, D. Sex stereotypes and self-concepts in college students. *Journal of Consulting and Clinical Psychology*, 1963, *32*, 287-295.
8. Selcer, B. How liberated are "liberated" children? *Radical Therapists*, 1972, *2* (5), 14-15.

33. *Children and Fathers**

Robert S. Pickett

The Motherhood Myth has clearly hit the skids. The most casual observer passing through the turnstiles of his neighborhood super-market or favorite discount drugstore cannot help detecting titles such as "Motherhood: Who Needs It? " and "The Obsolescence of Motherhood," gracing the covers of even the most middle-of-the-road publications. The reader need not resort to Philip Wylie, that faint voice from the Forties, or underground periodicals of obvious Marxist persuasion to discover that "Applehood and Mother Pie" are no longer sacrosanct. Articles in the *Saturday Review* and *Harper's* will do well enough for those who wish to discover the Ameri-can Mother's current low estate.

It could be argued, however, that Mom is still considered impor-tant enough to be a fit subject for discussion. No such thing can be said for Father. In my most recent trip to the store, I uncovered no headlines shouting forth, "Fatherhood: Who Needs It?" or "Down with Dagwood." True, I did run across a copy of Myron Brenton's *The American Male* bedded down in the pornography section, but, on the whole, Fatherhood, or its absence, seems not to have been considered particularly newsworthy.

After completing my field investigation, I went back to the family hearthside to discover whether or not that part of me known as Father still existed. Fortunately, I was informed that I existed, but there seemed to be less agreement among the members of my family whether or not the concept of Fatherhood, as they understood the historical meaning of the term, applied to my activities or had any-thing to do with their own life.

Shaken, but determined, I climbed the stairs to my study, to ponder the problem of possible obsolescence. Somewhere, deep in the recesses of my imagination, I pictured the possibility of return-ing to the steam heat days of Miss Witham, my old sixth-grade class-

---

*Reprinted with permission from The PTA Magazine, April 1972.

mates, and the poet of my youth, Henry Wadsworth Longfellow. Could it be that the familiar "pause in the day's occupations" would now have to be read as an intrusion by Father and his concerns upon the comings and goings of wife and children?

Sitting in my study, I reflected on the sorry state of a once majestic patriarchy. In a burst of resentment at my lost glory, I seized the nearest instrument to begin what I perceived as the necessary task of rebuilding the badly broken image of Father. Since my field of inquiry is the study of the American family structure, it seemed as if there should be much material at hand. I reached for a copy of one of the most recently published books on my shelf to see what it said about fathers and fathering. It happened to be a recent reader, *Family in Transition,* by Arlene and Jerome Skolnick (Little, Brown and Company).

At first glance, I found articles on sex differences among primates, sex-role stereotyping, and homosexuality, along with an excerpt from Friederich Engels' classic work, "On the Origin of Family, Private Property, and State." The closest I could get to what one might expect of contemporary fathers in our culture was an excerpt describing the miserable family lives of black street corner men from Elliot Liebow's *Tally's Corner* and Robert Jay Lifton's malicious little essay, "Protean Man." Against these savage portrayals, the editors juxtaposed several articles on women and the already mentioned "Motherhood: Who Needs It?" After rummaging back and forth through the pages I discovered what I really had known all along. Fatherhood, whatever it might have meant to Old Testament Joseph and to Freud, Longfellow and me, was dead . . . along with God!

Heavy Lies the Head

When one thinks about the many tasks historically related to the concept of Fatherhood, it is very likely that one might be glad to be rid of the whole business. The role of judge or chief arbiter that fell to the Hebrew patriarchs in the days before King David, for example, was a difficult one. Most modern men probably would not enjoy it. In the midst of the complexities of contemporary society, such a role would seem to involve many quandaries unshared by the ancient desert patriarchs. Judgments as to what is "right" and "wrong" seem considerably harder to make than formerly.

Also, the modern man is likely to appreciate the fact that other functions filled by fathers gone by have never been his to carry out.

The roles of educator as one who passes on accumulated wisdom, and of religious tutor, as one who carefully instructs the young (particularly boys) in spiritual and moral matters, have long since been turned over to school and church. While the results of the historical transfer of such functions have not always been impressive, most fathers would probably be frightened beyond measure if they caught a glimpse of the precarious position these institutions occupy today, and were told that fathers must suddenly assume the academic and religious nurture of their own offspring. Such a state of affairs might, in fact, lead to a sudden influx of financial and "moral support" into our existing schools and religious institutions.

It has, of course, been a long time since fathers, in any great number, worked beside their children in the fields. Perhaps the recent enthusiasm for rural communal living attests to a return to the ideal of nurture through common labor, but more likely such endeavors can only be regarded as an atavistic minority's approach to the grinding complexities of modern society.

A more universal problem is that faced by adult males and, increasingly, by adult females, in relation to the practice of working for wages. One key assumption in all this is that work, as we know it, will exist in the future. One must be modern enough in his outlook to realize that he is, indeed, teetering on the edge of what has been identified as a postindustrial society in which the male role of "breadwinner" is an anachronism. The average father could become very insecure when he realizes that the role which he has historically occupied most of his days on earth is rapidly vanishing.

Luckily, the adult male has options if he is willing to scrap the particular masculine category of father. If he is willing to be addressed as a parent who happens to be male, he can still receive attention. Although contemporary parents appear to be maligned by spokesmen from both the left and the right, it seems that the function of providing emotional and social nurture at least merits the dignity of discussion. Unlike Fatherhood, Parenthood is not ignored. In *Family in Transition,* Alice Rossi and others deal with parenting in an article entitled the "Mystique of Parenthood." Although this remaining possibility is a long distance from Longfellow's lofty position, it seems to be the only viable alternative left.

As I considered the actuality of the male parent, as opposed to the historic notion of Fatherhood, I was moved to examine what kind of entity it might represent. Since I could not become an ancient patriarch, it was necessary to consider what my lot in life really was. The following pages contain my initial findings on this matter.

Life Without Father

The role of the male parent has changed rapidly in recent years, as contemporary social science literature attests. Within the middle class, in particular, not only are decisions being increasingly shared by both sexes, but household jobs formerly designated as specifically male or female are now likely to be performed by either spouse. Chores usually equated with parenting, for example, are as likely to be carried on by the father as by the mother. For example, the task of disciplining in middle-class homes is, happily, less likely than formerly to be "saved up" for father to deal with at the end of the day. Whoever happens to be nearest at the time disciplines the child.

This concept has been extended in communal settings, where it is sometimes the practice to have any adult parent any child. Even in working-class homes, where the pattern has been traditionally authoritarian in terms of male dominance, a convergence of styles seems to be occurring. In the so called black matriarchy, where it has been assumed that black women do all the parenting, black males now appear to have played a greater role in parenting all along.

When adult males have shown warmth and affection toward the young, whether or not their role has been legally sanctioned, children have prospered even in adverse economic situations. The white father who believes that no black male can love and discipline children would do well to look closely at the largely unwritten history of the "man behind the door". Some white upper-middle-class fathers were clocked in a recent study as having spent an average of twenty-six seconds a day in direct interaction with their own infants. These fathers might well take particular heed as to when or where "fathering" is taking place.

In sex education either the father or the mother may inpart information or knowledge. And it has been recently argued that *both* fathers and mothers have wisdom, as well as feelings, to share with their young. Not even the best school curriculum in sex education can achieve much without the supplemental support and example of concerned parents.

It is understandable that fathers have often abdicated their roles as sex educators, but past ignorance is no excuse for present timidity. Those who sire children must be able to do more than they are now doing in this matter. If they feel ignorant and inadequate, let them jointly pick up the gauntlet with parent educators and children in community-wide sex education programs. There they may yet learn alongside their children and their children's teachers. Failure to do so is likely to have one of two results. The first is unrelieved ignorance, with its side effects of unwanted pregnancy and continued sexual inadequacy. The second result is constricted sex education curriculums that are both perfunctory and irrelevant.

In any event, fathers have an obligation to consider what knowledge from their own past is worth the consideration of their sons and daughters. For example, is it not fitting for a father to communicate the anxieties of his adolescent past to his growing son? A father is also in a position to help his daughter learn what it means to be a person in the eyes of a man who loves you as child, growing woman, and person.

I unabashedly hold that what is now sex education will increasingly be a part of education for life. In the country of the young, fathers as well as mothers must teach their young what they themselves have found out and will go on finding out in various painful ways.

Since fathers are increasingly denied the opportunity to claim their chief masculine identity from their jobs, they will have to define masculinity in new terms. The *balance* of vocation, avocation, and recreation in the life of adult males will have to be achieved against a new background—that of nonexploitative maleness. The physiques of males vis-à-vis females are, as has frequently been pointed out, probably less fitted for participating in the late twentieth century's automated world. Nevertheless, the continued trend for nondiversified task accomplishment will be worked out by entire families. Whoever is handy will operate the implement, whether it be eggbeater, hoe, plow, vacuum cleaner, dishwasher, or power mower.

Dad Shall Have His Day

In a world where the price of aggression has become too great, the notion of what it means to be a man of compassion and love, yet of vigor and determination, will require careful articulation in word and deed. Women have been the truly conservative force in society in that they have traditionally tended the hearth and nurtured the child while men have gone forth to procure food and make war. It is abundantly clear that these historic functions are in a state of rapid change, and that the social being known as the father will not return to past ways any more than the mother. If he would truly remove himself from the category of obsolescence, planned or otherwise, the man called Father, or the parent who happens to be male, will have to operate in future times as a conserving yet generative force in society.

To do so will mean to cease lamenting for lost glories and to seize the challenge of the hours and days ahead. The sole alternative is oblivion.

34. Family Planning in the 1970s— A Dynamic Force Affecting the Status of Children*

Naomi Thomas Gray

The social work profession is committed to helping relieve the pressures and deprivations suffered by children and their families. As the profession and its institutions consider factors affecting the status and general welfare of children in this decade, they must not fall into the trap of believing that family planning is the sole or even major solution to some of the economic, social, physical, and emotional plight of children. Planned Parenthood World Population estimates that there are at any one time about 5.3 million fertile American women between the ages of 15 and 44 living in poverty or near-poverty, not pregnant or seeking pregnancy.[1] A Planned Parenthood analysis of a U. S. Census Bureau study showed that 70 percent of these women—the population needing family planning services—are white, two thirds live in cities, and only 14 percent are recipients of public welfare.

Yet some social workers, like other well-meaning members of other professions, continue to express stereotyped ideas about the poor and especially those dependent on public welfare for minimal income. For instance, many, among them far too many professionals, oppose a guaranteed minimum income because of fear that this would encourage women to have more out-of-wedlock children. There is no evidence to support this fear. Schorr says that a rigorous scientific demonstration has not been provided to show that income maintenance either will or will not lead to a higher birth rate. A new income-maintenance program would in all probability lead some people, including some who are poor, to have additional children.

*This paper was presented at the CWLA Southwest Regional Conference at Fort Worth, Texas, 1970. It is reprinted with permission from *Child Welfare*, 1971, L. #3, 143-149.

But this effect would probably be insignificant in relation to other concurrent developments, and not discernible in subsequent population figures. Balancing any such small effect, a substantial income-maintenance program would significantly improve the circumstances of many families. In their children's generation, at least, it may provide the competence and climate to achieve the family size that the generation wants.[2]

Another study of fertility behavior among the lower class supports this thesis by concluding that there is one central norm about family size: "One should not have more children than one can support, but one should have as many children as one can afford."[3]

Podell, in a study of families on welfare in New York City, says that six of every 10 mothers on welfare would have only one or two children if they could begin again. Of those for whom birth control was applicable, 40 percent reported practicing it. More likely to do so were women who (a) were younger (b) had more children, especially preschoolers, (c) had husbands in the households, (d) were independence-oriented in their attitude, and (e) were exposed to the information media. Two-thirds of the women for whom birth control was applicable knew of the contraceptive pill. and seven out of 10 of them knew where to go to obtain free advice about family planning.[4]

These findings bear out what other researchers have found: Low-income Americans, when compared with higher socio-economic groups, show a preference for having as few or fewer children.[5] In fact, several authorities in the demographic field attribute the "population explosion" in the United States to the third "wanted" child among middle-class families.[6] The middle and upper classes are producing 70 percent of births in this country.[7]

Generally, when people, including professionals, think of birth control for the poor, they think of blacks and other minority groups, which has brought on a charge by some black nationalists of attempted genocide. Seldom is priority given to the needs of poor whites for family planning services. This is discrimination in reverse. Birth control is, of course, no substitute for the alleviation of poor housing, hunger and malnutrition, unemployment, and inadequate education, health, and welfare resources; however, it must be considered along with the other services and information made available to clients.

Indications for Family Planning As It Affects the Status of Children

As child welfare workers, we are aware of some of the problems affecting the healthy emotional and physical development of children. We are aware of the tragedy of the unwanted child and of the fact that, as urban pressures increase, the number of unwanted births both in and out of wedlock is likely to rise unless adquate options to space and limit pregnancies are offered. It is important to make a distinction between an unplanned pregnancy and an unwanted child. Unplanned pregnancies do not invariably result in unwanted babies. Probably most "accidental" babies are loved as much as planned ones.[8] However, a tragic percentage are born into homes without love, supervision, or systematic care.

Indications to the social worker for family planning include:

(1) *The rejected child.* Numerous studies have pinpointed the emotional and psychological damage to the child who is unwanted and rejected by one or both parents. Many end up in institutions or foster homes. They may develop problem behavior destructive to themselves and others.

(2) *The battered child.* The "battered-child syndrome" is getting increasing attention from health and welfare professionals, the courts, and public media. According to Kempe, at least 700 children are killed every year in this country by their parents or parent surrogates. Thousands more (estimated at 10,000 a year) are permanently injured, physically and mentally.[9] Kempe believes that child abuse is psychodynamically determined.

His experience at the Colorado General Hospital has included cases involving parents who are lawyers, ministers, army officers, engineers, and doctors. But he points out, on the basis of his personal experience, that child-abusing behavior may be affected by poverty, rapid urbanization, overcrowding, by unemployment, by the number of doors that can be closed between the parent and the injured child, and, of course, by the number and quality of lawyers the parent can hire if he gets into trouble. Unquestionably, with this disease, one is better off rich than poor.[10]

Some studies have shown that child neglect and abuse are much more common in white families than in black families. Child neglect is much more common among lower-class white families than among lower-class black families.[11]

(3) *Health hazards to mothers and infants.* The health risks involved in too frequent pregnancies have been well documented by medical authorities. For the children, these risks include prematurity, mental retardation, infant deaths, particularly in the perinatal period; and for the mothers, the dangers of illegal abortions and a high incidence of morbidity and mortality. It has been noted by physicians and health workers that successful family planning enables mothers to regain full physical and mental strength between preg-

nancies, reducing what is known medically as the "syndrome of depletion." Reduction of prematurity through 2-to-3 year intervals between pregnancies also decreases the incidence of infant deaths and birth defects, since both are closely associated with premature births.[12]

(4) *Family size and its relations to family fuctioning.* In a recent article, Dr. James Lieberman, a psychiatrist and consultant at the Center for Studies of Child and Family Mental Health at the National Institute of Mental Health, stated that family size is only one of the factors in child development and mental health. But it appears to be more important than most people realize.[13] He cited new research showing that a child requires a tremendous emotional investment on the part of his parents. (I suspect that low-income large families would express astonishment that research was needed to document this.) Behavioral scientists have found that a child's emotional health is strongly affected by the number of brothers and sisters he has. Several studies of elementary and high school children have shown that the youngster in a small family gets along more happily with brothers and sisters, as well as with parents, than youngsters in large families. He is less likely to suffer emotional upsets and much less likely to end up in a mental hospital. The child may be loved as much in a large family, but most parents, like most budgets, can be stretched only so far.[14]

(5) *Teenage out-of-wedlock pregnancies.* A quarter of a million babies (one baby in 17), are born each year to unmarried American mothers. Forty percent of these mothers are between 15 and 19 years old.[15] Services for these young mothers and their children are totally inadequate. And if the mother is a member of a minority group, especially if she is black, the chance of having her baby adopted is almost nil. It has been estimated that 90 percent of middle-class white girls who get pregnant out of wedlock have abortions or get married, and 90 percent of lower-class black girls who get pregnant have babies. Although the vast majority of white girls who have their babies place them for adoption, the vast majority of black girls keep their babies. It should be obvious that the choice of using or not using adoption and abortion services, under competent medical and social supervision, should be open to all.[16]

Pregnancy exacts a high toll from the teenager in increased physical hazard, interruption of education and possible dropout, and dependency, and often means tragedy for the mother, her baby, and her parents. The increase in the number of teenage out-of-wedlock pregnancies has reached such proportions that numerous special programs are being developed or carried out to provide comprehensive health and social services, including contraception if the girls wish it. The middle-class teenager is able to obtain birth-control counseling and service more eaily than her lower-class counterpart. Some college and university health services are beginning to provide birth-control guidance and service, usually as a result of student demands. But again, it is the adolescent girl from a low-income family who suffers from lack of knowledge and resources for meeting this social and health need.

Providing contraception to teenagers is a sensitive matter and must be handled with great care and skill. If the teenager is pregnant, family planning should be offered as part of a comprehensive service through the prenatal and postnatal period. In order to know how to handle discussions about contraception with individual girls, it is important to have knowledge of the circumstances surrounding the pregnancy. Is the girl sexually active? Is it a wanted or unwanted pregnancy? Accidental? Rape? Incest? One must be careful not to assume that the solution to all out-of-wedlock pregnancies is contraception. This is too simplistic an approach, and the result may be failure.

A major failure in working with pregnant teenagers lies in the way services are delivered to them. Services are not always offered when and where they are convenient. Voluntary agencies are often primarily concerned with middle-class clientele, leaving the poor to governmental agencies, whose services—staff and other resources —are often inadquate. As agency caseloads increase and manpower decreases, many of the professional workers' frustrations are passed on to the clients. Unless the unwed adolescent parent is treated as a whole person, solutions to problems will continue to be elusive. Let us not be fooled into thinking that birth control alone will solve the problem of successive pregnancies. Counseling of a more comprehensive character is needed.

San Francisco Program

Several experimental family planning programs for teenagers are being carried out in locations throughout the country under private or public auspices. In San Francisco for the last 3 years "sexually active" teenagers have been seeking and getting contraceptive counseling and services at a planned parenthood clinic of their own. The clinic, set up to curb out-of-wedlock births among the very young, uses a multidisciplinary team approach—social worker, psychiatrist, physician, nurse, psychologist—to advise young people on their sexuality.

During the first 2 years of this program, the clinic reported, almost 600 girls under 18 used its services. Less than 2 percent went on to unplanned pregnancies.[17] This is a preventive service. The clinic offers counseling and contraceptive service, under medical supervision, based on each girl's needs, to provide the insight and the tools to permit them to manage their sexuality intelligently. Any girl who walks into the clinic is helped. Some are referred by a school nurse or social worker; some by a parent; some by friends or relatives who have heard about the clinic. No appointments are necessary, but if the girls call in advance, they are told that boyfriends are welcome at the group discussions. The clinic meets twice a week in the after-school hours. Of the almost 600 girls who have taken part in the group discussions on sex and birth control, about 475 have been helped with contraception. Seventy percent of the girls are white; 20 percent black; 5 percent of Spanish ancestry and 5 percent Oriental. Eight percent of the patients had a prior pregnancy, and a history of induced abortion was not uncommon. Twenty-two girls of the 475 who wanted contraception help stopped using the method because they were no longer sexually active. Two girls stopped in order to become pregnant. There were ten unplanned pregnancies, two because of failure of the contraceptive method, and eight because of patient failure to use the method or to use it correctly. Five of the girls obtained therapeutic abortions; the others continued their pregnancies.

Only 11 percent of the girls dropped out of the program in the first 2 years of its existence. This includes girls who were lost to followup, but may be continuing as contraceptors. Eight percent of the girls were found to be infected with gonorrhea, and arrangements were made for treatment, either through private physicians or by the veneral disease clinic of the San Francisco Health Department.

Explaining the nonjudgmental attitude of the clinic, Dr. Sadja Goldsmith, its director, pointed out that the "job of helping the girl set standards for her conduct has generally been done earlier in her life by her family environment . . . We feel these girls will be more receptive to a straight message of responsible contraception than a mixed message such as, 'Don't do it, but if you do it, do it with this.'" At the same time, the clinic is alert to the girl who is being pushed into sexual activity and contraception by a boyfriend, peer group, or parent when this is not what she wants for herself. In many such instances, the clinic has helped the girl delay or discontinue coitus.[18]

The San Francisco program places its emphasis on primary prevention, whereas most other programs require as the "ticket of admission" at least *one* pregnancy. In other words,the price of getting contraception help in some programs is to get pregnant first and then apply. Surely we need not be chained to that absurdity any longer.

Program Implications

Family planning has different meanings to different people:
- To a mother overburdened with a large number of children, it can mean no more babies for her or her family's sake. It can mean improving her own physical and emotional health and well-being.
- To a father, it can mean improving his ability to provide for his family with·in the limits of his income.
- To a teenager, it can mean preventing the first or second unwanted pregnancy.
- To those concerned about population control, it can mean limitation of family size among the poor to cut down on the welfare rolls, or family limitation for all people, regardless of race, creed, income, or education, in order to improve the quality of life for rich and poor alike.

Whatever the motivation, it is obvious that family planning must be *voluntary* and acceptable to the individuals involved. I emphasize "voluntary" because there are people who believe that only coercive measures will stem or stabalize population growth.

Mrs. Helen P. Stanford, director of the Mid-Atlantic Region of Planned Parenthood World Population, has outlined five points for program planning for family planning services. They bear repeating here:

(1) Programs and services should be tailored to the needs of the clients and the society in which they live.

(2) Traditionally, programs for family planning services, as for other services, have been developed by administrators. If these services are to reach those who need them, they must be programmed to serve the women, rather than attempting to program the women to the administration of services.

(3) Parenthood and family planning are based on a partnership between male and female. Therefore, should not programs include the male? Can any family planning service that persistently excludes or simply fails to recognize the male and his role be a true family planning service? In many instances welfare has, although inadver-

tently, pushed the father out of the home. In doing so, it has created even greater problems than those it is trying to solve.

Society is very concerned about the unwed mother and her baby, and rightly so. Is society concerned about the unwed father? Does society assume that parenting for the unwed human male is always a casual thing and of no concern to him? If society does assume this, does this affect the male's ability and freedom to show interest and care? To whom does the unwed teenage father turn for help?

(4) Research and evaluation should be part of family planning programming. Such research should be geared essentially to finding ways of providing effective services, rather than studies that merely pry into the live of the poor. There are still many unresearched questions awaiting answers. Those who have labored long in the vineyard hope further research will be pertinent to the delivery of quality and comprehensive family planning services.

(5) Discussion of family planning, especially as it concerns the unwed, often arouses anxiety and even disapproval among those who are supposed to be offering help. Projections of unworthiness onto the poor seem to be intensified whenever sex enters. A focus on the health of the mother and child, on strengthening family life, and through the family the community, can sometimes help trainees in the field to place greater value on these goals and to give up personal, judgmental attitudes. Staff needs to be well informed about birth-control methods, patient fallacies, and areas of patient concerns. Staff, including all professionals and nonprofessionals, should be taught the overriding value of sensitive perceptive contacts with patients.[19]

The social work profession is only beginning to develop competence in family planning counseling. Some workers have more sexual "hangups" than their clients. To help clients achieve competence in family planning practice, the worker must be knowledgeable about and comfortable with human sexuality. For most men, the ability to impregnate, and for most women, the ability to become pregnant, are significant factors in their lives. A social worker must be capable of teaching clients a vocabulary to facilitate communication in this area.[20]

If family planning is to be an effective and dynamic force for enhancing the welfare of children in this and the next decade, the social work profession must step up its involvement in the provision of these services. Family planning must not be viewed as a panacea for all the problems of poverty and dependency, but rather as one important first step. As social workers, our motives should be positive ones, based on the sure knowledge that it is the human right of

each individaul—rich or poor—to decide these matters for himself.[21]
human right of each individual—rich or poor—to decide these matters for himself.[21]

Family planning counseling and services should be handled within the context of other problems of the individual and family, and not as an isolated phenomenon. These services must be dealt with in a sensitive manner to avoid any hint of coercion or implications that these programs and services are directed primarily to any one racial or ethnic group. If social workers are committed to the belief that children are our most precious heritage, the profession must continue to make available a wide range of services, including family planning, so that future generations will not suffer the results of society's neglect and indifference in this decade and the next.

References

1. George Varkey, Frederick S. Jaffee, Richard Lincoln, and Steven Polgar, *Five Million Women—Who's Who Among Americans in Need of Subsidized Family Planning Services* (Austin, Texas: Planned Parenthood World Population, 1967).

2. Alvin Schorr, "Income Maintenance and the Birth Rate," *Social Security Bulletin,* XXVIII, No. 12 (1965).

3. Lee Rainwater, *Family Design* (Chicago: Aldine, 1965).

4. Lawrence Podell, *Families on Welfare in New York City,* (New York: Center for the Study of Urban Problems, Bernard M. Baruch College, 1969), 43-45.

5. Pascal K. Whelpton, A. A. Campbell, and John E. Patterson, *Fertility and Family Planning in the United States* (Princeton University Press, 1966), 37-44.

6. Lincoln and Alice Day, *Too Many Americans* (Boston: Houghton Mifflin, 1964), 106-107.

7. E. James Lieberman, "The Case for Small Families," *New York Times Magazine,* March 8, 1970, 86.

8. Alan F. Guttmacher, "The Tragedy of the Unwanted Child," *Parents Magazine* XXXIX, No. 6 (1964).

9. C. Henry Kempe, "The Battered Child and the Hospital," *Hospital Practice,* IV, No. 10 (1969), 44.

10. *Ibid., 46*

11. Andrew Billingsley, "Family Functioning in the Low-Income Black Community," *Family Casework, L*, No.10 (1969), 567-568.

12. Drs. Helen Wallace, Edwin M. Gold, and Samuel Dooley, "Relationships Between Family Planning and Maternal and Child Health," in *Advances in Planned Parenthood, Vol. V* (Amsterdam and New York: Excerpta Medica Foundation, 1970), 58-59.

13. Lieberman, *op. cit.,* 86.

14. Lieberman, *op. cit.*
15. Guttmacher, *op. cit.*
16. Andrew Billingsley, "Strategies for Expanding Services to Negro Unwed Mothers," Charles N. Crittendon Memorial Lecture, University of California (Los Angeles) School of Social Welfare, April 1968.
17. Sadja Goldsmith, "San Francisco's Teen Clinic," in *Family Planning Perspectives,* I, No. 2 (1969).
18. Goldsmith, *op. cit.*
19. Helen P. Stanford, "Program Planning for Family Planning," in *Family Planning* (New Brunswick, N. J.: Graduate School of Social Work, Rutgers—The State University, 1968).
20. Margaret J. Bernstein, "Social Work Practice Toward Enhancing Competence in Family Planning," in Florence Haselkorn, ed., *Family Planning: The Role of Social Work* (Garden City, N. Y.: Adelphi University Graduate School of Social Work, 1968), 138.
21. Naomi T. Gray, "Family Planning and Social Welfare's Responsibility," *Social Casework* XLVII, No. 7 (1966).

35.   Second Thoughts about
Sex Education in the Schools*

Sol Gordon

Those who argue for increasing public knowledge about sex have
consistently emphasized the role of the schools. Sex education
classes have been set up in many schools and usually are conducted
as a separate course or as a sequence in the health education curriculum. The theory has been that such courses offer the best hope of
reducing the rate of unwanted pregnancies and venereal disease, and
at the same time are helpful in developing more satisfactory sexual
adjustment among youth.

I think it is time we started having second thoughts about the role
of schools in sex education. If by sex education we mean not just
reproduction, but "the broader" aspects of human relationships
which revolve around sexuality, then it is difficult to believe that the
schools can be a pre-eminent force.

Many of us feel that schools have a great tendency to turn kids off
in general. Sex can be made just as dull as any other subject if it is
taught in an uninteresting and evasive manner. Often schools are
teaching sex in just that way—dealing with the plumbing rather than
with what students really want to know.

Schools in many areas have been notoriously unsuccessful in
teaching such basic skills as reading and writing. How can we
assume that they will be able to teach sex any better? Certainly,
schools are not qualified to run birth control clinics or abortion
counseling services.

Sex education is perhaps appropriate in a school with high morale,
where the students enjoy the time they spend there. In an environment which is emotionally reinforcing, schools may be able to help
adolescents develop a better awareness of their own sexuality along
with a greater sensitivity to others. But in a school with low morale

*Reprinted from *Clinical Child Psychology Newsletter,* Vol. X, Nox. 2 & 3, 1971.

—and many of our public schools fit this description—it is doubtful that sex education can be a positive influence on the students' emotional development.

In schools with high rates of pregnancy and venereal disease, it can be beneficial to supply information on contraception and V.D. prevention. But considering that these schools are generally the ones with low morale, "traditional" sex education which seeks to influence attitudes and sexual behavior is not likely to produce significant results.

The advocates of sex education in the schools have seriously overstated their case. They have thought that schools should assume the role of trying to improve the students' sexual and emotional adjustment. Schools, no matter how high their morale, cannot be expected to clear up all the personal problems which affect relationships. *A sound knowledge of the physical aspects of sex can serve to reduce the anxieties and misunderstandings which result from ignorance*, but it cannot significantly change basic personality orientations. The quality of a person's sexual relationships depends less on his knowledge of sex than on his own self-concept and personality adjustment. School authorities are generally too immature to handle the broad issues of morality and sexuality, but this does not mean that they should not work intensively to improve their status so that they can become a more effective force in the education of our youth, including dealing with sensitive and controversial issues like sexuality.

Instead of teaching sex education as a separate subject, the crucial facts should be taught in already existing courses. Human reproduction should be taught well and not evasively in biology. In health classes, venereal disease can be discussed in the same way as any other communicable disease, but with complete candor about its causes and treatment as well as its prevention, including mention of the use of condoms.

Ideally, the models for healthy sexual behavior should be the parents. Unfortunately, most parents fail to carry out this task adequately, both because of their own behavior and because they are not good sources of information. The sexploiting media certainly do not do much in sex education either.

We must begin to place greater emphasis on the role of community services. Churches could be very influential in developing counseling and information centers. Ideally, birth planning or Planned Parenthood centers would be set up in every community. They should be completely open to adolescents. Community members should be trained as workers to talk to people in their own peer, ethnic or language groups.

Colleges and high schools should have courses teaching students how to be effective sex educators as parents. There should be a major curriculum expansion in sex studies in all the schools which prepare people for community service, including the medical, nursing, and social work schools. It is incredible that clinical psychologists are not being educated in the field of human sexuality and family planning. Professionals and paraprofessionals educated in human sexuality would not only be better parents themselves, but would be able to give sound advice to other parents about how to educate their children.

Birth control programs, population education as well as sex information in general must avoid being associated with "the establishment." Political authority has little effect in influencing an area as personal as sexual behavior. People will only do what they can see to be in their own interest. The government of the Soviet Union has been unsuccessful in its efforts to persuade couples to have more children, simply because Russians do not wish to have more than one or two children. This is true despite the ready availability of day care centers and other incentives such as tax relief. It is also interesting that the pill is not generally available and birth control is not encouraged. We know from other experiences that the mere availability of birth control does not mean people will use it.

And, in this country, government warnings about the dangers of drugs are more likely to be met with youthful derision than acceptance. The young are particularly likely to reject anything pushed at them by the establishment, *including* birth control and V.D. prevention. This can be avoided by having birth control clinics run by community members interested in communicating with the young—which means being completely candid and straightforward about sex. Adolescents will accept informaiton which they can use to their own advantage, but they are not likely to readily adapt their behavior to the moralizing platitudes of their uninformed elders. If there were more acceptance about sexual matters, there would not be so many people whose ignorance about sex cripples their ability to relate to others and exposes them to the risk of veneral disease, unwanted pregnancy or sexual hangups.

One popular misbelief interferes with intensive community efforts to offer sex programs to adolescents. This is the idea that girls who become pregnant actually wanted to become pregnant. This myth is largely based on a series of false assumptions documented by research. The studies have asked girls who are already pregnant whether or not they had wanted to become pregnant. A large percentage of the girls reply "yes." This is more likely to be post-facto rationalization than an honest response. When the same question is asked of a comparable group of sexually active non-pregnant girls, the response is almost invariably negative.

Unwed girls do not want to become pregnant, but unfortunately this is not enough to prevent pregnancy. If present rates of out of wedlock (mostly unwanted) birth continue during the next ten years, we can expect one and a half million mothers to give birth to a total of two million children. The reasons are complex, including inadequate knowledge about sex, lack of emotional stability, and a high degree of risk taking. All these conditions are characteristic of young people growing up in our povery-stricken areas. When the environment offers little emotional reinforcement, sex becomes one of the few ways of asserting a person's individuality and escaping from the misery and boredom of life. As a result, a young person is likely to have sex, no matter what the risk.

Next to "risk taking", perhaps the single most important cause of both teenage pregnancies and venereal disease is lack of knowledge. In one high school, 50 per cent of the students thought girls could become pregnant only during menstruation. In the July 28, 1970 issue of *Look Magazine,* Thomas and Alice Fleming reported on "What Kids Still Don't Know About Sex." They cited the fact that more than half of the sexually active girls who were studied at Oberlin College had not used contraceptives. They also included evidence that among unwed teenage girls who were studied at Sinai Hospital, Baltimore, 25 per cent had not even considered the possibility that they would become pregnant.

These are the problems to which we must respond. We must tell adolescents what they really want to know. Here are some typical written questions asked by high school students (unedited):

- I heard after having intercourse you enter a bottle of cola in your vagina you won't become pregnant. Is it true?
- I heard that if a woman doesn't have sex until she's married when she does get married she'll want to have sex with other men to see if all men give the same feeling. Is this true?
- Is it nessesary for a man to use a rubber during sexual intercourse if the woman is taking birth control pills?
- Why can't a man reach climax time after time during sexual intercourse like a woman?
- What causes homosexuality and why?
- Is it good to have sex with a 19 year old if your fifteen?

- How often should you have sex?
- How do a person masturabate?
- If a normal man have sex with another man, is he a homosexual?
- During your 1-2 months of pregnancy when you have a laxative can you get rid of the baby?
- If you have a I.U.D. put inside you to prevent pregnancy, can your boyfriend knock it out of place?
- How would you know when your pregnant—how would you feel, sick or what?
- How can you tell if a girl has VD if she or you does not no?

And most plaintively:

- Where can I get an abortion?

Schools hardly ever answer questions like these!

It is imperative that we relay elementary facts. For example, most teenagers do not know *that all thoughts are normal* and that consequently there is no need for guilt feelings about socially unacceptable desires that spring from the unconscious. They need to be made aware that there is a distinction between a thought and actual behavior, for which they must accept responsibility. Can you imagine how much better a kid would fee if he knew this one simple fact?

Teenagers should also know things like:

- *Masturbation* is a normal and common practice among adults and teenagers (no matter what parents do about it) and that it is not physically harmful, no matter how frequent. It should be explained that it is a healthy expression of their sexuality except when it becomes a compulsive, mechanical behavior with the aim of avoiding life, rather than enjoying it.
- *"Perversions,"* such as oral-genital relations, though technically outlawed in many states, are normal methods of foreplay and normal substitutes for intercourse among many couples.
- Agonized doubts about *penis* size disturb adolescent boys. The average size when erect is four to six inches, but whether smaller or larger, the pleasurable effect during intercourse, in both partners, remains the same, despite legends to the contrary.
- A few *homosexual* acts and/or sexual thoughts about a person of the same sex are common to many girls and boys. These acts and thoughts rarely are signs that a person is becoming a homosexual. The "fear" is what worries young people. Further, homosexuality is not necessarily inherently abnormal. In Ancient Greece, for instance, it was acceptable; in our culture it generally isn't. The problems related to homosexuality decrease when adolescents are helped to overcome secret fears of the opposite sex. Also, being a "he-man" is no indication of sexual preference. In any case, there

should be no laws discriminating against sexual behavior between two consenting adolescents or adults.

- The more objective investigators have found that *pornography* is not harmful and that rather than stimulating sexually aggressive behavior, it acts as an alternative and thereby as a deterrent. Anyway, most people, young and old, get bored with even the most explicit pornography after awhile.

- Without proper medical treatment, *venereal disease* can cause tremendous damage, including sterility, insanity and death; the first symptoms often disappear even while the disease continues to progress internally. V.D. spreads through homosexual or heterosexual sexual contact.

Adolescents need to be told outright how and when girls can get pregnant and how and when they are most likely to avoid pregnancy.

We should remember that, whether or not society likes it, many teenagers engage in sexual activity. And if we think that by not telling them about birth control we can prevent this, we are wrong.

For this reason, they should be aware that condoms ("rubbers") usually prevent pregnancy and vastly reduce the chances of V.D. contamination. Boys need instruction in their correct use. Girls need medical guidance in the correct use of the birth control pill and the facts about foams, and insertion of intrauterine devices (IUDs). Emphasis should be placed on what adolescents can secure easily without prescription or medical controls. For instance, the combination of the foam and the condom will greatly reduce the risk of V.D. and unwanted pregnancy.

They should be aware that in the event of unwanted pregnancy there are states, such as New York, where abortion is safe, legal and professional. They should know that if an abortion if performed in the first 20 weeks of pregnancy, there is less chance of maternal injury or death than in childbirth.

Information like this is of *immediate* help. It will do much more to resolve some of the basic problems associated with sexuality than will school courses which deal only in plumbing or, on the other hand, spend most of their time emphasizing how to build rewarding human relationships.

Perhaps one of the most hopeful approaches to education for healthier attitudes toward sex can be found in the Women's Liberation movement. It is getting across the message that women are human beings, not creatures existing only to be exploited by males. Contraceptives could free women from the restrictions of bearing children primarily and allow them to pursue different directions in life. With women and men relating as equals, hopefully many of the anxieties which have arisen out of the traditional male-female role-games can be avoided. If women can see opportunities existing for them outside the home, they will be more likely to use contraceptives.

In the effort to reduce the rate of unwanted births, both inside and outside marriage, and to reduce the incidence of venereal disease, we should, of course, devote the major part of our efforts to the factors which have the greatest impact on these problems—education and economic well-being. The lowest birthrates are consistently found among those at the higher education and economic levels. Examples can be found in college-educated women, Jews, and middle-class blacks, who all produce children at a rate well below that of the national average. In the problem of unwanted births, like many other problems, the greatest enemy is poverty. These problems are likely to continue until all Americans can expect a fair income and a decent education. Obviously immediate efforts—even if they be stop-gap—are needed to help poor families plan their families, but the only real solution is a total national commitment to ending poverty.

Sex education should teach young people how to relate to each other as responsible and responsive human beings. Sex education is meant to have an impact on the whole personality, to make people more self-confident, more sensitive, more open about their feelings and more understanding about the feelings of others. *And there should be widespread dissemination of the crucial facts about sex.* Adolescents are particularly in need of information in order to counteract the anxiety they often feel as their sexual awareness and experience increases.

We must give second thoughts to the matter of sex education! Schools cannot handle the entire job and parents have failed in it. The community must take on the job of setting up services and distributing information. Community service people should be educated in human sexuality so that they can carry out this function. Eventually, sex education of the young will go back to the parents where it has been assigned traditionally. The goal of all of us should be to educate so well that as people become parents, they will assume the task of sex education gladly and successfully.

Instead of depending on the schools, we should concentrate on the community, setting up the services and distributing the information which people need to meet their problems. Parents as well as young people need to be better informed. Our goal must be that all parents will become qualified to fulfill the duty traditionally assigned to them—the sexual education of the young.

Part Eight

PROFESSIONAL TRAINING

In this section, the manifold training issues of the young profession of clinical child psychology are explicated.

36. The Training of Clinical Child Psychologists

Loretta K. Cass

Issues in the Training of Clinical Child Psychologists

The founders of the Section on Clinical Child Psychology (Section I) of Division 12 had, as one of their first priorities, bringing to the attention of the parent organization their conviction that clinical psychologists who work with children require education and training in that specialty. In fact, the Interest Group for Clinical Child Psychology, the precursor of Section I, wrote in its very first *Newsletter,* "It is thought that our Interest Group can offer a real service to our profession by clarifying the issues involved in the training of psychologists for clinical work with children, particularly by crystallizing our own thinking in this area and offering our recommendations as a group to relevant national groups such as our own APA and others." (*17*, p. 2). Even while this conviction was being voiced, however, and increasingly in the decade thereafter, the specialty itself had proliferated into so many professional roles that the question of setting standards for training is now a question of training for *what.*

The central issue in the training of clinical child psychologists is how to provide the didactic and experiential background for the many professional roles which have arisen, without design or protocol, out of community needs. Related to this, and equally important, is the issue of whether or not there exists a *core* of knowledge and skills which can serve as a common denominator for all or most of the developing professional roles. Finally, there is the question of the locus of professional training—in the university or in the practicuum setting. More specifically, can the university define and provide that theoretical and technical background which will provide the solid base for the widely diversified needs of the practicuum settings?

The Changing Scene in Professional Psychology

Clinical child psychology is caught up in the rapid changes which have characterized the last twenty years of professional clinical psychology and which have set committees of national accreditation bodies and university programs to work to identify and to prepare psychologists for these innovations in the field. The changes in practice are·clearly outlined by Hersch (*13*) as changes in the definitions of who is the *patient,* who is the *therapist,* what is the *process* of treatment and what are its *goals,* what *theory* guides professional work and, finally, what is the role of the mental health professional. "The overall changes in the mental health field represented fundamentally a shift from a clinical to a public health frame of reference. The move was from an intensive preoccupation with the individuals to a concern over large populations. Programs came to orient themselves not only to intrapsychic pathology, but to focus on the community. Attention was placed on the prevention of disability, not only upon its cure." (13, p.912). This latter emphasis on prevention of disability and on the "optimizing of human development" was a highlight of the Report of the Joint Commission on Mental Health of Children in 1969 (15, p.6).

The Committee on Standards and Professional Practice of Section I, faced with this proliferation of roles in the children's field, finally decided to start with the current scene and work from there, i.e., to find out what is the work of practicing clinical child psychologists, what education and training are now provided, and what else is needed to prepare them to do that work effectively *(8).*

Several recent surveys reveal a bold excursion of the clinician into new terrain. In one such survey, conducted by the Joint Information Service of the American Psychiatric Association (11) in 1970, clinical child psychologists, in addition to their "traditional" clinical settings, were found in the schools, in welfare departments and juvenile courts, in housing projects and settlement houses, in well-baby clinics, in "crisis" and walk-in clinics. Their work included discussion groups for teachers; group therapy with children in school settings; identification and remediation of children with learning disabilities; consultation or direct service in drug addiction programs; discussion with mothers in housing projects; consultation to group workers in inner-city recreational programs; training indigenous workers, paraprofessionals, and other mental health workers; conducting research on outcome of therapy; and administering a large community mental health center. Specifying what all these roles might have in common with academic coursework and with earlier practicuum training is as difficult, for the clinical psychologist, as describing a preferred base of operation for his practice. Some clinical child psychologists still stick fairly close to their traditional home in the clinic or private office; others retain this home base but roam out into the community for varying proportions of their work-week, while others have deserted their clinic or private offices altogether and find their work-space in the agencies they serve.

Background of Training in Clinical Child Psychology

The prospects for formal training in the new functions of the clinical child psychologists are quite disheartening if one looks only to the history of the recognition of the specialty itself within APA and university settings. By a fortuitous set of circumstances, largely the employment of psychologists in World War I and, more importantly, in World War II, "clinical psychology" was born as clinical *adult* psychology. The psychologists who were called in to develop selection and performance tests during those wars and, later, to provide treatment for soldiers and veterans were the group out of which academic clinical psychologists and the APA Education and Training Board (E and T) members came. Even though there were many psychologists already practicing in children's clinics and in school settings by 1950, the clinical training programs in the universities began with few courses in child development, learning disorders, or children's behavior problems, and the E and T Board has never developed requirements for specialized child training. It was actually an organization of children's clinics called the American Association of Psychiatric Clinics for Children which recognized the specialty of clinical child psychology, first through specifying supervised experience with children as one of the qualifications for Chief Psychologists in its member clinics and, in 1966, through setting standards for its training programs in clinical child psychology, the only standards on a national scale formulated to date for the specialty. This organization of clinics staffed by psychologists, psychiatrists, and social workers, responding to the expansion of clinical services into the community, changed its name, in 1970, to the American Association of Psychiatric *Services* for Children. (AAPSC).

It is worthy of note, moreover that it was not the American Psychological Association but the psychiatry, directed APSC which supported the development and administration of standards for the specialty of clinical child psychology.

Present State of Clinical Child
Psychology Practicuum Training

Present-day practicuum training in clinical child psychology has grown, for the most part, through a succession of graftings of various kinds of innovations onto the traditional Boulder model of clinical training. This model, described in Boulder in 1949 and reaffirmed at the Chicago conference in 1965, sees the clinical psychologist as a scientist-professional "trained in a Ph.D. program as both a professional psychologist and a research scientist." (*14*, p. 92). The Chicago conferees insisted that the clinical psychologist should be a psychologist first and a clinician second. They recommended core content areas in learning and developmental and social psychology, and stressed the need for research training that is "so embedded in the program that research orientation becomes an integral part of the clinical psychologist's mode of professional behavior." (*14*, p. 89). In the years immediately after the Boulder conference, predoctoral practicuum training was confined largely to the Veterans' Administration hospitals or United States Public Health Service agencies. The universities taught techniques in psychodiagnosis and in therapy as their chief contributions to the "professional" half of the scientist-professional model.

Many of the Chicago conferees came to the 1965 meeting with the conviction that training for professional practice would have to take cognizance of socially-oriented developments in the field of mental health. After heated debate on this issue, the Conference adopted this statement:

"This conference recognizes the development in recent years of new methods in clinical psychology. Among these we note behavior therapy, milieu therapy, community psychology, group therapy, and new approaches to individual therapy.

"We recognize, also, the ever-widening opportunities for clinical psychologists to render professional services. New opportunities are continually developing in hospitals, clinics, private practice, community mental health programs, schools, work settings, the various components of the poverty program, and in many other areas of life. It is clear that, in addition to added skill in the established techniques of assessment and therapy in dyadic relationships, clinical psychologists need new knowledge and skills to meet the every-changing challenge presented by these service opportunities.

"For this reason, we strongly recommend diversification of training opportunities in doctoral programs in clinical psychology. The objective of such diversification would be to provide the opportunity for different students to stress different knowledge and methods in their professional preparation." (*14*, p. 93).

The newly revised Accreditation Procedures and Criteria of the American Psychological Association incorporates this position as its training model (*3*, p.10):

> "The prototypic training model for programs in clinical, counseling and school psychology has been the scientist-professional model initially proposed by the APA Committee of Training in Clinical Psychology (Shakow, 1947). As previously noted, major national conferences on graduate education and professional preparation in psychology have continued to reaffirm this model as the best approach to training. Over the past five years, however, a need for diversity and innovation in training program development has been increasingly expressed by those planning clinical, school and counseling training programs.
>
> "The model of training must unify the divergencies of research and the service-oriented practice of psychology. It must also be flexible and viable enough to meet the diverse needs of various regions and communities in which programs are located and to respond to changing standards for training as well as to sub-specialty differences. Training models must also permit a diversity of philosophies, goals, and practices from program to program and from individual student to individual student."

One grafting onto traditional models of professional training was this diversification in clinical approaches and clinical settings. Others had to do with extension of practicuum training over a longer period of time in the doctoral sequence and the inclusion of new types of client populations. Still another was the development of entire internships specifically in the children's field, with or without correlated academic programs in this specialty.

Although the AAPSC clinics are the only centers with formal accreditation procedures for clinical child psychology programs, there are now many additional centers which offer training in clinical psychological work with children. A concerted effort by Section I to compile a complete directory of such training opportunities resulted, in 1970, in a listing and description of 154 centers which offer some kind of child training and seven more in the planning stage (21). This listing is probably incomplete, especially in listing municipal, county, and state agencies, since this category of agencies was not as likely to be reached by the survey procedures.

Within the 154 different centers in the Section I Directory, 134 centers list predoctoral and 31 list postdoctoral internships while 34 of the centers offer clerkships either alone or in combination with predoctoral and/ or postdoctoral training. Of a total of 139 centers listing pre- or postdoctoral internships or both, 70 are APA approved; 73 are AAPSC members and 33 claim both APA approval and AAPSC membership. Up until 1971, the Committee on Evaluation of the E and T Board of APA granted an "S" type of approval to those internship programs which, although more restricted in patient population than the "G," or general-type internship, were outstanding examples of their (special) kind. While most of the 25 S-type programs of 1970 were internships in clinical *child* psychology, a few S programs specialized in other restricted populations. The S and G differentiation was discarded in 1971 and the new guidelines for evaluation of internship programs call, instead, for effective matching of agency specialization with trainee interests and talents" and that "the agency develop descriptive material in which the goals and content of the training program are explicitly formulated and which are made available to prospective trainees, directors of professional training programs, etc." (*3*, p. 24). This document also makes reference to the need for a student to "choose research topics (dissertation and otherwise) that are relevant to and support his area of specialization" and to the provision of instruction in research methodology appropriate to such topics (*3*, p. 12).

The list of 110 programs which have *either* APA approval or membership in AAPSC, or both, probably represents the best estimate of the number of concentrated and monitored traning programs in clinics serving children. But standards for clinical *child* psychology internships specifically have been set up only within AAPSC and only thirteen of its own programs had been approved by 1970 by the AAPSC Committee on Psychology.

These statistics point up the paucity of training resources for the specialty of clinical child psychology. They are even more disconcerting in the light of the burgeoning growth of clinical and community services to children. Although still far behind those provided for adults and shockingly inadequate for the nation's needs, "psychological" services of all kinds are being delivered to children in all kinds of settings and by personnel whose training runs the gamut from no formalized training at all to clinical child psychologists with several years of postdoctoral training. In some cases the group at the former end of this continuum claim that they are providing some of the same services (especially in "therapy") that highly-trained psychologists at the other end of continuum provide. Well-trained psychologists have often accepted this state of affairs and moved into administration, into consultation, and into training and supervising this new therapy personnel. A report of the First Institute on Innovations in Psychological Training found that "psychologists were generally not engaging in those kinds of activities for which they were best trained, namely, research, intensive individual psychotherapy and diagnostic evaluation" (5, p. 16), and that "in a number of facilities lay workers were doing almost all of the direct treatment which that agency was providing (5, p.17). It should be noted that the installations visited by this Committee were chosen because they were sites in which innovative practices had been going on for a sufficiently long period of time for the program to have a reasonable degree of stability. (The Committee's chief interest was not evaluation of children's services, but some of the installations they visited had these units and were included in the report.)

There still remain those clinical child psychologists who do diagnostic evaluations and therapy and who want interns to be trained both academically and in practice in these techniques both for their own professional service and research needs and to prepare them for teaching and supervising those functions in others. Generally, even these "traditional" psychologists have greatly expanded the scope of "diagnosis" to include the use of a wide variety of measures such as interviewing, observation of family interaction, and the addition of tests other than the traditional intelligence and projective test batteries. Therapy now includes, in addition to psychotherapy, newer approaches such as behavior modification and a return to "guidance"; in addition to individual treatment, psychologists are doing parental, family, and group therapy and consultation to various kinds of group constellations. It bears repeating that even where the professional career of the clinical child psychologist will involve mainly "on-the-job" teaching of diagnostic and therapeutic techniques, supervising, and consultation, training in the clinical interactional process is still a logical prerequisite. In doing diagnostics and therapy and in being supervised in the process, the clinician learns to use himself as an instrument to evaluate, weigh, and organize diagnostic data and, in therapy, to understand, interpret, and respond to another's communications. Too often the Ph. D. in clinical psychology, with little or no additional experience, is the certificate for teaching others what one has not learned to do.

Present State of Academic Clinical Programs

From the published reports available, it appears that academic growth in clinical child psychology is lagging far behind current needs. The state of education for this specialty within the university clinical programs was included as part of Simmons' comparison of these programs in 1968-9 and 1964-5. In 1968-9, forty-seven of the 74 programs reviewed, or 63½%, had "offerings in child-clinical" (*23*, p. 719). These "offerings" are presumably courses in child development, behavior disorders, child therapy, etc. A *general psychology* "core sequence" was required in 54% of the programs and a *clinical* core sequence was prescribed in only 18% of the programs. In addition to courses in traditional psychotherapy, 75% of the programs provided training in behavioral therapies and 36% included training in community psychology. These figures give only an indirect view of the inclusion of education for clinical *child* psychology in the university curricula. They represent the addition of various child courses in the curriculum rather than the development of comprehensive clinical child programs. From her work on the Joint Commission of Mental Health of Children, Engel (*10*, p. 6) estimated, in 1969, that of the 67 university clinical training programs currently supported by the National Institute of Mental Health, "41 include some training with children and *ten can be said to have a distinct emphasis in child clinical psychology.*" Representatives of NIMH told Dr. Engel that the increase in interest in the establishment of clinical child psychology training programs which they had expected has not developed over the past few years.

A survey of academic clinicians in the 72 university training programs holding approval in 1969 confirms the support of the Boulder Model of training (*24*). Over three-fourths of the 179 academicians who responded ranked diagnosis, research, and therapy high in terms of receiving emphasis in their programs while reporting that administration, consulting, and teaching were receiving little emphasis. The respondents were generally satisfied with this emphasis on research and therapy, somewhat less enthusiastic but still in favor (64%) of emphasizing diagnosis and quite dissatisfied with the (small) amount of training in consulting and teaching. It is interesting that therapy and research shared about equally in being currently promoted and highly valued now and for the future of the profession.

Clinical Child Psychology Defined

While the roles in which the clinical child psychologist practices continue to divide and multiply, the central question for both the university and the practicuum agency remains, "Is there a core of theoretical knowledge and professional skills which can serve as a common denominator for all these roles, i.e., is there, still, a definable clinical child psychology?"

The answer to this question leads back to a consideration of the basic functions of a clinical psychologist, functions which are as essential to the innovative programs of community psychology, consultation, and social change as they are to traditional roles in the clinic office. Ross (22) has called these the two main concerns of the clinical psychologist. "One is the prevention of psychological disorders, the other the treatment of these disorders. The focal question of the former enterprise is, 'How does disordered behavior come about?' For the latter endeavor, the question becomes, 'How does one bring about change in behavior?' " (22, p. 2). In this formulation lies the common denominator which ties together the variety of "bags" which the psychologist has chosen or which others, recognizing his professional expertise, have handed to him. Academic learning and practicuum training must be fashioned to help the clinical psychologist to answer these two questions no matter what the setting in which it is asked or whether it is asked of an individual, a group, a society, or a research sample. *These* two concerns differentiate the psychologist from the social welfare worker, differences sometimes overlooked in present-day eagerness to do something about mental health needs. While it may, indeed, be possible and even economical to develop new types of personnel as agents of behavioral and social change, the specific prescription for change must be based on professional diagnosis, and the process of change must be purposefully directed according to psychological principles such as those of learning theory and personality dynamics.

The two main concerns of clinical psychology are easily expressed in terms of clinical *child* psychology. As Ross points out, both are questions about development. The first becomes, "How is the *development* of human effectiveness enhanced and safeguarded?" and the second, "How does one help people with impaired effectiveness develop more adaptive behavior?" (22, p. 2). The core of theoretical knowledge, the common denominator for training in clinical child psychology, and, ideally, for all of clinical psychology, is the concept of development.

The Application of the Developmental Concept of the Training of the Clinical Child Psychologist

A New Approach to Academic Course Requirements

The content areas recommended by the APA Education and Training Board for its doctoral internships (1, 3) and the courses they generate can readily incorporate the developmental orientation toward personality development. Its omission is analogous to ignoring, in physiology, the study of physical growth and, in medicine, the study of disease etiology. It is only reasonable that courses in perception as well as courses in projective techniques should trace perception and projection from their beginnings. This genetic approach is essential to the understanding of perception in general and to projection whenever it occurs. This understanding is as essential to the clinical *adult* psychologist as it is to the child psychologist. Moreover, many of the perceptive and projective manifestations which are considered, in adults, to be pathological are available, during childhood, as ordinary, developmentally-appropriate behaviors which the child can and does report readily. The primitive fantasies of the psychotic adult are, at one stage in childhood, fairly ordinary Rorschach projections. Adult defenses can only be understood in terms of their value as anxiety-reducers at various conflict points in psychological growth. It should be a matter of course to introduce the diagnostician to intelligence and personality testing through the test protocols of children where one can trace the changes in these functions with age. Similarly, the study of children's productions in therapy provides a basis for understanding the later, more obscure meaning of the adult's therapy material.

In addition to this basic orientation toward total personality development in both "core" and clinical coursework, the academic programs may need to add education in specific areas such as the study of social systems including the school, program evaluation, and principles of administration. *The most important academic change needed, however, is not so much in the courses required but in their orientation toward useful application to the current scene.* Theory, and especially the principles of development, must be integrated with professional experience through planned interweaving of the two.

The Clinical Child Psychology Internship in the New Scene

Clinical child psychologists, especially those in clinics such as AAPSC who employ an interdisciplinary "team" approach and a child-within-the-family orientation to diagnosis and therapy, have always been attuned to the child's environment as an important force in his personality development. The natural settings of personality growth—the family, the school, and the neighborhood—have traditionally been a part of the subject matter of these clinics' study of the child. It is a relatively short step for the psychologist with this background to move out of the clinic into the community to work first-hand with the agents who are entrusted with "enhancing and safeguarding human effectiveness" in the developing child. Is is noteworthy that the only children's facility (as contrasted to all-purpose facilities) which has been funded to date as a Community Mental Health Center by NIH is directed by a clinical child psychologist who has his professional and paraprofessional staff working within a residential treatment unit, a day care center, an out-patient child guidance clinic, and out in the community in a variety of education and settlement installations. Their *psychological* orientation is the same in all these settings (*11*).

Although the clinical child psychologist may work more frequently now with adults, and often with groups of them, his basic knowledge about the genesis of disordered or problem-inducing behavior and how to help change it is still relevant and receiving increasing acceptance as prevention becomes an ultimate goal.

These considerations suggest the outlines for the child psychologist's internship training. Upon the base of knowledge of principles of development and change, the internship must build skills in old and new techniques of assessment, treatment and research, and in ways of relating to community problems. In addition to individual therapy, the trainee needs to learn family and group therapies, behavior modification and crisis intervention and to select and then to evaluate the treatment best suited to the child and family.

While it is desirable that the intern should have some of his experience in an extraclinic setting, such as in a school, it is certainly impossible and probably unnecessary to include experiences in all the types of social settings in which he may work as a professional. Fortunately, there are basic characteristics of social systems and, more importantly, common characteristics of interactions between people that can be learned and transferred across experiences. Again, the need is to introduce the trainee to core concepts, in this case those of personal interaction, and to demonstrate their application in varying social contexts.

This latter principle has been reiterated in the recent recommendations to APA of the Psychotherapy Curriculum Consultation Committee of the Division of Psychotherapy (*9*). This Committee's recommendations are outlined in 22 principles having to do with faculty qualifications, practicuum settings, and curriculum for the teaching of psychotherapy. One of the guidelines is for experience in a "one-to-one" psychotherapy relationship plus one or more other approaches on the premise that "it is in the dyadic situation that the student is likely to have the best opportunity to observe the deeper nuances and complexities of the human interaction" and that "it is a baseline with which to compare other approaches to effecting change in persons" (p. 153). This viewpoint is also expressed by the APA's Committee on Training in Clinical Psychology. The recommendations of the Division of Psychotherapy go on to stress the need for training in long-term therapy in order to include all phases of the psychotherapeutic process. Other recommendations include exposure to the broader social context in which psychotherapeutic practice exists and experience in treatment situations in which the aim of the work is preventive or oriented toward maximizing human potential. These recommendations, formulated in this age of rapid role change, seem to embody the experience of the past with a progressive awareness of social needs.

AAPSC Standards for Predoctoral Training in Clinical Child Psychology

The guidelines established by the American Association of Psychiatric Services for Children are the only formalized set of standards for the specialty currently in operation on a national scale. The actual setting of standards for clinical child psychology internships can be considered as a kind of midpoint in the process leading to an eventual definition of "clinical child psychologist" and the professional training required. Admission of a clinic to AAPCC membership carried with it requirements for its chief psychologist. These requirements, which related to academic degree, experience, and supervised experience, were revised in 1963 to ensure that the degree should be specifically in psychology and the clinical experience and supervision specifically in work with children.

When, in the early 1960s, a group of AAPCC psychologists decided to tackle the job of formulating standards for training in their specialty, they soon came to the decision that they would need first to outline the qualifications for training supervisor. This decision rose out of the conviction that a training program depends most heavily on the background and capabilities of the person who directs it.

After much discussion within this "grass roots" group[1] and, later, among AAPCC psychologists in general, the qualifications for training supervisor were agreed upon and, in 1964, were put into effect. The requirements include clinical training beyond the Ph.D., experience and training in supervision of students, and some experience in administrative responsibilities. The guidelines they set up provide enough structure to ensure basic requirements such as staff-trainee ratio, length and quality of training, proper supervision, major content areas (e.g., training in diagnosis, therapy, and research), provision for training seminars, and collaboration with the other professions, especially child psychiatry and psychiatric social work. On the other hand, the guidelines allow for and encourage flexibility in regard to particular emphases and innovations in the programs. For example, there is no specific allocation of time for training through experience in extraclinical agencies such as schools, courts, pediatric settings, etc. The specific items covered in the standards for training are only summarized here.[2] In brief, these are the requirements:

1. The center must be an active member clinic of AAPCC: Its internship program must meet the APA standards for practicuum training, its training director must meet specified AAPCC qualifications, the training center must accept as primary a commitment ot the intern's training needs, and the center must provide its staff with the opportunity for research.

2. The training center must have at least one full-time clinical child psychologist, child psychiatrist, and psychiatric social worker.

3. The professional disciplines must utilize a meaningful interdisciplinary approach in administration, service, training, and research.

4. The training program must provide the intern with supervised experience in diagnosis, psychotherapy or behavior modification, and research and (as a recommendation) experience in other roles such as consultation with community resources, pediatric settings, etc. It must provide (specified) training seminars and contact with a broad scope of clinical problems and age groups. It must involve child psychiatrists and psychiatric social workers in the intern's training experience so that he will understand their unique work, skills, and background.

---

[1]The Committee on Clinical Psychology, which initiated the task of defining the specialty of clinical child psychology and setting training standards for it, was chaired by Alan O. Ross and consisted of Theodore Leventhal, Lovick Miller, and Sebastiano Santostefano.

[2]A copy of the complete *Manual for Predoctoral Training in Clinical Child Psychology* may be obtained for $1.00 by writing to AAPSC's central office: American Association of Psychiatric Services for Children, 250 West 57th Street, New York, New York 10019.

5. The qualified clinical child psychology training director must maintain responsibility for all aspects of the intern's training, even though he may delegate the actual supervision to other staff. The proportation of time devoted to the intern's service-experience and time for supervision shall be such as to maximize his training; the staff-intern ratio shall be such as to maximize training.

6. The intern must participate in the training program full-time for one year.

The standards are administered by a Committee on Training in Clinical Child Psychology of AAPSC and site visits are made to clinics within the organization who apply for training status in psychology. To date 13 programs have been approved.

The AAPSC standards probably represent an ideal envisioned by one group of clinical child psychologists rather than a goal to which most child training programs could or, even, *would* choose to aspire. The standards have been criticized for retaining the traditional emphases by *requiring* the team approach which tends to perpetuate the "medical model" while only *recommending* the inclusion of experience in extraclinic roles and settings. AAPSC psychologists are criticized for not having gone far enough in promoting a new professional model, more independent of psychiatry and more attuned to the community's needs. This would certainly seem to be the direction that clinical child psychology should be going, but AAPSC may not be the organization which can foster the independent psychologist. AAPSC has, nevertheless, performed an extremely valuable function by drawing up standards which provide the first tangible description of a "clinical child psychologist."

The requirements that the training director should have training and experience in the specialty of clinical child psychology and experience in supervision and administration, which seem to be logical even as minimum requirements, are beyond many clinics' job specifications as is also the length of the internship period devoted to work with children. Shortage of manpower is given as the reason for the employment of psychologists without training in the children's field as child psychologists but it is also true that there has been, up to now, little effort by APA to exert pressure to remedy this situation in training.

Postdoctoral Training in Clinical Child Psychology

Postdoctoral education in clinical child psychology is confined almost entirely to clinical settings. The thirty-one postdoctoral internships listed in the Section I Directory (*21*) probably represent a fairly complete list of comprehensive training centers. There are a few other programs which offer postdoctoral training in specific areas such as research, psychotherapy, or behavior therapy.

Of the thirty-one postdoctoral programs in the 1970 Section I Directory, nine do not require a predoctoral internship for admission and these programs are often quite similar to predoctoral programs but placed in a postdoctoral year. In the 1967 Directory, of the twenty postdoctoral internships listed, sixteen required predoctoral interships for admission. Of the thirty-one listed now, twenty-six post doctoral settings also have pre-doctoral internships devoted fully or in part to clinical child psychology.

Of the post doctoral training programs in the Directory, 20, or approximately 65%, are completely child-centered. In the other 11 centers, 25% to 85% of the training is devoted to children with the exact percentage only infrequently stated. The duration of training varies from six months to two years. Half of the 24 centers who state a definite period of intership require one year; 8 require two years; and the other 4 require from six months to "one to two years."

It is difficult, from the literature available at this time, to differentiate the content of these postdoctoral programs from predoctoral training. It appears that postdoctoral programs fall roughly into the following categories (with some overlapping): 1) "predoctoral" clinical child training offered in postdoctoral years to those who have had no internship or whose internship was not child-centered; 2) advanced training in child-centered clinical skills and/or in supervision techniques for those who have had a predoctoral internship, preferably in a child-centered program; and, 3) training in *skills* different from those acquired in predoctoral internship such as clinical research, supervision, and administration and/or in *settings* not included in predoctoral settings such as in community agencies, residential treatment centers, etc. A few of the postdoctoral training programs have as their stated goal intensive training in psychotherapy and diagnosis to prepare psychologists for a professional career in clinical child psychology. The Menninger Foundation exemplifies this position: "Post-doctoral training in clinical psychology begins where the university program and the clinical internship leave off" (*16*, p.71). Even these "traditional" centers include research, newer treatment procedures such as short-term therapy, and clinical experience out in the community. More frequently, the postdoctoral program includes, in addition to advanced training in traditional skills, such "innovative" activities as psycho-educational diagnosis and remediation, school consultation, community mental health development, administration, etc. One center, that of the University of Colorado Medical School, has developed two subspecialties or "directions" for its fellows, a "clinical intensification" focus and a "school consultation-community mental health focus." (16, p.70).

The nature of supervision in postdoctoral training may differ somewhat from predoctoral programs and the average amount of supervision per intern is higher in the postdoctoral programs listed in the 1970 Section I Directory (approximately 7½ hours per week postdoctorally versus 5 hours in the predoctoral programs). Treatment is listed as the priority in 16 or 55% of the postdoctoral programs which list priorities and diagnosis is given the most emphasis in the other 13 programs. It is interesting that neither consulting or research is listed alone as first choice in any of the postdoctoral programs although consulting is listed in first place along with diagnosis and treatment in 2 centers. Research fares no better. It is usually listed last in emphasis. The Directory data give no further information as to actual content of the programs but they do seem to indicate that treatment and diagnosis are still the chief subject matter in postdoctoral programs, as they are in predoctoral programs.

A few of the well-established postdoctoral programs have combined didactic coursework and clinical training much in the nature of a professional school. In these settings advanced trainees from several disciplines usually attend the courses together. The Reiss-David Child Study Center, for example, admits, in addition to postdoctoral psychology interns, social workers who have had a minimum of three years casework beyond the Master's degree and fellows in child psychiatry who have completed two years residency in psychiatry. The emphasis in this program is on training in intensive child psychotherapy but the Center also offers the psychologist "additional training in diagnostic testing," counseling of parents, and research (19). The Center has, in fact, a permanent research department and several long-term research projects are available for the trainee's participation. The Reiss-Davis brochure lists some twenty formal courses and seminars, at least half of which are conducted by staff psychologists. This program also has regularized training resources outside the Center itself including clinical experience in the court, in a center for retarded and other handicapped children, in a nursery school, and in a pediatric setting. Their community education programs include teachers, pediatricians, and social agencies of various kinds. Although such highly formalized postdoctoral programs in clinical child psychology are few in num-

ber, their existence points up the wide divergence in current philosophies as to the training required to diagnose and treat children. At
one end of this continuum is the Ph.D. from a clinical psychology
program who participates in two additional years of internship and,
at the other, the child psychologist with a few months of on-the-job
training and little or no academic background related to the clinical
function. The discrepancy could be understood if the intensive and
prolonged education of the postdoctoral graduate was to equip him
for a specialized career of teaching, administration, and research but
the fact is that many postdoctoral graduates are engaging in practice
which may differ, on the surface and in the eyes of the public, only
in length of service to the individual and in the class of people served.

An Overview

The evolution of national interest in the training of clinical child
psychologists comes from at least two important developments in'
the field of mental health within the last two decades. One is the
birth and growth of an organization of clinical child psychologists,
the Section on Clinical Child Psychology of Division 12 of the
American Psychological Association. The other is a rapidly changing social scene with a new awareness of children's mental health
needs springing up in all classes and institutions of society and new
demands for the psychologist's time and expertise.

The Section on Clinical Child Psychology publicized its conviction that those who work clinically with children should have special
training for their profession and that standards for this training must
be set up. As the first step toward this goal, the Section has compiled a Directory of the existing Practicuum Training Resources in
Clinical Child Psychology (21), a list of 154 Centers which, in 1970,
are offering some kind of child training to predoctoral and post doctoral clinical psychologists. The only *standards* for interships
specifically in clinical child psychology are, however, those set up
by psychologists of the American Association of Psychiatric Services for Children. These standards are tailored to the medical
model of the AAPSC centers and are not likely to be adopted by the
profession as a whole.

The recognition of the need for specialized training in clinical
child psychology brought with it the task of defining what clinical
child psychology is and if there is, indeed, a core of theory and professional skills which could form the basis for training in the field.
This issue, crucial for the future of the profession, stems directly

from the second main trend of the last two decades: changes in the social scene in mental health which brought about a proliferation of roles and expectations for which clinical child psychologists often found themselves poorly prepared. This state of flux and increasing demands has forced universities and practicuum facilities to take a new look at their programs in order to provide more adequate training.

The core concept which can tie together the many professional roles and point the way for academic and professional preparation of the clinical psychologist is that of development. As Alan Ross has clearly pointed out, the many functions of clinical child psychology in today's scene coalesce in these two endeavors: 1) how to enhance and safeguard the development of human effectiveness and 2) how to help people with impaired effectiveness to develop more adaptive behavior (22, p.2). These aims are germane to clinical child psychology in its research, in the reform of its academic curricula, and in fulfilling its many professional responsibilities including both the recently accepted ones of the prevention of mental illness and the maintenance of the mental health of children as well as the more traditional ones of the diagnosis and treatment of already existing children's disorders. University programs and practicuum training can be integrated on the basis of this core concept.

It is likely to be several years before actual APA standards for training in clinical child psychology can be formulated. The Committee on Standards and Professional Practice of Section I has decided to begin this task by conducting a survey among practicing clinical child psychologists to determine what they are *doing* and to develop training guidelines from their findings. This approach to the problem represents a healthy return to the considerations upon which clinical psychology was initiated: relevance to social need.

References

1. American Psychological Association, Education and Training Board. Criteria for evaluating training programs in clinical psychology or in counseling psychology. *American Psychologist*, 1958, 13, 59-60.
2. American Psychological Association, Education and Training Board. The evaluation of university programs in clinical and counseling psychology. *American Psychologist*, 1967, 22, 153-155.
3. American Psychological Association. *Accreditation Procedures and Criteria*, 1971.
4. Boneau, A., and Simmons, W. APA accreditation: A status report. *American Psychologist*. 1970, 25, 581-584.

5. Bloom, B. L. Training the psychologist for a role in community change: A report of the first institute on innovations in psychological training. Mimeographed material, 1969.

6. Cass, L., Cain, A., and Waite, R. American Association of Psychiatric Clinics for Children training standards for predoctoral internship in clinical child psychology. *Professional Psychology,* Winter, 1970.

7. Cain, A., *et al*. AAPCC Committee on Clinical Psychology. *Report to Council*, 1970.

8. Dingman, P., *et al*. Report of the Section I Committee on standards and professional practice. *Clinical Child Psychology Newsletter*, 1969, 8, No. 1, 7-8.

9. Division of Psychotherapy, American Psychological Association. Recommended standards for psychotherapy education in psychology doctoral programs. *Professional Psychology*, 1971, 2, 148-154.

10. Engel, M. Ideologies and financial support in clinical child psychology. *Clinical Child Psychology Newsletter*, 1969, 8, No. 4, 4-7.

11. Glasscote, R. Report of Joint Information Service of the American Psychiatric Association survey of children's services in community mental health centers, 1972.

12. Goodstein, L. D., and Ross, S. Accreditation of graduate programs in psychology. An analysis. *American Psychologist*, 1966, 21, 218-233

13. Hersch, C. From mental health to social action: Clinical psychology in historical perspective. *American Psychologist*, 1969, 24, 909-916.

14. Hoch, E. L. Ross, A., and Winder, C. L. *Professional preparation of clinical psychologists*. Amer. Psychol. Assn., Washington, D.C., 1966.

15. Joint Commission on Mental Health of Children, Inc., *Crisis in Child Mental Health: Challenge for the 1970's*. Joint Commission on Mental Health of Children, Washington, D.C., 1969.

16. Matulef, N., Pottharst, K., and Rothenberg, P. The revolution in professional training: A review of innovative programs for the training of professional psychologists. National Council on Graduate Education in Psychology, 1971.

17. Newsletter, *Interest Group for Clinical Child Psychology,* Vol. I, No. 1, Mar. 1962.

18. Raimy, V. C., (Ed.) *Training in clinical child psychology*. Prentice-Hall, New York, 1950.

19. Reiss-Davis Child Study Center, Los Angeles, California. *Brochure*, 1966.

20. Rie, H., and Catullo. Practicuum training in clinical child psychology. Publication of Section on Clinical Child Psychology, Division of Clinical Psychology, American Psychological Association 1970.

21. Rie, H., and Poutakoglou, A. S. 1970 Director of practicuum training resources in clinical child psychology. Publication of Section on Clinical Child Psychology, Division of Clinical Psychology, American Psychological Association, 1970.

22. Ross, A. General or special? *The Clinical Psychologist*, 23, No. 4, 1-2.
23. Simmons, W. L. Clinical training programs, 1964-65 and 1968-69: A characterization and comparison. *American Psychologist,* 1971, 26, 717-721.
24. Thelen, M., and Ewing, D. Roles, functions and training in clinical psychology: A survey of academic clinicians. *American Psychologist,* 1970, 25, 550-554.
25. Williams, G. J. The death and rebirth of clinical psychology. *Clinical Child Psychology Newsletter*, 9, No. 4, 1-3.

Part Nine

CLINICAL CHILD PSYCHOLOGY REASSESSED

Every profession must examine itself and occasionally declare itself obsolete. Paradoxically, the declaration of obsolescence generates the potentialities for rebirth.

37. Is Traditional Clinical Child Psychology Obsolete?[1]

S. Thomas Cummings

Introduction

In an epoch marked by a pervasive sense of uneasiness about the integrity of many of our primary social institutions and about ambiguity in national purpose, it is not surprising to find many traditional features of American culture being challenged. That the methods of traditional clinical child psychology are among those institutions whose utility is being questioned is not unexpected, especially in view of increasing public awareness of inadequacies in our health maintenance systems and continuing severe manpower shortages in the traditional mental health disciplines. The challenges to traditional clinical service methods have come largely from a strongly government-funded community mental health enterprise and from applied neobehaviorism. Characteristic of vigorous competition in the American marketplace, the claims and counterclaims for superiority of both new and old products have sometimes reached a degree of stridency and overstatement which could further obscure the difficult task undertaken here: evaluation of the usefulness of traditional methods in clinical child psychology for helping children.

Several other factors increase the difficulty of trying to reach an essentially rational answer to the question. We confront at the outset uncommonly great problems in definition of terms. Merely attempting to define something called "traditional clinical child psychology" (abbreviated TCCP) is a difficult task in itself. The term, TCCP, implies both a high degree of consistency of essential elements and their existence over a long period of time, neither of

[1]I appreciate the careful reviews and suggestions given this paper by Dorothy Fuller, Martin Leichtman, and Sydney Smith of The Menninger Foundation, none of whom, of course, is responsible for the opinions expressed.

which is true for TCCP over the period of its relatively brief history. The spawning grounds of early clinical child psychology, the multidisciplinary child guidance clinic, have been in existence since 1909 when Healy established the Juvenile Psychopathic Institute (Healy and Bronner, 1948) but it was not until the late 1940s that university curricula in clinical psychology regularly began to include training in the three core content areas: psychodynamic concepts, comprehensive personality assessment via a test battery which included projective techniques, and psychotherapy. The "typically used" techniques and procedures for evaluating and treating children with behavior deviations have actually shown considerable diversity, as review of three texts which have appeared over the past quarter-century reveals (Louttit, 1947; Ross, 1959; Palmer, 1970.)

How to give precise meaning to the term "obsolete" is another vexing problem, when the term is applied to the effects of patterns of complex behavior (clinical techniques) on other patterns of complex behavior (children's disorders), when the former are filtered through clinical practitioners (intervening personality variables) and without specification of a uniform time interval for determining the effects. Were we to confound our notions of work settings (and our value preferences for these) with our notions of patterns of clinical psychological operations, which may be found in a wide variety of work settings, we would add further confusion to our efforts to deal rationally with the central issue. My focus is on the clinical methods themselves rather than the settings in which they are employed.

How can we distinguish the essential from the inessential differences between the two diverse sets of events comprising TCCP and non-TCCP? Some interpreters of this comparison would claim that the essential differences rest in differences revealed in the positions taken on several philosophical issues: humanitarian versus utilitarian values; the proper distribution of power between patient and clinician; the clinician's moral responsibility for awareness of the countertransference aspects of his interventions. While acknowledging the importance of working towards clarification of the differences in philosophical positions distinguishing the two camps, I make my primary focus a comparison of more palpable dimensions, i.e., differences in character and style of clinical activities performed with patients.

For the purposes of this essay, I will assume that the essential elements of TCCP are present in clinical psychological practice with children which emphasizes: (1) comprehensive diagnostic studies (including psychological testing) leading to inferences about the nature of a child's disorder and its determinants, which formulation becomes the rationale for a treatment plan with that child; (2) practice of individual psychotherapy in order to remedy what are conceived of as the psychogenic determinants of a given child's disorder. In contrast, non-TCCP, a considerably more diverse group of practices, will be assumed to have in common an emphasis on relatively brief diagnostic efforts before attempts at change of a child's behavior are undertaken, and in treatment interventions, a deemphasis on individual psychotherapy. Naturally, some overlap in clinical practices used exists between traditional clinic settings and nontraditional settings (community mental health centers, storefront clinics, behavior analysis and therapy centers). I assume that TCCP includes the two elements specified above as standard and predominant practice and that non-TCCP includes them infrequently, if at all.

Obsolescence: How to Know When to Change Tools

What constitutes obsolescence in TCCP?

By analogy, one might ask oneself while undertaking a carpentry project entailing cutting boards to fit a new pattern, does the handsaw one has traditionally used for such work still serve? Or should a different tool be used? Do changes in the material dictate a new choice? Are there better available ideas about the relationship between the application of a serrated cutting edge to wood fiber and the likely effects of this procedure? Does one's saw still cut acceptably? Has another tool been proven more rapid and efficient? Should apprentice carpenters still be taught manual sawing, even if their subsequent work as journeymen may require little of this skill? Has the community changed its ideas about sawing, and, if so, how much of that old activity should be allowed to go on? Or, are there simply more boards to be sawed than one can comfortably acknowledge? Or fewer skilled answers?

Without straining the analogy any further, within it are most of the relevant issues which need consideration in approximating an answer to the question heading this essay. In brief, the principal questions to be faced in determining the degree of obsolescence in TCCP in meeting the mental health needs of maladjusted children and their families are:

A. Have the deviant children changed? In numbers? In their patterns of deviance?

B. Have the concepts from TCCP about the nature and origins of the children's behavior disorders changed significantly?

C. Have TCCP methods been proven ineffective?

D. Have non-TCCP methods been proven more effective?

E. Does the contemporary social-political scene significantly lessen the acceptability of TCCP methods?

TCCP Obsolescence and the Children

How has our clientele changed? Are there changes in the "basic psychological processes" through which children organize their experience and mediate their adaptations? Are there significantly more or less clients? Do the children present distinctively different patterns of disorder? If a "yes" answer follows to any of these, how does this conclusion raise questions about the relevance of thorough diagnostic studies and the use of individual psychotherapy in clinical practice with children?

The number of clients has changed. There are more—especially poor ones. Not simply through population increase, but through broadened governmental support of health and welfare services which have created eligibility for mental health service for many people with low incomes who were not previously so covered. Many children of low-income families, a large proportion of them black, are finding they have access that they did not previously have to health care and some other services supported by the national mental health enterprise.

As they arrive for services in the clinic, neighborhood center, community mental health center, or school special services department, we are impressed with their durability in the face of multiple adversities, and with their appearing to share some behavioral features (impulsivity, high activity level, low verbal fluency) which are not as frequently found in disturbed children of middle-class parents, be they white or black. But beyond some few similarities of this order in the low income group, we are impressed, also, with their great variety and complexity. How much can we risk stereotyping the care given them, now that we are beginning to shake the national stereotype of them?

In harmony with the implications of research findings of Hirsch, Borowitz, and Costello (1970) on individual differences in black ghetto children, can we afford not to pay attention to the complexity of the lives of individual children such as the two black lower-class children briefly described below?

Gus, 13, had been increasingly disobedient to his 41-year-old mother and to the teacher, when brought for help. His school grades had dropped markedly, and he had been spending long hours watching television. His father had died a year previously in an industrial accident, leaving Gus, his mother, and his eight-year-old brother only tiny insurance benefits. A 24-year-old second cousin rented a room in their small home for a while after his father's death, but now only visits the family occasionally. Gus improved after a half year of psychotherapy for him and casework interviews with his mother. The therapeutic work with the boy was gauged to help him mourn his father and integrate his threatening feelings and fantasies of intimacy with his mother. Casework help to his mother was oriented toward assisting her with bereavement and the management of her guilt about a temporary sexual liaison, the termination of which was followed by her making disturbing demands for closeness on Gus, concurrent with her relaxation of disciplinary controls on him.

Henry, 9, did failing work in school in spite of having above-average intelligence test scores, and constantly provoked fights with both peers and school authorities. His father, on military duty away from home during most of Henry's life, beat him severely when he was home, but also helped him with his homework. His mother, foreign born, was constantly in fear of their house being assaulted and the family attacked; she denied their skin color. Examination also established that Henry had a perceptual-motor disorder which appeared to complicate his school achievement, but to contribute little to his near-paranoid view of interpersonal relationships. Casework with the father encouraging his becoming a more palpable model of masculinity and reason, psychotherapy with Henry oriented to assist him in understanding and controlling his counterphobic aggressive maneuvers and rejection of his black identity, referrals to a boys' social club and to a reading clinic offer early promise that Henry will not need to synthesize a deviant adult identity.

Certainly, no "scientific proof" exists that the traditional clinical methods used with Gus, Henry, and their available parents are comparatively more effective in getting them back on their respective developmental tracks than alternative methods would have been. Briefer methods might have picked up Henry's perceptual-motor problem, but that seems doubtful. What seems even more doubtful is that these families could have turned the corner toward more helpful and appropriate family relationships without the immediate experiences of being valued and of being understood, which was reflected in the careful diagnostic work and highly individualized therapeutic work done with them.

What the relative efficacy of alternate clinical methods, in particular brief service methods, would have been in trying to help these two youngsters and their families is unknown. Different methods might well also have yielded similar beneficial results. What does seem certain is that these families experienced a careful evaluation which helped them to care for themselves, individually and collectively, in a better way than they had previously.

How else has the caseload changed? Very clearly in the large number of so-called "alienated youth," drug-oriented or not, who are dumped at the clinic door or who somehow manage to find a clinic back door. Their mistrust of most adults, of anything supportive of conventional societal values, their emphasis on action and immediacy, on casual sexual relationships, and their ambiguous work ethos, seem clearly antithetical to the value structure inherent in traditional clinical work. Much of the rehabilitative work attempted with them to date seems to recognize this in its flexible variation of structures and situations for providing a sustaining contact through which disaffiliation may be challenged. Group methods with peers have been most frequently offered and are considered by some professionals as the only appropriate structure for an attempt at "reaffiliation."

Implications for TCCP? Clearly a demand for flexibility in the structure of clinical contacts. But I would strongly question the suggestion that, thorough diagnosis and an individual therapeutic approach should be abandoned. My individual therapy experiences with several anomie-burdened adolescents offer me encouragement about the responsiveness of many of them when certain aspects of a real relationship (rather than a therapeutically neutral one) can be offered and some facility in moving quickly back and forth along the supportive-expressive therapeutic-operations continuum can be demonstrated by the therapist.

Have the children changed so as to outdate or render useless the methods of TCCP? Essentially not, not the majority of them. They continue to require, whether or not it is available now, through diagnostic studies and a variety of therapy options including individual psychotherapy.

Changes in Concepts of Children's Disorders Relative to the Question of TCCP Obsolescence

Have there been significant changes in clinicians' concepts of the nature and origins of children's behavior disorders which dictate changes in clinical practice with them?

TCCP starts with a heritage of a multifactorial model from A. Meyer (Lief, 1948) and the Freuds (father, 1932, and daughter, 1965). The model asserts that personality formation occurs through a process of transactions between a biological structure, socializing agents, and the self. Within the structure of the most common form of this model, the quality of the individual's experience as he seeks to satisfy his motives is given special etiological weight in determining the qualities and structure of his personality, be it one with either high or low adaptive value. The psychoanalytic variant of this model emphasizes conflict between the child and his socializers as he seeks motive satisfactions, the conflict at first expressed externally in the interaction, ultimately being internalized but manifested in the child's symptomatology, object relations, and ego-defense patterning. Therapeutic efforts put forth under this aegis stress the importance of the patient's conscious experiencing of unconscious conflicts and the fear derivatives they have generated. This psycopathological model held sway during the flowering of the American child guidance clinic movement (1920-60). It continues to have considerable currency, reflected in the contemporary literature of clinical child psychology and child psychiatry, in spite of its many latter-day challenges.

The past two decades have seen a salutary ferment in the conceptual vat of childhood psychopathology. Claims have been made for the need to give greater recognition to constitutional factors; e.g., the child's temperament pattern (Thomas, Chess, and Birch, 1968) and subtle forms of cortical dysfunction termed "minimal brain damage" (Clements, 1966). Family unit research has emphasized the factor of pathogenic communication patterns within the family (Haley, 1964; Mishler and Waxler, 1968). Neobehaviorism has burgeoned forth with a flurry of therapeutic applications (Krasner and Ullman, 1965), nearly all of which demonstrate a simplistic emphasis on the environmental response to a child's overt behavior. The excellent recent compendium edited by Rie (1971) reviews the contributions of many of these recent alternatives to and refinements of the conflict-model of psychoanalysis.

What is the distillate of these conceptual variations in the form of implications for changing diagnostic and treatment methods with deviant children? It soon becomes apparent that the varying answers to this question reflect more accurately the colors of the old school ties being worn by the respondents than their use of veridical data base. There does not exist the empirical research of the scope and duration necessary to making a reasoned choice among these alternative conceptual emphases and the clinical methods derivative of them. Nor is it ever likely in the ideal sense to develop. Clearly, the choices made will be based on other than hard data in the forseeable future.

Obsolescence and the Questionable Effectiveness of TCCP Methods

Have the traditional tools lost their cutting edges? Or, some would ask, "Did they ever have them?" What is an "appropriate" balance between diagnostic effort and therapeutic effort with children?

A discussion devoted to these issues alone would trace the development of clinical methods within the history of child psychiatry, clinical child psychology, psychiatric social work, and of the child guidance movement,[2] it would review the few systematic evaluative studies that have been completed of the effectiveness of clinical methods with children. The focus adopted here is considerably more limited. I start with an assumption that the high demand for his diagnostic testing skills in a wide variety of agencies serving children establishes an acceptable operational criterion of the relative effectiveness of the clinical child psychologist's diagnostic contribution.

TCCP has most often been challenged, not for the essential validity of its diagnostic methods and report documents, but for its implicitly wasteful "overdiagnosis" of children. This quaint term means most commonly that its user believes that less of the psychologist's time should be spent in evaluating children's disorders in some setting, relative to the proportion of time the psychologist spends in some form of treatment effort.

Wherever clinical service to patients is considered to be the sole function of the clinical work (i.e., excluding some concurrent training or research function), conservation of treatment time directs that the elaborateness of the diagnostic examination take account of the variety of the treatment alternatives available to a given patient. Theoretically, diagnosis would be largely obviated if only a single uniform treatment method were known and available for all patients, regardless of the nature, duration, and severity of their disorders. In actuality, of course, this is never the case and the decision to treat or not to treat is always present. However, my impression is that traditional clinics have revealed in varying degrees oversimplification and

---

[2] Informative summaries of material in several of these areas may be found in chapters by Rie (1971) and Rosenblatt (1971) in the book edited by Rie (1971).

stereotypy of the treatment alternatives which they have conceived of and made available. Institutions appear to be especially vulnerable to these limitations when they face an incessant and insistent knock on the door to services and where their programs are not floodlighted with built-in evaluation studies.

The question of whether individual therapy with children is effective in improving their behavior disorders sounds naive to the experienced child therapist, whose professional life is replete with therapeutic "success stories" of his colleagues and his own. The doubt and disbelief which greeted Levitt's (1957) essentially negative conclusions from his survey of the effects of child psychotherapy appeared to derive, not merely from the acute abrasions to experienced therapists' narcissism, but from a failure to account for the limitations of his methodology in reaching his conclusions, when other available "evidence" would have encouraged any but the more obtuse and myopic experimentalists to acknowledge that such a conclusion required tempering. That the "crucial experiment" in therapeutic outcome has not been completed is apparent to those who read this literature. That it is not likely to be completed soon, if ever, is also apparent to those who have confronted the full complexity and decades-long laboriousness of attempts at well-controlled outcome research. (What currently constitutes proof under these limitations on what can actually be known empirically is an interesting epistemological problem, expecially in a culture which apparently has begun a renaissance of humanitarian values. Bakan (1967, 1972) has made a cogent critique of the adverse effects on the development of psychology which have been imposed by its nearly exclusive preoccupation with experimental method.)

A related question to which devoted practitioners of individual therapy with children may prove to be vulnerable is: Has individual psychotherapy been given a priority of choice among various treatment interventions, which sometimes has failed to take adequate account of contextual and other constraints on the likely responsiveness of a child to psychotherapy; e.g., converting id to ego probably should be postponed with a child who has a chronically empty stomach. The substantial diversification of treatment alternatives which has occurred in well-established clinics,. most notably since the Community Mental Health Centers Act has been promulgated, suggests the possibility that, at least in the past, individual psychotherapy has sometimes been given too high a priority.

Individual psychotherapy, the voracious consumer of professional time, is a treatment option indicated under certain conditions which permit optimism about a favorable therapeutic response and contraindicated when these are not present. Most clinicians who have earned a few hash marks in traditional community child guidance clinics can recall some examples from their experience where individual therapy for a child might have been at least prematurely, if not inappropriately, applied: for example, where a trial of a combined remedial-reading and casework-with-parents approach before initiating individual therapy would have been appropriate to a third-grader with focal reading disability, or where casework only, individually or in a group, might have been an apt and economical first attempt at helping the mother of a three-year-old with night fears and mild asociability.

Some recent changes in traditional clinic procedures have made for a slight reduction in the great discrepancy between the high demand for clinical therapeutic services for children and its relatively limited availability. A reduction in rigid role specialization among clinic team members, so that various treatment modalities may more rapidly and flexibly be made available and larger numbers of individual therapy hours provided, is an avenue which many clinics are successfully traveling. Expansion and quality control of paraprofessional training offer another partial answer to the numbers problem, once professionals manage their status-sensitivity more comfortably.

As valuable as these procedural changes in personnel utilization can be, they offer little hope of solving the basic problem: an acute shortage of fully qualified professionals. Unless we solve this problem, so clearly stated by Albee (1959) and recently restated by the Report of the Joint Commission on Mental Health of Children (1970), through maintaining strong budgetary support for the training of mental health professionals and through improving the quantity and quality of graduate education in the mental health professions provided by universities and practicum training centers, the vast majority of the children who during this century will need the clinical services of the professional in order to avoid or remove the crippling effects of a psychological disorder will be unable to obtain such services.

Obsolescence and the Comparative Effectiveness of non-TCCP Methods

Are the shinier new tools from the non-TCCP foundries (crisis interviews, multiple family group intake and follow-through, behavior therapy, etc.) doing the job of improving the behavior disorders of children more effectively than was done before? What effects are these new tools having on the discipline and its potency for making contributions in the future?

The experience of going over Niagara Falls in a barrel probably cannot best be evaluated while in transit—especially with the band playing so loudly that it is difficult to hear oneself think and when the captain of the "Maid of the Mist" may prove to be a helmsman of uncertain expertise. At this point we are too close to the entire exciting experience to reach carefully reasoned judgments about what the positive or negative outcome trends will be in the use of the newer methods of non-TCCP, much less to be able to predict accurately the comparative yield relative to TCCP. In evaluating the effectiveness of all the latter-day innovations except the behavior therapy methods (which excel in the short-term outcome data they provide), we are further handicapped by the complexity of the criteria and the apparent lack of interest in outcome evaluation among most of the practitioners. In the face of the lack of a solid body of substantive data regarding the effectiveness of non-TCCP methods, little can yet be generalized. Instead, some brief impressions of the positive and negative yield for children and for clinical child psychology of the broadened application of non-TCCP methods are offered.

Some clearly socially constructive gains have been effected in bringing some form of mental health service to segments of the total population of children in need who were not well served previously: the poor, the family in crisis, the suicidal patient, and many of the so-called delinquents or delinquency-prone children.

A by-product of this expansion of services has seemed to be an increased sense of relatedness to, identification with, and responsibility for the larger society on the part of many members, members of the populations only recently being served. Those who value democratic ideals welcome changes of this order.

Contributions made largely by the behavior therapy contingent have included a valuable emphasis on clear definition and measurement of the outcomes of interventions and successful programs for developing social and self-help skills in the mentally retarded.

Balanced against these contributions are several kinds of essentially negative fallout: hazardous underdiagnosis, minimal conceptual clarification and research impetus, and the likelihood of the attenuation of the quality of training in clinical child psychology.

While it is not being claimed that every disturbed child requires an evaluation with the thoroughness described recently as a typical evaluation conducted by the Staff of the Children's Divison of The

Menninger Foundation (1969), abandonment of a serious effort to evaluate the nature and sources of a child's adaptive difficulties potentially places that child at risk and creates a condition encouraging mistrust of mental helath services on the part of the child and his family. Among partisans of this viewpoint, who also have extensive familiarity with brief service methods, Small (1970, 1971) has been one of the more articulate in pointing out the dangers inherent in minimal diagnostic efforts, especially for those who are likely to receive only brief service.

A ·decade of mushrooming of community mental health center-generated brief service methods and expansion of behavior therapy applications has added little to the conceptual framework of childhood psychopathology. This seems to be a natural consequence of having a clinical service orientation emphasizing immediacy and activity, rather than deliberation and conceptualization. However, if these newer methods are ever to be noted as more than minor temporary technologies in a phase of the history of abnormal psychology, some substantial conceptual additions leading to testable research hypotheses will need to be developed. (Although behavior therapies based on operant conditioning principles offer a few clearly stated constructs, such constructs deal with only a small fraction of total human experience and do not furnish a valid model of human psychological functioning.)

My concern is greatest about the third of these issues: the effects on the next generation of clinical child psychologists of their being trained primarily in the methods of non-TCCP. Will they have mastered the essential developmental tasks of the competent new clinician with children? That is, will they be able to assess the nature and determinants of a given child's disorder; to make appropriate choice and application of a combination of therapeutic resources for alleviating the child's disorder; and to perceive accurately their own personal strengths and weaknesses as clinicians in offering services to patients? It is difficult to be optimistic. The gray-haired tailors of most of the community psychology and behaviorism-oriented training programs, who for the most part learned TCCP methods before opting for non-TCCP methods, seem remarkably shortsighted about the manner in which their training in TCCP has prepared them for making the transition to a type of non-TCCP practice where rapid diagnostic assessments and brief therapy refinements are called for. If one expects to be able to offer one's patients diagnostic and individual therapeutic services of quality, is it inappropriate to expect that large amounts of supervised training will be devoted to these activities during the training period? Unless one gains confidence with diagnostic testng while opportunities for study, reflection, and supervision are maximal, is not truncation in diagnostic skill development likely? Unless a trainee in long-term individual-therapy carried out under supervision learns the meaning of the psychopathological terms he has been verbalizing and the varieties of distortions that he and his patient attribute to each other, his position on the community mental health firing line is a very vulnerable one. Sustained uncertainty in the face of the need to decide complex issues quickly is the kind of affective burden which often seems to include young clinicians toward trying to learn how to manage other people rather than how to emphathize with or help them.

Social Climate, Politics, and the Viability of TCCP

We are comonly reminded by sociologists that in a democratic society, social institutions such as occupational specialties, schools, and sanctioned methods for influencing other persons' behavior endure so long as their values remain within certain tolerance ranges of discrepancy with the dominant social values of the era. The possibility exists that recent social and political changes may have significantly narrowed the tolerance range for the methods of TCCP, considerations of their efficacy notwithstanding. A systematic coverage of this broad issue lies beyond the province of this paper[3]; as illustrations of the issue, two examples representative of the spectrum of relevant issues are mentioned.

It is highly likely that the recent trends in enfranchisement (actual and symbolic) of groups not previously afforded a full stake in our socity, i.e., 18-20-year-old youths, blacks, and women, has implications for the structure and durability of many social institutions, including the mental health enterprise. To the extent that these newly enfranchised groups differ in their modes of valuing and experiencing and are able to make their newly found power felt, changes in many societal ways are predictable. There are suggestions in the current literature that all three of these groups—youth, blacks, women—occupy positions on a hypothetical continuum of "preferred mode of experiencing" which are more toward the immediate and affective rather than the delayed and cognitive when they are viewed relative to the "establishment." Over the next century it is likely that these preferred experiencing modes of the

---

[3] Some valuable material supplying further context on this issue may be found in Slater (1970), Grier and Cobbs (1968), Gutmann (1965), and Silber (1971).

recently enfranchised will shape public institutions, including legis lation and budget support for mental health programs, towar greater conformity with their own values (given the assumptior no new countervalent force occuring). The effects of these hypothe-sized changes on TCCP and non-TCCP methods are difficult to predict. It seems likely that there will be increasing pressures on TCCP to shorten its procedures and to provide more opportunities for pleasure for more people sooner.

Political factors clearly influence the climate of support for dif-ferent varieties of mental health services. Since the implementation of the Community Mental Health Centers Act of 1963, an increasing proportion of the total expenditures for mental health has come from federal and state government treasuries. Concomitant with this trend has been the creation of a new orthodoxy of service patterns, dictated by government authorities to not only publicity funded agencies but also voluntary agencies for those parts of their pro-grams which are supported by government funding. "Treatment" of "sick communities" through political activism has been a frequently adopted feature of mental health agencies. Cost accounting in terms of dollars per service unit, urged by government management experts, has been used to replace accounting in terms of the relief of human suffering in many of these centralized programs (Goldsmith and Schulman, 1971). Paradoxically, the new machinery for extend-ing improved health services to individuals who have long needed them creates the risks of a reduction in quality of service, of rigid standardization of service patterns insensitive to individuality, and of loss of support for the heterodoxy necessary to constructive growth of the field of treatment techniques. With the gradual attribu-tion in private philanthropy which has been a major support of the bastions of traditional clinical methods, the voluntary agencies, TCCP may well find its methods altered more by political forces than by professional opinions regarding its relative efficacy in clinical service and training.

Contemporary *Weltschmerz*, Vicissitudes in the Identity Development of the Clinical Psychologist, and Pseudo-Obsolescence

Perhaps the obsolescence imputed by some to TCCP is more apparent than real. Consider the possibility that certain strains in the national ethos now accentuate for many of us that doomful mode of experiencing events termed *Weltschmerz*. Consider the additional possibility that certain strains in the identity development of many clinical psychologists lower their thresholds for self-repudiation and in interaction with the Weltschmerz mode create an aura of pseudo-obsolescence about TCCP, i.e., an inclination to discard the methods of TCCP on other than purely rational grounds. The sense of urgent need for rapid corrective action (*"Do* something, don't just *stand* there!"), highly plausible and infectious, may at first produce responses which have more of an abreactive, tension-draining function than a problem-solving function.

As a nation, we have recently become aware, as never before, of our tolerance of violent aggression. With repugnant regularity we experience: the dramatic violence of Vietnam, of assassinations of national leaders and protesting college students, and of murderous assaults on ordinary citizens on our city streets; there is also the quiet violence of racial prejudice and of intractable poverty which blights the lives of children even before they are born. The discrepancy between such violence and the ethical values most of us verbalize defies denial and inculpates most of us.

The failure of a significant portion of our political and industrial leadership to place national interest before personal interest has raised gnawing doubts about the integrity and viability of our principal institutions and about our capacity to rehabilitate ourselves rapidly enough to prevent national disaster. The phenomenon of a large body of alienated young people no longer surprises us. "If it feels good, do it," and "Action now!" are entirely comprehensible persuasions when one confronts the mind-boggling discontinuity between the window dressing and the actuality in many of the places where we live.

Populated largely by those who have acute awareness of human distress, the mental health enterprise is inevitably influenced by these strains. Sight may be lost temporarily of the fact that the inadequacies in our social institutions and the deprivations of the millions adversely affected by these can be only minimally altered via the mechanisms available to the mental health clinic. Use of mental health professionals to staff political action programs of community mental health centers ironically imposes further attenuation of the specialized manpower force needed for clinical services—that is, unless one is committed to the simplistic notion that political action always carries top priority and that individuals or families undergoing acute decompensations must always recognize this in regulating the depth and pace of their decompensations.

Strains also show clearly in the identity development of clinical psychology since mid-century. The version of the scientist-professional model of the clinical psychology adopted by most of our universities has been found inadequate to the goal of helping clinical students acquire the clinical skills they seek. Many academic departments of psychology, highly ambivalent about accepting educational responsibility for their rich but soft-headed clinical cousins, assuaged their guilt about accepting the budget support which the clinicians' presence afforded by providing the clinical psychology graduate students with surplus training in research methodology (which the clinical students wanted little of) and deficient training in clinical theory and method (of which they had requested a large amount). This not uncommon state of affairs in the educational histories of many current clinical psychologists has accentuated their identity-consolidation problems in several ways: by enhancing vulnerability to self-repudiation derived both from a failure in synthesis of the markedly different values of clinic and laboratory and from disapproval of career choice by the university "fathers"; by contributing measurably to the realistic fear that convocation day had been reached before any reassuring sense of clinical competence had been approximated. That this system for training clinical psychologists, through intensifying the frustrations of occupational identity synthesis, has produced no more casualties in the form of broken careers than it has is surprising. That it has not, provides more evidence for the extremely great manpower needs of the national mental health establishment and greater testimony to the high levels of ego strength and skillful use of dissociation among successful trainees in clinical psychology than it provides assurance of the coherence and quality of training in clinical psychology provided by the majority of graduate departments.

A related strain on the identity development of many clinical psychologists has been their difficulties in developing therapeutic competence. The training programs of the Forties and Fifties pushed large numbers of clinical psychologists onto the psychotherapy stage with little more to cover their therapeutic nakedness than the flimsy veil of eclecticism or a pair of ostrich-feather fans from nondirective method, "um-hmm" and "you feel - - -." The situational requirements for the bursting of bubbles of naive therapeutic omnipotence were well met. The scar tissue residual to these narcissistic injuries has been an accentuation of occupational identity diffusion for many of the walking wounded. The pathways to survival for the wise and the fortunate who survived this trauma typically have included one or more of a variety of postdoctoral therapy training sequences and/or curtailment of practice to a less demanding band on the spectrum of therapy patients. Not all survived. Many of the less wise and/or less fortunate failed to develop skill as psychotherapists and either, subsequently, shaped their careers to exclude it or rejected psychotherapy wholesale as an ineffective treatment method. Some of the least fortunate live out their therapeutic lives in the limbo of endless twiddling with the latest therapeutic fad.

The historical contingency of medical hegemony in serving emotionally troubled people also has complicated the course of identity synthesis for clinical psychologists. Growing up in Older Brother Psychiatrist's house has not been easy. It has occasioned a degree of reciprocated sibling rivalry and competitiveness at times which has penalized not only both adversaries but also many patients. The youngster who finds it necessary to make a bootstrap definition of his autonomy usually deprives himself of both the opportunity to learn from, and the opportunity to teach, the particular relative whom he perceives as tyrannizing him; and thus it has often seemed to be for clinical psychology vis-a-vis psychiatry. Several unfortunate consequences for the development of a comprehensive theory of psychopathology have ensued: slavish conformity to the disease-model of psychopathology on the part of some clinical psychologists; rejection of psychodynamic theory which is either unknown or at least ill-understood on the part of some others.

The proposition is entertained here, then, that some measure of the perceived obsolescence in the methods of TCCP may derive from strains within us as citizens as we experience a critical reappraisal of many of our basic social institutions and from difficulties in our professional identity consolidation as clinical psychologists. That these strains interact with certain elements of national character—an action-orientation, idolatry of the novel, repudiation of the ancestor and the aged—so as to reinforce the inclination to "change for change's sake" also seems likely to me. Nothing in this sentiment denies the incompleteness and imperfections in the concepts and tools of TCCP or the inappropriateness of their applications in certain clinical situations. It does suggest, amidst making the many radical changes called for in national social organization and in our professional training programs for clinical psychologists, that in rationally determining obsolescence in clinical tools it might prove advantageous over the long haul to rephrase the familiar dictum to read, "Don't just *do* something, *stand* there a little while—and *evaluate*."

Conclusion

Is TCCP obsolete?
Do deviant children no longer require the diagnostic skills of psy-

chologists who can accurately differentiate: the constitutional from the experiential determinants of their disorders; the recurrent inner patterns of emotion-laden ideas about themselves in relation to others and the alterability of these; how their patterns of thinking disturbances will change their abilities to learn under different educational regimens?

Do the emotionally disturbed child and his family no longer need the therapeutic skills of a psychologist who can: use the relationship with the child to help the child see the difference between his anxiously overdetermined anticipations of others' responses to him and the actuality of their responses, or use the complicated affective complexes which the child stirs in him to tailor a pattern of treatment experience accurately attuned to the highly personal logic of the child's regnant needs?

In the extent to which these questions are viewed as relevant and the answers to these are negative lies the essence of the reader's answer to the question heading this essay. By now, I have made my negative answer plain: Children with behavior disorders will be better served professionally with the procedures of TCCP, thorough diagnostic assessment and individual therapy which accounts for intrapsychic phenomena, than without these procedures.

This belief is held in a context of other beliefs which might appear at first to be incongruent with it:

a) that the concepts and methods of TCCP have not been "scientifically validated";

b) that some misapplications of TCCP methods are made in traditional settings;

c) that many of the brief treatment and group methods of non-TCCP offer the promise of making worthwhile additions to the conceptual base of childhood psychopathology, have clinical value, and should be included within the therapeutic armamentarium of traditional settings;

d) that the continuing shortage of mental health manpower urges a variety of attacks on the problem at several levels simultaneously: through social reorganization, through support for training of the traditional mental health professions, through innovations in service methods and through further additions to the differentiations of the traditional mental disciplines.

However, it would be unfortunate if we ended in confusing an extremely taxing problem in the logistics of mental health manpower with our evaluations of the effectiveness of various procedures for understanding and altering the patterns of behavior disorder in children and if we shaped the education of future clinicians in accord with this confusion. Likewise, it would be unfortunate, as Cain (1967) has eloquently argued, if the promise of the contributions of preventive mental health principles were attenuated in hasty applications which reject the utility of traditional approaches where they have proven useful, simply to preserve the purity of the new ideology.

Implied in these views is a further belief regarding TCCP training: that the constructs and procedures of TCCP constitute the appropriate core training (minimum essential) for those clinical child psychologists who aspire to achieving full professional status. A corollary would be that training in many of the methods identified with non-TCCP (group methods, brief therapy, consultation to gatekeepers, behavior therapy) represents a set of potentially valuable additions to basic training in TCCP, but that these variants are unable to take the place of the thorough grounding in the assessment and treatment of the complexity of human personality which comprises training in TCCP.

A final argument in support of TCCP: its relative potential for contributing new knowledge. In its conceptual differentiation and articulateness, in the scope of human complexity which it attempts to comprehend, and in the suitability of its methods for further refinements and syntheses of that complexity, it continues to offer substantial promise for contributing to new knowledge, be it by itself or in conjunction with other competing systems.

Tomkins (1971) offers us some wise counsel here:

> "Psychology has to deal with the most complex system in the world and has permitted itself, in my opinion, to be persuaded with increasing velocity of several absurdities: that the key to understanding human beings is to be found in one or another of many different specific places, each of which has been overly inflated. First in his drives, in his Id, in his unconscious, and thus to be partly controlled through its interpretation. Then, in observable, manipulable behavior and that the key to heaven is through behavioral technology. Then again, that the key was to be found in cognition, in man's priceless information processing capacities and that the computer and computer simulation would illuminate as it saved man. That the key was to be found in feeling, affect and emotion and that sensitivity training, encounter and catharsis would illuminate as it saved man. That the key was to be found in society, hence community psychology, or in the family, hence family therapy, or in the individual, hence individual psychotherapy. It is my belief that the individual will not be found in any of these places for the very simple reason that he is in all of

them at once and in varying degrees at varying moments in historical time. And if clinical psychology is ever to become a cumulative science and profession it must stop inflating its very special visions at the expense of other deflated visions. A human being is all of the things that clinical psychologists and psychiatrists have accused him of being, all of them at once, and the only way in which, it seems to me, we can save ourselves (if the theological metaphor is appropriate) is in fact to confront that very simple fact and to begin the very hard work of dealing with this complexity as it exists . . ."

There is ample room in the American mental health enterprise for experimentation with different clinical methods derived from various conceptions of psychopathology. Within the next century, it is to be hoped that refinements in concept, diagnostic methods, and treatment techniques will lead to much more rapid and effective modes of getting disturbed children back on their respective developmental tracks. My personal view is that the needed empirically based refinements (contrasted with administrative or "armchair" refinements) will not occur as rapidly with the application of brief service or group methods which minimize assessment of the particulars of an individual child's disorder, as they will with the typically used elaborate assessment methods of TCCP.

In sum, I believe that we shall make the most of our little time to 'set things right' when we are able to control our tendencies to oversimplify that which is complex, to value our heterodoxy rather than disparage it through either a hollow washout of our true differences or in self-aggrandizing exaggeration of those differences, and to channel the energies of our intramural conflicts into unremitting assault on our collective ignorance.

References

Albee, G. W. *Mental health manpower trends*. New York: Basic Books, 1959.

Bakan, D. *On method*. San Francisco: Jossey-Bass, 1967.

Bakan, D. Stimulus/Response: Psychology can now kick the science habit. *Psychology Today*, 5, No. 10 (March, 1972), p. 26ff.

Cain, A. C. The perils of prevention. *American Journal of Orthopsychiatry*, 1967, 37, 640-642.

Clements, S. D. *Minimal brain dysfunction in children: Terminology and identification*. NINDB Monograph No. 3. Washington, D. C.: U. S. Government Printing Office, 1966.

Freud, A. *Normality and pathology in childhood*. New York: International Universities Press, 1965.

Freud, S. *New introductory lectures on psychoanalysis*. New York: Norton, 1933.

Goldsmith, J.M., & Schulman, R. The politicalization of mental health. Paper presented at the annual meeting of the American Association of Psychiatric Services for Children, Beverly Hills, Calif., November, 1971. In *Psychosocial Process*, 1972, *2* (No. 2).

Grier, W. H., & Cobbs, P.M. *Black rage*. New York: Basic Books, 1968.

Gutmann, D. L. Women and the conception of ego strength. *Merrill-Palmer Quarterly*, 1965, *11*, 229-240.

Haley, J. Research on family patterns: An instrument measurement. *Family Process*, 1964, *3*, 41-65.

Healy, W., & Bronner, A. F. The child guidance clinic: Birth and growth of an idea. In Lowrey, L. G., & Sloan, V. (Eds.) *Orthopsychiatry 1923-1948: Retrospect and prospect*. Menasha, Wisc.: American Orthopsychiatric Association, 1948.

Hirsch, J. G., Borowitz, G. H., & Costello, J. Individual differences in ghetto 4-year-olds. *Archives of General Psychiatry*, 1970, *22*, 268-276.

Joint Commission on the Mental Health of Children. *Crisis in child mental health: Challenge for the 1970's*. New York: Harper & Row, 1970.

Krasner, L., & Ullmann, L. P. (Eds.) *Research in behavior modification*. New York: Holt, Rinehart & Winston, 1967.

Levitt, E. E. The results of psychotherapy with children: An evaluation. *Journal of Consulting Psychology*, 1957, *21*, 189-196.

Lief, R. (Ed.) *The commonsense psychiatry of Adolph Meyer*. New York: McGraw-Hill Book Co., 1948

Louttit, C. M. *Clinical psychology of children's behavior problems* (Rev. ed.). New York: Harper, 1947.

Menninger Foundation Children's Division. *Disturbed children*. San Francisco: Jossey-Bass, 1969.

Mishler, E.G., & Waxler, N. E. *Interaction in Families*. New York: Wiley, 1968.

Palmer, J. O. *The psychological assessment of children*. New York: Wiley, 1970.

Rie, H. E. Historical perspective of concepts of child psychopathology. In H. E. Rie (Ed.), *Perspectives in child psychopathology*. Chicago: Aldine-Atherton, 1971.

Rie, H. E. (Ed.) *Perspectives in child psychopathology*. Chicago: Aldine-Atherton, 1971.

Rosenblatt, B. Historical perspective of treatment modes. In Rie, H. E. (Ed.), *Perspectives in child psychopathology*. Chicago: Aldine-Atherton, 1971.

Ross, A. O. *The practice of clinical child psychology*. New York: Grune & Stratton, 1959.

Silber, J. R. The pollution of time. *Bostonia* Boston University alumni magazine), September 1971, 2-8.

Slater, P. E. *The pursuit of loneliness*. Boston: Beacon Press, 1970.

Small, L. Psychodiagnosis and "quality" psychological services. Paper presented at the annual meeting of the American Psychological Association, Miami Beach, Florida, September, 1970.

Small, L. *The briefer psychotherapies*. New York: Brunner/Mazel, 1971.

Thomas, A., Chess, S., & Birch, H. *Temperament and behavior disorders in children*. New York: New York University Press, 1968.

Tomkins, S. S. Remarks upon receiving an award for Distinguished Contribution to the Science and Profession of Clinical Psychology from the Division of Clinical Psychology, American Psychological Association at the annual meeting of the American Psychological Association, Washington, D. C., September, 1971. Printed in *The Clinical Psychologist*, 1971, *25*, p. 3ff.

38. Is Clinical Child Psychology Obsolete? Some Observations on the Current Scene

Ira Iscoe

Introduction

Prudence dictates a consideration of some of the background factors before confronting what undoubtedly is a controversial issue. We are in the midst of profound changes in our entire conceptions of mental health and ways of preventing and coping with so-called mental illness. The mental health field today can best be described as fluid with disciplinary boundaries becoming less clear. The knowledge explosion has generated much "action," and in an increasingly technological world, there is hopefully rising concern for humanity and the problems confronting humanity. Established institutions such as universities, religions, and the family are finding it very difficult if not impossible to cope effectively with the problems they are presented with. Some of the most cherished beliefs regarding psychopathology, its origins and its treatment, are being changed as a consequence of not meeting the challenges presented. Despite the confusion there should be optimism and hope. We may very well stand at a point where robust mental health, effective interventions, and the improvement of strategies in meeting the emotional needs of children are not too far in the future. Looking about and seeing how far we have yet to go can, however, generate some despair.

Background Factors

The publication of *Action for Mental Health* (Ewalt, 1960) climaxed five years of work of the Joint Commission of Mental Health and Mental Illness. Today the report is viewed as conservative, although for its time, many of the recommendations it con-

507

tained were exceedingly bold and formed the antecedents of programs that are widely accepted today. In 1963, President John F. Kennedy made history by delivering a congressional message dealing with the topic of mental illness and mental retardation. The Mental Health Facilities Act was soon passed by Congress leading to the development of community mental health centers, to general improvements in institutional settings, innovations in mental health training, and a general encouragement for the development of new strategies in planning for the more effective delivery of mental health services at all levels of severity and at all ages. Services to children were generally implicit in planning, but no revolutionary steps were proposed.

It is appropriate also to mention changes in the field of special education, in which various types of classroom approaches for the education (and treatment) of emotionally disturbed children have been developed. This movement had proceeded for the most part independent from clinical child psychology. Teachers have been trained to deal more or less effectively with emotionally disturbed childen in classrooms as compared to clinical settings. A variety of skills developed by psychologists have been employed, such as various forms of behavior modification, and clinical psychological consultation is being increasingly employed. However, clinical child psychology and special education of emotionally disturbed children are not as closely linked as one would hope. To the advantage of emotionally disturbed children and their parents and despite some definitely negative developments, school resources for the emotionally disturbed have increased enormously in the last ten years, and it is most unlikely that this facet of special education will be less emphasized in the years to come.

Why the Lack of Emphasis on the Mental Health of Children?

Despite general agreement (at least on the surface) among educators, psychologists, psychiatrists, social workers, social planners, parents, and politicians as to the need to improve mental health services for children, especially in the area of primary and secondary prevention, it is most disappointing to note the current lack of emphasis on mental health services to children at all levels. What accounts for this indifference in a supposedly child-centered culture?

A position paper of the American Psychological Association (Smith and Hobbs, 1966) on community mental health centers recommended that at least 50% of the services to be offered by these centers be geared to the needs of children. This certainly constitutes recognition, and as a matter of fact, this position paper was the first in APA history. Obviously, then, American psychology voiced its concern about children (at least to its membership). The recommendation was never followed by those in charge of setting up community mental health centers. Perhaps it was the lack of experience in community settings or more likely the absence of a workable model designed to offer new types of services to emotionally disturbed children in community settings, especially the economically disadvantaged. Psychologists were, and to a great extent still are, strangers to communities.

Disappointment is heightened by the *Report of the Joint Commission on Mental Health of Children* (1970), in which a bleak picture is painted of the current status of mental health of children, especially severely disturbed children. McCall *(Contemporary Psychology,* 1972) points out in his review of the report that "one cannot help but be appalled by the detailed accounting of the unsatisfactory, ugly status of child mental health service in the United States. Mentally disturbed children share a common fate with some minority groups and with the poor. At every White House Conference since 1930, the serious nature of this problem and noble recommendations for its solution have been offered to the federal and state governments, yet it would appear from the Joint Commission's reports that things are getting worse rather than better."

Some of the fault (but certainly not all) can be laid to the Ph.D. level training programs from which the great bulk of clinical psychologists have graduated in the last twenty years. Dealing with children and their problems is difficult indeed. Treating children gets enormously complicated; in their naivete and simplicity they destroy the defenses and avoidance techniques that clinical psychologists employ so effectively in dealing with adults. The writer estimates that only about one of every ten psychologists competent with adults has the ability to competently deal with children and their problems, including the families of the children. Using parents as whipping boys is easier than looking for assets in admittedly inadequate adults as far as child rearing is concerned. Clinical child psychologists have always been in short supply and never really in positions to take the lead in the setting up of innovative services for children. The so-called clinical team of the past has usually resulted in a fairly comfortable alliance between the social worker and the psychiatrist with the psychologist usually more in the diagnostic testing role. Another factor has been the relative lack of emphasis on childhood psychopathology and clinical child psychology in Ph.D. clinical psychology requirements. Experience with children and their families has been limited, resulting in an unfortunate lack of appreciation of how even seemingly inadequate parents may be helpful to children who have problems and how community resources can be better employed for the benefit of the child or children concerned. In the area of adolescence, the scarcity of psychological resources for children is probably worse. Even in the metropolitan area, experienced psychologists know how difficult it is to find facilities for adolescents and their families, especially hostile acting-out adolescents.

From the clinical child psychology graduate school view, increase in the number of Ph.D. child clinicians may very well not be the answer. In planning to deal with problems one must always avoid the "more of the same" philosophy. One of the best ways to test whether a discipline is conceptually on its toes is to ask what it needs most. If the answer is essentially more manpower in the same mold then the discipline is moribund. The Ph.D. child clinician, trained to deal with individual face-to-face psychotherapy with a full armamentarium of child diagnostic instruments, may very well be a vanishing breed. This does not imply that he should not and will not be active in the treatment of child psychopathology and child mental health. It does imply, however, that resource deployment is called for and clinical child psychologists must be newly and differently armed. How such personnel are to be trained and what should constitute the bulk of their armamentaria is a crucial issue.

Is Clinical Child Psychology Obsolete?

Given that above, how does one answer such a question? Who is to pronounce the judgment! What criteria should be used? Of what concern is it for the mental health of children if clinical child psychology is obsolete or not? Would they be better off without it? Is clinical child psychology being blamed for what is really a failure of American clinical psychology to "get with it" and develop comprehensive forward-looking mental health programs with appropriate preventive and intervention methods? How long will we continue to moan over the inadequacies of the medical model? Have we overdone our attacks on traditional clinical approaches?

Judgment of obsolescence of a profession or technology is not to be done lightly. One cannot ignore the intellectual and emotional investments of the professionals working under a certain system and in many cases doing highly creditable work. No group likes to be told that "they have had it." The ascription of obsolescence also has certain consequences. What alternatives are to be proposed? Are certain renovations needed, or must the entire technological and theoretical underpinnings be scrapped?

The term obsolete has several meanings, and although it is not customary for clinical psychology types to produce clear definitions (what consternation we would cause our colleagues in more exact areas of psychology), a sample of dictionary definitions puts the matter in some perspective. One definition says "no longer in use or in fashion." Another says "no longer used or useful because of outmoded design or construction or because of hard wear, e.g., an obsolete locomotive." A third says "from a biological standpoint increasingly vestigial or disappearing in each succeeding generation." The first definition referring to use or fashion has been mentioned. Clinical psychology is in use today although, as has been noted, it is undergoing various types of transformation such as moving from the medical to the community model, less emphasis on diagnostic testing, and more seeking of its own identity. It seems reasonable to predict that the sheer demands on the field will make traditional clinical psychology somewhat of a luxury and that financial realities will introduce "competitive obsolescence" wherein many of the good things that it has done can no longer be afforded financialy within an agency setting. It may, however, be possible to go "Cadillac class" in private settings, via insurance and the like. The second definition implies outmoded design and construction and has direct implications for strategies in the delivery of mental health services to children and of course their families. From the writer's point of view, this is the crucial issue. There are emerging needs and new demands for services. Clinical child psychology must find ways to deal with these demands and needs, or some other approaches will fill the void. The public need not wait for the professionals to get in gear. This warning, although oft given, is never considered seriously by the professionals. However, it is here given again. Competition in mental health services should not be viewed as duplication of services. It serves to keep the surveyors of services on their toes and prevents the security that was once engendered by long waiting lists and full appointment books.

School psychologists are undertaking new roles including contingency management and mental health consultation within the school system. Special education, as has been mentioned, is much involved with emotional disturbances of children. In some states an M.A. level educational diagnostician writes an "educational prescription" based partially on the results of psychological tests. Many of these tests have not been administered or interpreted by psychologists, let alone clinical child psychologists. Diagnostic testing, once considered part of the heavy artillery of the clinical child psychologist, is being looked down upon by Ph.D. clinicians and is being increasingly relegated to M.A. level psychologists. Added to the ferment there is a definite activist flavor somewhat disconcerting to the traditionally trained clinical child psychologists. They are urged from several sides to "move out into the real world," variously defined as the ghetto, the community, in fact any place except the office or usual agency location. The reception given psychologists in community settings is not generally a friendly one. This is understandable since the public conception of a psychologist is a narrow and generally unflattering one indeed.

Educators (mostly teachers) are becoming increasingly disenchanted with the contributions made by traditional clinical child psychologists. Extensive diagnostic testing followed by a long case conference in which it is revealed that the child is emotionally maladjusted or has a learning disability or is suffering from some personality disturbance does not sit well with the teacher who is being pressured for answers and an action plan. The chances are that the teacher already knew that the child was emotionally upset or had a learning disability or had some personality problems. This was the reason for the referral. The teacher's activist orientation means that something has to be done and implies "at least help me as a teacher to do something or let's do something together, but stop already with the fancy terminology, the inspired notions as to causality, and unrealistic recommendations such as a teacher spending more time with the child" or "the provision of all invironment designed to provide the child with a degree of security which will permit him to constructively experiment with interpersonal relationships designed to further his emotional-social growth," or similar bunkum. Much of the same holds for child guidance centers. The "do something" pressure cannot be answered by the recommendation of individual psychotherapy of the longer term variety. It has not proven that effective, and the resources are simply not there. The emphasis is more on crisis intervention, the initiation of action, the utilization of resources of nontraditional sorts, and finally on the development and training of resources that may not presently exist within school or community settings. These types of demands are difficult for the traditional clinical child psychologist to meet at present, and it is doubtful that a drastic reconceptualization will take place on the part of those who have a large investiment in what they have been doing (and most likely doing well) in the past. There is

clear need for the clinical child psychologist to become more sophisticated with regard to new skills and the utilization of community
resources. These new techniques are not presently taught in graduate schools and are not readily available in most clinical child
internship settings.

Towards a Viable Clinical Child Pshchology

Clinical child psychology, as the writer knew it and was trained in
it, with prolonged and inspired diagnostic testing, in-depth case history, psychoanalytically-oriented individual face-to-face therapy for
at least a year, plus interviews with parents, is obsolete as far as its
employment within community settings is concerned. This does not
mean, however, that it is not effective; it does imply that given the
market place of human needs it does not compete effectively, it is
too expensive, and is limited in the range of populations it can help.
The competition from other disciplines, the increasing need for services, the pressures for "action," all mitigate against the clinical
child psychology of the past. The question is therefore answered.
Clinical child psychology as most of us knew it twenty, fifteen, or
even five years ago, it not viable and capable of dealing effectively
with the many problems of children and their families.

Good sense should dictate an ending of this paper at this point.
However, the pronouncement of such a judgment means that something has to take the place of so-called traditional clinical child psychology, and indeed several things are already taking place. There is
an expected continuity where the old blends with the not-so-old.
Whether the new will be called clinical child psychology or not will
depend on a variety of factors including whether the field can be
flexible enough and adapt new procedures and reconceptualize its
goals. Most likely there will be a split. The older child clinicians will
continue to do their thing in the way they best know how, and no
one should fault them for their efforts. The younger child clinicians,
hopefully exposed to new training programs and experience, may
lead clinical child psychology to new heights of viability and even
scientific validity. In order for this to take place it is necessary for a
new knowledge base to be established independent of child psychiatry, employing behavioral science findings, and adopting more of an
ecological rather than a development model.

The possibilities for a new clinical child psychology are great
indeed. Recent issues of the journal of *Clinical Child Psychology*
furnish perhaps the best clues as to areas that could be entered with

excitement and profit. We can look forward to the treatment of entire families rather than individual children. More of this treatment will take place in the public rather than the private sector. Strategies will be more intervention-oriented and less protracted in terms of contact. Clinical child psychologists will most likely spend less time in direct contact with children and more time in consultation program planning, evaluation research, and the translation of research findings into treatment and preventive programs. It may very well be that the term "clinical child psychology" will have to be abandoned for one that is more suitable to the wider range of activities that will be encompassed. There will always be children who are severely disturbed and who will need the help of mental health professionals. Nevertheless, more and more children and parents have difficulties in dealing with the "problems of living." From the writer's point of view, the competent clinical child psychologist should be active in community planning and in school settings rather than being the more or less passive recipient and treater of the victims of inadequate social systems and mentally unhealthy milieus. A pipe dream? Of course. The greatest detriment to the emergence of a new clinical child psychology is the so-called "practical" view. A call for practicality may be interpreted as a put-off for innovative planning. Pipe dreams, when adequately implemented, have a delightful habit of coming true. The problems of redeployment of resources are admittedly enormous but the opportunities are greater than most dreamers will concede. From the R.I.P. for traditional clinical child psychology should emerge the L.I.V. (live in vitality) of the new.

39.   The Death and Rebirth of Clinical Psychology—Tragicomical Reflections*

Gertrude J. Williams

Death reapeth all, and hath no shame:
A day will come, the whole world shall sate its greed.
All this is truism; what need
To say it? Yet as oft as it comes true
It startles us anew.[1]

In an incredible application of the medical model he so vehemently repudiates, George Albee—brow furrowed, stethoscope tensed—has pronounced clinical psychology dead.[2] In what has to be the pre-eminent redundancy of all time, he has further stated that clinical psychology has an uncertain future.[3] Reactions to the news of death were fairly typical of the early work of mourning: shock, bewilderment, incredulousness, rage, grief, guilt, despair, surreptitious chortling among the tough-minded mourners, anger at the bearer of bad tidings. But the initial tumult and the shouting have subsided, and now we are impelled to ask straightforward questions. Does clinical psychology have an uncertain future? Has it died? If so, should its loss be mourned? Above all, what is the fuss about? Why have psychologists responded so excitedly to Dr. Albee's statements? As a guardian of one of the putative orphans, *Clinical Child Psychology*, we feel moved to share our reflections on these moribund matters with our fellow alleged bereaved.

Titilating Titular Trauma

To begin with, the provocative titles of Dr. Albee's presentations were bound to cause a stir. Still, what's in a name? One is struck by

*This essay is a slight revision of an editorial published in *The Clinical Child Psychology Newsletter*, 1970-71, IX, No. 4, 1-3.

the jarring imbalance between the sensational titles and the non-polemic, almost lacklustre tone of the texts. The titles do assert that clinical psychology is dead, but the texts contain unconvincing obituaries without proof of death. The stimulating titles to which many clinical psychologists are responding with excitement are but verbal teases that make promises which the anti-climactic texts fail to keep. The situation is all so reminiscent of that earnest poem by E. V. Rieu:

MEDITATIONS OF A TORTOISE DOZING
UNDER A ROSETREE NEAR A BEEHIVE AT NOON
WHILE A DOG SCAMPERS ABOUT
AND A CUCKOO CALLS FROM A DISTANT WOOD
So far as I can see
There is no one like me.

So much for titular verbal foreplay and its overly heightened arousal value for frustrated clinical psychologists.

The Certainty of Uncertainty

We will graciously refrain from postulating uncertain futures for postulators of uncertain futures as we now consider the postulation that clinical psychology has an uncertain future. To this assertion, we can only shrug, "So what else is new?" Especially in these times of instant change, the future of everything including even futurology is most certainly uncertain. That clinical psychology is also included in the domain of universal uncertainty hardly inspires further reflection. What is worthy of at least brief consideration is the remarkable attention psychologists are paying to the uninspiring assertion that clinical psychology shares the fate of everything else.

The inappropriately intense reaction to the view that part of psychology has an uncertain future may be symptomatic of serious problems within our discipline. At a time when "the problem with existing societies is not how to stablize them but how to change them"[4], at a time when "we are the first generation absolutely certain that tomorrow will not be like today"[5], is it not significant that large numbers of psychologists assume fixity of social process and irrationally repudiate uncertainty in psychology? Why? Who are we? Are we elitist isolationists in the global village, exempt from natural forces? Are we non-risk-takers closed-mindedly rejecting change and threatened by the ambiguities of existential reality? Research on the sociology of psychology and on the psychology of psychologists recommends itself.

In short, it is obvious that clinical psychology has an uncertain future. That such a reminder even needs to be presented and *then* is viewed as controversial is an important commentary on the forzen adaptive potential within the profession. Inadvertently, George Albee has done the field a service by his presentations. In the words of Oliver Herford:

> *The Smile of the Walrus is wild and distraught*
> *And tinged with pale purples and greens*
> *Like the Smile of a Thinker who thinks a Great Thought*
> *And isn't quite sure what it means.*

No matter that the important message may have been unintended. The Great Thought, change-shock in the field of clinical psychology, remains.

In the Wake of Clinical Psychology

Let us boldly confront the matter of the so-called demise of clinical psychology and the impact of its autopsy report and requiem on clinical psychologists. Our own association to the aftermath of death is the Jewish mourning period known as *sitting shivah.*[6] At this time, the mourners sit on wooden boxes, their feet bare, their garments rent, preoccupied with memories of the deceased and with their own grief. The austerity of the *shivah* ritual is always relieved by the offering of sweets to the bereaved by neighbors and a visit from a member of the local Society to Comfort Mourners. Now, if anyone is a close relative of the deceased, it is certainly Dr. Albee whose active concern and professional attention (albeit non-medical) helped keep clinical psychology alive. He, a loving nurturer of the now dead and proclaimer of the demise, must surely be mourning too. Yet he receives only bitters, not sweets, from his compatriots in grief; and what is even more touching, he seems to be sitting alone and uncomforted on his wooden box. As unofficial representative of the Society to Comfort Mourners, we would like to examine some bases for this poignant state of affairs.

Three possibilities come to mind. The first relates to Dr. Albee's audacious violation of the taboo against denouncing the deceased. The initially shocked reactions were to be expected, but the intensity of the furor and the continued righteous indignation has a me-thinks-thou-doth-protest-too-much quality. Quite possibly, the unpersuasive denials of Dr. Albee's candid critique of the dead may represent unacknowledged *déjà vu* reverberations in the fainter hearts of the survivors. Secondly, certain lapses in the formal thinking of Dr. Albee's critics are suggested by their outraged reactions to his declarations of the death of clinical psychology. They are behaving as if the deliverer of the funeral oration is also, word-magically, the assassin. Finally, the tumult may relate to the mind-blowing possibility that Dr. Albee is both correct and incorrect in his statements that clinical psychology is dead. On the one hand, in view of the vast numbers of people practicing, preaching, and producing something called clinical psychology, it does seem that Dr. Albee has somewhat exaggerated the occurence of its death. On the other hand, it appears that processes within something called clinical psychology are stagnant, useless, not only dead, but in need of burial. How can we resolve the cognitive dissonance created by these apparent contradictions? Which clinical psychology is dead, and which clinical psychology is alive? Will the real clinical psychology please stand up (and then lie down, if need be)!

The full name of the deceased has been misheard. The name of the corpse is *Medical-Model, Elite-Type Clinical Psychology*. A *Medical-Model* is used by certain duly certified panacea-pedlars to designate disease, pathology, or sickness within a person branded "mentally-ill-patient' with little or no regard for environmental circumstances or social realties in the person's life; this definition is contained in the "clinical" portion of the name of the dead clinical psychology. *Elite-Type* refers to an isolationist ideology, under the guise of true scholarship, in which work in the laboratory and lecture hall which frequently makes no social contribution whatever is viewed as infinitely superior to work in the public sector which frequently does; this definition is contained in the "psychology" portion of the name of the dead clinical psychology. The entire House of Clinical Psychology has not fallen, merely two of its ancient relatives whose ghosts continue to haunt us. To equate clinical psychology with these dubious ancestors is an irrational *pars pro toto* inference on the part of both Albee and his critics. Dr. Albee has beaten a dead horse or rather, a dead profession. Current clinical psychology, however inchoate and uncertain in its flounderings, is not dependent on either the medical model or an elitist tradition for its existence and viability.

> *I tell you, it is not me you are looking at,*
> *Not me your confidential looks*
> *Incriminate, but that other person, if person,*
> *You thought I was: let your necrophily*
> *Feed upon that carcass..*[7]

Come, let us bury the proper dead.

The Wake and the Awakening of Clinical Psychology

Just as it is a delusion and a snare to keep defining psychology solely as the science of behavior, so it is a delusion and a snare to keep defining clinical psychology solely as the application of the science of psychology to the diagnosis and treatment of pathological behavior. While rudiments of such traditional functions do remain and contribute in many ways to knowledge and human welfare, the rubric of clinical psychology is no longer the triad of testing, treatment and—uh—oh, yes—uh—research. These roles have not died; they have been overshadowed by our desperately needed acceptance of newer roles which require a changed philosophy of clinical psychology.

Mass media technology foists on our once unwilling consciousness man's inhumanity to man. As the profession uniquely concerned with furthering knowledge about man and applying this knowledge to the solution of human problems, clinical psychology cannot fail to become involved in the actualization of man's potential for humanity. We are impelled by our intellectual and ethical values to play our part in the awesome responsibility of providing the greatest good for the greatest number. Only in memory can we recapture the short, *happy* life of that young clinical psychology once exhilarated by each mastery and advance, however slight, during it first enthralling falterings toward professionalization. Time and the times have vanquished that precious youth. It has aged. Having willed us an inheritance of knowledge to be treasured and used, it has died. The fruit of clinical psychology must fall if the seed is to be scattered and give rise to new forms in our field. If the fruit does not fall to the earth, it will decay on the branch. Nostalgic conservatives of clinical psychology, you must not longer act as if the rotting fruit of clinical psychology is still in the bud! You are powerless to transubstantiate phantoms of past, less tormented times. You must discard pretense; you must do the renunciative work of mourning and assimilate the reality that the dead can never be brought back to life.

Come, let us bury the dead clinical psychology. Let us know that its immortality is assured by its contributions in life. As a mite in the midst of the mighty medical profession, clinical psychology invented itself out of social necessity. At a time when elitist detachment was the hallmark of our discipline, clinical psychologists explicitly committed themselves to humanistic and democratic values and built a bridge to the real world by willingly accepting public responsibility. This birthright shall never die.

Having eulogized by the graveside of clinical psychology, let us also pay our last respects to the dead by offering it the incisive courtesy of candor. As we inter *Medical-Model, Elite-Type Clinical Psychology*, perhaps we can learn from the losses we do *not* mourn. We shall hardly miss the clinical psychologist in the role of Uriah Heep or Count von Masoch in his relations with medical colleagues. We bid farewell to that unenlightened, vacuously asocial view that an intrapsychic exploration constitutes the only authentic means of liberating human beings. *Au'voir* to that grim *Weltanschauung* which characterizes the one, called therapist, as omnipotent psycho-microbe-hunter and the other, called patient, as diseased, disordered and devoid of irreductible potentialities for selfactualization and transcendence! Goodbye, O normality, mindlessly portrayed as a Norman Rockwell illustration of the white, rosy-cheeked, college kid as control subject! Another goodbye to the relegation to miscellaneous multitudes of experimental groups variously labelled abnormal, disturbed or deviant if they departed from this inane, inspid pseudo-standard! So long, institutionalization of cowardice engendered by a dogma which implicitly affirmed that a psychologist could not be both a scholar and a change agent and of course, chose to be a scholar because it was infinitely superior! O perish, proliferation of drivel by promotion-pushing professorial practitioners who placidly published while people perished! Ah, relics of clinical psychology, the good you have done will surely live after you. May the evil be interred with your bones! Amen.

Our post-morten is completed. We have come full circle. The antiquated models and doctrines of clinical psychology die hard for whatever "is most like the dead shrinks from death."[8] But what if clincial psychology shrinks from burial and clings to past remnants hoping to find a half-life in its own remains? Probably, the world will continue creaking on its axis. Clinical psychology will be merely set aside, placed in limbo like alchemy, phrenology, and other extinct disiciplines that meant well but outlived their usefulness. In a footnote, future historians can say of the fossilized clinical psychology of the Seventies that with it or without it, the world was pretty much the same, that its quasi-existence really made no difference whatsoever.

If it rises from the ashes of inertia and anxiety, clinical psychology can be reborn. Are we not already suffering the birth pangs of a New Clinical Psychology? We are made dizzy by the kaleidoscope of new roles thrust on us once *again* by social necessity: daycare planning; the training of psychological technicians; sex education; the development of creative potential; school consultation; population control; construction of curricula for indigenous paraprofessionals; advocacy of children, the poor, the despairing, the homosexual, the retarded and others for whom social justice and mercy have been denied.

"Give us new models!" we demand as we reel in confusion. They have yet to be created. First, we must clear the debris and wash away the stagnation. Then we will be able to reconceptualize, revitalize, renourish and give birth to the New Clinical Psychology!

> *Deep in the earth I rested now:*
> *Cool is its hand upon the brow*
> *And soft its breast beneath the head*
> *Of one who is so gladly dead.*
>
> . . . .
>
> *O God, I cried, give me new birth,*
> *And put me back upon the earth!*
> *Upset each cloud's gigantic gourd*
> *And let the heavy rain, downpoured*
> *In one big torrent, set me free,*
> *Washing my grave away from me!*[9]

L'ENVOI

Reflective investigation, actualization of ethical principles, the promotion of human welfare — these, our eternally shared values, sustain our profession amidst the terrifying vicissitudes of social reality. Though we venture in fear and trembling, our vital, glowing ideals illumine the darkness of the ever-present uncertainty of clinical psychology and will resurrect it in its future deaths. Clinical psychology is dead. Long live Clinical Psychology!

References

1. LaFontaine, *Death and the Dying* (a fable). Quoted in Vischer. A.L. *On Growing Old,* Houghton Mifflin Co., 1967.
2. George W. Albee, The short, unhappy life of clinical psychology (Clinical Psychology—R.I.P.) *Psychology Today,* September 1970.
3. George W. Albee. *The Uncertain Future of Clinical Psychology.* Presidential Address. American Psychological Association Convention. Miami, September 1970.
4. Everett Reimer, quoted in Miller, S. M., Alternatives to schools. *New York University Education Quarterly,* Summer 1970.

5. Walter Lowenfels. *The Writing on the Wall* (poems of protest). Double-day and Co., 1969.

6. See Leo C. Rosten, *The Joys of Yiddish*. McGraw-Hill Co., 1968.

7. T. S. Eliot, *Family Reunion* (a play).

8. Op. cit.: reference 1.

9. Edna St. Vincent Milay, *Renascence*. Quoted in *One-Hundred One Famous Poems,* Cook. R. J., Editor. The Cable Co., 1929.

Index

A (vitamin), deficiency in, 283-84
AAPSC (American Association of Psychiatric Services for Children; American Association of Psychiatric Clinics for Children), 465, 467, 468, 472, 474-76, 479
A-B-A-B design for data gathering, 83
Ability Structure Project, 72
Abortions, 433-34, 458
Academic performance, preschool education and, 313, 314
Academy for Educational Development, 375
Acceleration techniques of behavior modification, 87-88
Action for Mental Health (Ewalt), 507
"Action for Mental Health" (report of the Joint Commission on Mental Health and Illness; 1961), 36, 39, 40, 42
Activities in Family Style Program, 216-17
Ad Hoc Committee on Advocacy, 47
Adams, P.L., 197
Adaptation to environment, intelligence as, 192
Adaptative growth, conditions of, 121-22
Adelman, Howard S., 258-65
Adler, Alfred, 249
Adolescence
  work and, 381-89
    naturalistic studies of, 381-85
    as therapy, 385-88
  See also Identity Group Psychotherapy; Teenagers; Youth
Adolescent development, psychological identity and, 318
Adoption laws of New York State, 25
Adoptions, subsidized, 25
"Adult Behaviors in Caregiving" (ABC scale), 158
Adults
  dialogue between youth and, 19-20
  drug use among, 99
  role of work for, 381
Advocacy, *see* Child advocacy
Affects in contextualizing of behavior, 339

Aggressive behavior
  of boys and girls, compared, 230-31
  mass media stimulating, 22
Agriculture, women in development of, 426
Aid to Dependent Children, 60, 127
Alabama, infant mortality rate in, 268
Albert, S., 248
Albee, George W., 53-66, 494, 515, 517-18
Alienation of youth, 19-20, 363-64
Allen, K.E., 83
Allport, G.W., 394
Alternate Approaches to Graduate Education, Panel on, 378
Alternatives Model to drug use, 101-5
  implementing, 105-8
Altman, Charlotte H., 19-34
American Association of Psychiatric Services for Children (American Association of Psychiatric Clinics for Children; AAPSC), 465, 467, 468, 472, 474-76, 479
American Male, The (Brenton), 437
American Medical Association (AMA), 55
American Orthopsychiatric Association, 198
American Psychological Association (APA), 35, 64, 198, 423
  Ad Hoc Committee on Children and Youth, 45
  advocacy concept and, 48
  1968 Convention of, 42
  1971 Convention of, 26
  pediatric psychology and, 112
  position paper of, 508-9
  training of psychologists and, 463-65, 467, 468, 471, 473, 479, 480, 482
American Psychiatric Association, 55
Amidon, E.J., 255
Amphetamines, 99
Anderson, E.L., 281
Anemia among socially disadvantaged infants, 280, 281
Angel, E., 394
Angyal, Andras, 126

Antisocial behavior of adolescents, work reducing, 387-88
Antonov, A. N., 274-275
Anxiety
  memory and, 189
  reduced by RET, 248
APA, see American Psychological Association
Appalachian Regional Commission, 145
APPROACH (numerical coding system), 157
Arbitrary representation, symbols as, 186
Arneil,G.C., 281
Arbolino, Jack, 376
Ashton-Warner, Sylvia, 233, 234
Aspiration levels of adolescents, 384
Assaults in state institutions for mentally retarded, 13
Association of Black Psychologists, 310, 320
Association of Psychologists for la Raza, 326
Association for Supervision and Curriculum Development, 254
Attention capacity
  of mentally retarded children, 74
  of socially disadvantaged children, 294
Autistic children, responses of, 231
Autobiography of Mary McLeod Bethune, The, 233
Automated teachers, human vs., 149
Ayllon, 39

B₁ (vitamin), deficiency in, 283-84
B₂ (vitamin), deficiency in, 283-84
Badger, Earladeen, 136
Bailey, J., 75-76
Baldwin, V.L., 77
Bandura. A., 86, 95
Barbiturates, 99
Barnes, R.H., 278
Barrera-Moncada, G., 286
Basic process of cognition, 182
Basic units of cognition, 181-82
Battered children, 445
Baumgartner, L., 268-70
Bayh, Birch, 30
Bayley, N., 156, 157
Bayley Scales, 125
B-complex (vitamins), deficiency in, 283-84
Behavior
  acceleration and deceleration techniques for modifications of, 87-88

Behavior (cont'd)
  aggressive
    of boys and girls compared, 230-31
    mass media stimulating, 22
  antisocial, of adolescents, 387-88
  assessed through psychotherapy, 82-84;
    see also Psychotherapy
  contextualizing of, 339-32
  disturbed or deviant 53-54, 56
  emotional, cognitive development and, 123
  public, 181
  sexual, 419-24
  as study of paradoxes, 6
Behavior Therapy (journal), 88
Behavioral deficits, defined, 82
Behavioral excesses, defined, 82
Behavior Research and Therapy (journal), 88
Beller, E.K., 161
Belmont, I., 72
Belmont, L., 72
Beman, A., 328, 329
Bender, L., 398
Bender-Gestalt Test, 203-4
Bennett, E.L., 126
Bennett, George K., 317
Berberich, J.P., 77
Bereiter, C., 151
Bessell, Harold, 254
Bettelheim, Bruno, 395
Bettis, Moody C., 56, 65
Biafra, starvation in, as example of inhumanity, 4
Biber, B., 145
Bijou, S.W., 67, 69, 77, 83
Bilingual studies programs, 299
Bill of Rights for Children (1930), 24
Billewicz, W.Z., 271
Binet, Alfred, 119
Binet Scales, 120, 157
Birch, Herbert G., 72, 74, 266-91, 491
Birnbrauer, J.S., 77
Birth control (contraception), 422-424, 427, 429, 433, 456-59; see also Family planning
Birthweight, distribution of, among whites and nonwhites, 269-71
BITCH Test (Black Intelligence Test Counter-Balanced for Honkies), 311, 314
Black Boy (Wright), 233
Black children
  genetic inferiority of, 343-46
  percentage of, in inner city schools, 301
  self-concepts of, 58-59

Black children *(cont'd)*
  testing of
    attacked, 309-11, 324-25
    defended, 315-20
    as intellectual genocide, 320-22
    viewed as secondary problem, 312-15
  as victims of racism, 60
Black Intelligence Test Counter-Balanced
    for Honkies (BITCH Test), 311,
    314
Blain, Daniel, 64, 238
BLAT (test), 319, 320
Blatt, Burton, 3-18, 25
Bloom, B. E., 127, 297
Boek, J. K., 276
Boek, W. E., 276, 279
Borowitz, G. H., 488
Boston City Hospital, 277
Boulder Conference (AAPSC, 1949), 466
Boulder model of psychologists training,
    466, 470
Bower, E. M., 227-30, 235, 238
Bowlby, J., 142
Boyd-Orr, Sir John, 272
Boys, aggressiveness of, 230-31
Brain damage
  mental retardation and, 70, 74-75
  learning disability caused by, 343
Brattgard, S. O., 126
Breadwinners, fathers as, 439
Breast feeding, social class and, 280
Brenton, Myron, 437
Brickman, Harry R., 57
Brock, J., 279
Bronfenbrenner, Urie, 33, 34
Bronner, A. F., 486
Brown, Claude, 233, 322
Brown, R. D., 235
Bryan, H., 281
Bruner, J., 151
Brunet, O., 142
Bug-in-the-ear system, 91
Bureaucratic Zombie Syndrome in Head
    Start programs, 204-5
Burlingham, D. T., 398
Burnham, J. R., 309
Butler, A. L., 145
Butterfield, W. H., 77
Byck, M., 78

C (vitamin), deficiency in, 280-84
"C" group, characteristics of, 255-56
Calcium deficiency, 283-84
Caldwell, Bettye M., 143, 145, 150, 154,
    155, 157

Caldwell, Edson, 255
California, external credit plans projected
    in, 374
*California against the California State
    Department of Education,* 327
California State Department of Educa-
    tion, 326
California Test of Mental Maturity, 327
Calmerde, 126
Campus-Free College, 375-77
Camus, Albert, 173
Cannabis drugs, 99
Caregivers, *see* Child care specialists
Cass, Loretta K., 463-82
Castro, Fidel, 9
Catholic Church, birth control and, 433
Cattell, R. B., 320
Cattell IQ scores, 154-55, 160
CCMHC (Comprehensive Community
    Mental Health Centers), 37, 57-58
Census Bureau, 443
Center Model for infant development proj-
    ects, 145-46
Center for Studies of Child and Family
    Mental Health, 446
Center Work Conferences, 206-7
Central nervous system, maturation of,
    126-27
Chandler, J. T., 326
Change, psychologists as agents of, 177
Chauvinism in testing of black children,
    312-15
Chess, S., 491
Chessman, Caryl, 364
Chicago Conference (AAPSC, 1965), 466
Child advocacy
  applications of, 46
  as instrument of child power, 45
  at state level, 43
Child Advocacy, Office of, 173
Child Advocacy Bill (S.1414), 43
Child Advocacy System, 42
Child care programs, 168-78
  background of, 168-70
  ecological approach to, 175-77
  lip service paid to, 180
  need for developmental, 171-72
  new concepts in, 170
  psychologists as lobbyists for, 177-78
  turned over to experts, 32-33
  urgently needed, 172-75
  See also Day care centers
Child care specialists
  funds for training, 31-33, 36, 41, 150-52

Child care specialists *(cont'd)*
  for infant development projects, 148-53
    assessment of, 158-59
    assignments, 152-53
    selection, 148-50
    training, 150-52
  for screening of emotionally handi-
    capped
  pre-school children, 238-39
Child development, need for research in'
    40
Child Development, Office of, 32, 34, 43,
    199
Child Development Art (1971), 43
Child Development Commission (Ha-
    waii), 43
Child Development Councils, 42, 45-46
psychologists' function in, 48
Child Development-Day Care Forum
    (White House Conference on Chil-
    dren; 1970), 171
Child labor laws, 381
Child Manifest Anxiety Scale (CMAS),
    327, 328
Childbirth among socially disadvantaged
    perinatal risk, 271-72
    prematurity and obstetric complica-
      tions, 268-71, 273-74, 445, 446
Childhood, experiences in early, and ef-
    fects on learning ability, 179-80
Childrearing
  cognitive development and, 132-33
  pediatricians' training in, 110-12
  between 10 months to 3 years of age,
    124-25
  varieties in, 180-81
Children
  autistic, 231
  in communes, 368-70
  disguised punitiveness against, 22-23
  disruptive, 296
  foster 24-25
  hyperactive, 229
  illegitimate, 22-23
  individual and social competence of, 227
  liberated, liberated women and, 425-36
  obsolescence of TCCP and, 488-90
  rejected and battered, 445
  status of, affected by family planning,
    444-67
  number of handicapped, 177; *see also
    specific forms of handicaps; for ex-
    ample:* Emotionally disturbed chil-
    dren; Mentally retarded children
  as psychotherapists, 86-87, 92-95
  sex roles as viewed by, 124

Children *(cont'd)*
  See also Black children; Educationally
    handicapped children; Emotionally
    disturbed children; Infants;
    Institutionalized children; Learned
    disabled children; Lower-class
    children; maladjusted children;
    Mentally retarded children;
    Mexican-American children; Middle-
    class children; Socially disadvan-
    taged
Children's Bureau, 177
Children's Reinforcement Survey, 83
Chitlins Test, 319
Christmas in Purgatory (Blatt), 25
Chronological age (CA), 119-20
Clark, Kenneth B., 305
Classroom situations
  for EH and ED children, 260-61
    implications of, 261-65
  freedom of movement in, 213-23
  personalized, 261
Clausen, Johns, 72, 73
Cleaver, Eldridge, 322
CLEP (College-Level Examination Pro-
    gram), 376
Clergy, mental health training of, 62
Clement, Paul W., 19-34, 81-97
Clements, S. D., 491
Clinical, defined, 67
Clinical child psychologists, *see* Psycholo-
    gists
Clinical child psychology
  death and rebirth of, 515-22
  defined, 470-71
  obsolescence of, 507-14
  See also Traditional clinical child psy-
    chology
Clinical Child Psychology (Albee), 515
Clinical Child Psychology (journal), 513
Clinical Child Psychology Newsletter,
    312, 318, 324
CMAS (Child Manifest Anxiety Scale),
    327, 328
Cobbs, Price M., 58
Code of Ethics of social workers, 47
Cognition (thought)
  motivation and, 122-24, 195-96
  pre-school learing and, 181-82, 185-91
  primary functions of, 181-82
  shaped by language, 119
"Cognitive Capability of Exceptional
    Children" (Newland), 320
Cognitive development
  adolescent, 381
  experience and, 126-27

Cognitive development *(cont'd)*
  Family-Style Program and, 221
  of mentally retarded children, 135-37
  motivational autonomy and, 124-26
  plasticity of, 131-33
    heredity and, 133-35
  prevailing notions of intelligence and, 119-21
  revised conceptions of intelligence and, 121-24
Cohen, Allan Y., 98-109
Cohen, L., 122
Cohen, Rosalie, 329
Cohen, T. B., 229
Coiner, B., 269
Coleman Report, 301-2, 382
Coles, Robert, 363
College Entrance Examination Board, 375, 378
College graduates, number of, in U.S., 371
College-Level Examination Program (CLEP), 375, 376
College Proficiency Examination Program (New York State Education Department), 375
Colorado, University of, 478
Colorado General Hospital, 445
Comic books for sex education, 351-61
Communes 363-70
  children in, 368-70
  life in, described, 363-66
  sexual matters in, 366-67
  work in, 367-68
Community
  effects of Head Start programs on, 27
  role of, in sex educationa, 454-55, 459
  schools and needs of, 21
Community Facility Act (Lanham Act; 1941), 169
Community Mental Health Centers Act (1963), 493, 498
Commmunity participation, 21
Community psychology programs, psychological sciences in, 197-209
  guidelines for, 199-201
  models of, 206-7
  to serve lower-class children, 197-98
  types of problems encountered in, 201-6
Community schools, 302-3
Compensatory education programs
  number of (1971), 293
  purpose of, 27
  See also Head Start programs
Competence
  defined, 125

Competence *(cont'd)*
  highly regarded by the culture, defined, 333, 334
  promotion of individual and social 224-35
    in children, 227
    as goal of Head Start programs, 27
    schools and, 227-28
    strategy and plan for action in, 235-39
    through symbols, 232-35
    teachers in, 228-31
    of youth, 225-26
Comprehensive Child Care Act (Mondale-Brademus bil!; 1971), 177-78
Comprehensive Child Development Bill (1970), 42-43
Comprehensive Community Mental Health Centers (CCMHC), 37, 57-58
Conant, James B., 128
Concepts, cognition through, 182,187
Conditioning
  learning by, 156
  public behavior acquired through, 181
Connecticut, external credit plans projected in, 374
Conservative force, women as, 441
Contemporary Psychology (McCall), 509
Contextualizing of behavior, 339-42
Contraception (birth control), 422, 424, 427, 429, 433, 456-59
Costello, J., 488
Cottingham, Harold F., 255
Counseling by clergy, 62
Courses
  credits without, 375-77
  without credits, 375
  elective, grading system for, 107-8
  for psychologists, 471-72
Cox, F., 336
Cravioto, J. DeLicardie, 267, 278, 285, 286
Creative-aesthetic experience, drug use and search for, 103
Creative Expression Room, 214, 216, 217
Credits
  courses without, 375
  guidance plus, 374-75
  without courses, 375-77
Crimes, perversions as, 422-24
"Crisis in Child Mental Health, Challenge for the 1970's" (Joint Commission on Mental Health of Children), 42
Criterion-referenced tests, 129
Cummings, S. Thomas, 485-506

Curricula
  average-child orientation of, 343
  developing self-understanding through, 253-56
  innovative, 299-301
Cutright, Phillips, 420, 421

Dachau (concentration camp), as example of inhumanity, 4, 18
Daly, S., 247
Dann, S., 144
Darby, W. J., 275
David, (King of the Hebrews), 438
Davidson, A. N., 278
Davis, A., 310, 319
Davis-Eels Games Tests, 310, 317, 319
Day care centers
  as adjunct to family experiences, 21
  background history of, 169
  beneficial effects of, 432-33
  in Child Development Act (1971), 43
  effects of, on infant development, 142-44
  function of, 33
  heterogeneity in future, 30-31
  lack of funds of, 35
  women's demands for, 429
Day Care Resources Project, 152
Dean, R. F., 275
Death rate, see Mortality rate
Deceleration techniques of behavior modification, 88
Decentralization
  of schools, 303
  of state institutions, 36
Deduction, cognition and, 182, 190-91
Dehumanization
  of black children through testing, 309-11
  of social environment, 59-60
DeLabry, T., 77
Delgado, G., 283
Delinquency
  identity crisis resolution 2nd, 401-7
  individual and social competence and, 224-26
  prevention of, 230, 387
Demands of women, 429-31
Dennerll, D., 247
Dennis, Lawrence E., 375
Dennis, W., 142
Densen, P. M., 268, 278
Deprofessionalization of psychologists, 343
Desocialization of institutionalized children, 64

Destructive forces of society, 59-60
Developing Understanding of Self and Others (DUSO; Dinkmeyer), 254
Development
  adolescent, psychological identity and, 381
  child, need for research in, 40
  concept of, applied to psychologists training, 471-74
  fetal, 273
  personality, environment and, 110
  physical, 278-81
  social, IQ and, 124
  of socially disadvantaged children, 29; see also Socially disadvantaged children
  speech, 181
  See also Cognitive development; Infant development projects; Language development
Developmental child care programs, 171-72
Developmental retardation, 67-68; see also Mental retardation
Developmental tests, 156
Deviant behavior, sickness model of, 53-54, 56
Dewey, J., 232
Dialect, nonstandard negro English as, 344
Diamond, Marian C., 126
Diana vs. the California State Board of Education, 307
Dibble, M. F., 282
Dickerson, J. W., 278
Diet
  prematurity and, 270, 273-74
  of socially disadvantaged childbearing mothers, 272-75
  See also Malnutrition
"Dietary and Nutritional Problems of Crippled Children in Five Rural Counties of North Carolina" (survey), 281
Dimensions of Personality (Limbacher), 254
Dinkmeyer, Don, 247, 252-57
Direct observation of impaired adaptive behavior, 69
Disadvantaged children, see Socially disadvantaged children
Discrimination along sex lines, 429, 430, 435, see also Racism
Disease model of labeling, Rumpelstiltskin Fixation derived from, 70, 71

Disillusionment of youth, 363-64

Disorganized, Indifferent Syndrome in Head Start programs, 202-3

Disruptive children, misconceptions about, 296

Distribution of psychiatrists, 55

Disturbed behavior, sickness model of, 53-54, 56

Dobbing, J., 278

Domination, freedom from, as women's demand, 429, 434-35

Donnelly, J.F., 270, 271

Doppelt, Jerome E., 317

Dreikurs, R., 247

Drillien, C.M., 269

Drucker, Peter, 372

Drug education, fear in, 105-6

Drug use, 98-109
  Alternatives Model to, 101-5
    implementing, 105-8
  myths about, 98-99
  reasons for, 100-1
  search for identity and, 407-11
  as widespread phenomenon, 99

Duerfeldt, P.H., 95

Duncan, E.H.L., 273

Dunn, L.C., 132

Dusewicz, R. A., 145

DUSO (*Developing Understanding of Self and Others:* Dinkmeyer), 254

Early Childhood experiences, effects on learning ability of, 179-80

Early Language Assessment Scale (ELAS), 157

"Eating Patterns Among Migrant Families" (study), 283

Economic Opportunity, Office of (OEO), 199, 205, 206

ED children, *see* Emotionally disturbed children

Edgarton, Robert B., 329

Educable mentally retarded (EMR), 72-74, 326

Education
  compensatory
    number of programs (1971), 293
    purpose of, 27; *see also* Head Start programs
  drug, 105-6
  higher, *see* Higher education
  malnutrition and lack of, 283-84; *see also* Malnutrition
  in parenthood, 33-34, 40
  persuasion as tool of, 196

Education (*cont'd*)
  purpose of, 23
  remedial, 296-99
  self-understanding through, 252-56
  sex, 351-61
  of socially disadvantaged children, 292-306
    in community schools, 302-3
    examples of wasted funds, 293-94
    false assumptions about, 294-96
    innovative curricula in, 299-301
    integration and, 301-2
    need to change approach to, 313
    remedial programs in, 296-99
  See also Curricula: Learning; Preschool education; Schools; Students; Teachers

Educational goals, of Head Start programs, 26-28

Educational institutions
  creating new, 374-77
  extensions of present, 373-74
  See also Schools

Educational opportunities, women's demands for, 429

Educational Policy Research Center, 377

Educational Testing Service, 376

Educational unrest, 305

Educationally handicapped children (EH), 258-65
  classroom situation and, 260-61
  implications of, 261-65
  defined, 259

Educators, fathers in role of, 439; *see also* Teachers

Eels, K., 310, 319

Effectance, defined, 125

Effectiveness
  of multiple approaches, intelligence as, 336
  relative to age peers, 333-35

Ego identity, 392-99
  identity confusion vs., 393-99

EH children, *see* Educationally handicapped children

Einstein, Albert, 233

Eisenhower, Dwight D., 60

ELAS (Early Language Assessment Scale), 157

Elective courses, grading system for, 107-8

Elegy Written in a Country Churchyard (Gray), 323

Elite - Type Clinical Psychology, 519, 520

Ellenberger, H.F., 394

Ellis, Albert, 242-51

Emotional behavior, cognitive development and, 123
Emotional experience sought by drug users, 102
Emotionally disturbed children (ED), 258-65
  classroom situation and, 260-61
    implications, 261-65
  defined, 259
  identifying, 228-29
  screening of, 235-38
Empire State College (State University of New York), 374-76
"Employement Problems and Issues Related to the Mental Health of Children and Youth" (Joint Commission on the Mental Health of Children), 383
EMR (educable mentally retarded), 72-74, 326
Enabling, advocating vs., 46
Engel, M. 384, 472
Engels, Friedrich, 438
Engelman, S., 151
English, nonstandard negro, 344
Environment
  disturbed or deviant behavior and, 54
  effects of, on personality development, 110
  effects of, on problem solving ability, 74
  home
    of black children, 313, 314
    cognitive development and, 128
  intelligence as adaptation to, 192
  learning ability and, 110, 126
  of maladapted children, 68-69
  social, dehumanization of, 59-60
Epstein, N., 398
Erhardt, C.L., 270
Erikson, Erik, 143, 381, 391-98, 403
Escala de Inteligencia Wechsler Para Ninos (Wechsler Intelligence Scale for Children), 72, 319, 321, 326
Escalona, S.K., 157
Eskimos
  child rearing practices of, 180
  visual and cognitive signs used by, 344
Establishment, the, social pathology as explained by, 60
Esteban, M. E., 126
Evaluation, cognition and, 182, 190
Evans, R.I., 395
Ewalt, 507
Executive processes, pre-school learning and, 182-84
Experiaction, defined, 339
Experience sought by drug users, 102-3

Experimental manipulation to assess behavior, 82
External Degrees by examination, 376
Eysenck, H.J., 89
Eysenck, M., 26

Fairweather, 39
Family, the
  adolescent ego identity and crisis in, 393
  alternatives to, see Communes
  functioning and size of, 446
  limits of, 21
  role and responsibilities of, 40-41
  See also Children; Fathers; Lower-class families; Middle-class families; Mothers; Parents
Family heads, women as, 432
Family life, changes in, 32-33
Family planning, 443-52
  implications of, 449-51
  indications for, as it affects status of children, 444-47
  San Francisco program of, 447-49
Family Planning Perspectives, 421
Family-Style Program, 213-23
  discussion on, 221-23
  preliminary findings on, 220-21
  program for, 214-20
Family in Transition (Rossi), 439
Family in Transition (A. & J. Skolnick), 438
Fantasy and Feelings in Education (Jones), 254
Farrell, James T., 233
Fathers
  changing roles of, 437-42
  meaning of family planning to, 449
Fazzone, R.A., 91
Federal Communications Commission (FCC), 58
Fear
  in drug education, 105-6
  in sex education, 351
Federal Commission on Population Growth, 433
Feinleib, M., 280
Feminine Mystique, the (Friedan), 428
Ferguson, G. A., 122
Fetal development, adequate diet for, 273
Fidelity, defined, 394
Filer, L.J., 280
Films (movies), aggressive behavior stimulated by, 22
First Institute on Innovations in Psychological Training, 469

Fischer, Constance T., 333-48
Fisted swiping, new evidence on, 131
Fitzgerald, H. E., 143
Flanders, N.A., 255
Fleming, Alice, 456
Fleming, Thomas, 456
Fleischmann Commission (New York State), 301
"Fleischmann Commission Report on Quality, Cost, and Financing of Elementary and Secondary Education" 304
Food, Health and Income (Boyd-Orr), 272
Forrester, B. J., 155
Foster children, legalized abuse and dehumanization of, 24-25
"Foundation Goes to School, A" (Ford Foundation report), 305
Fowler, W., 145, 154, 157
Frank Porter Graham Child Development Center, 145
Freedom of movement between classrooms in Family-Style Program, 213-23
French creche system, 154
Freud, Anna, 144, 491
Freud, Sigmund, 249, 365, 429, 438, 491
Friedan, Betty, 427
Friedlander, 149
Friedman, Erwin, 19-34
Friendship, psychotherapy as purchase of, 58
Functional illiteracy in U.S., 296
Future Resources and Development, 375

Gagne, R. M., 129
Galbraith, John Kenneth, 267
Gallagher, J. J., 71, 145
Garry, R. C., 273
Gathering economies, children in, 425
Gauguin, Paul, 191
Genetic inferiority, as artifact of psychometry, 343-46
Genocide, intellectual, testing of black children as, 320-22
George Peabody College, 237
George Washington University, 387
Gesell, Arnold, 120, 130
Gestational age, prematurity and, 270
Gibbons, Sam, 239
Giesy, R., 147, 151
Gilden, M. C. L., 225
Giles, D. K., 76, 77
Gilles de la Tourette's Syndrome, 88-91

Giorgi, A., 337
Girls, aggressiveness of, 230-31
Gjerge, C. M., 229
Glaser, R., 129
Glasser, W., 247
Glicken, M., 247
Glidenell, J. C., 208, 225
Global Electronic University, 376
Glossary of Psychoanalytic Terms and Concepts (APA), 423
Goal orientation of infants, 125
Goldberg, S., 150, 156
Goldsmith, J. M., 498
Goldsmith, Sadja, 448
Goldstein, B., 91
Gordon, E. W., 293
Gordon, Ira J., 34, 147, 155, 159
Gordon, Sol, 292-306, 351-61, 453-60
Gorman, Mike, 57
Gould, L., 123
Gould, Samuel, 378
Gourmont, Remy de, 196
Grading system, getting rid of, for elective courses, 107-8
Graduate Record Examinations Board, 378
Graduate Schools in the United States, Council of 378
Graham, K., 168
Grant, D., 386
Grant, J., 386
Gray, S. W., 34, 147
Gray, Thomas, 323, 443-52
GRE Test, 330, 331
Great Society programs, 37
Green, B. F., 130
Greenberg, D. J., 122, 131
Grier, William H., 58
Griesel, R. D., 279
Grotberg, E. H., 145
Group milieu, ego identity and, 377
Group play therapy, 93
Growth, conditions of, 121-22; *see also* Development
Growth Through Reason (Ellis), 247
Guidance plus credits, 374-75
Guilford, J. P., 128

Halley, J., 491
Hall, E. T., 344
Halpern, F. C., 324-25
Handicapped children, number of, 177; *see also specific forms of handicaps; for example:* Emotionally disturbed children; Mentally retarded children

Harper, R. A., 244
Harper's (magazine), 437
Harman, W., 372
Harris, Fred. R., 26
Hartsough, D. M., 309
Hartman, E. E., 276
Harvard Educational Review (magazine), 198
Havighurst, Robert, 310
Hawaii, 43
Hawkins, R. P., 77
Haynes, A., 268-278
Hayes-Binet Test, 319
Head Start Manual (guidelines), 199-201, 203
Head Start programs
    black children in, 344
    content of, 155
    effects of parent participation in, 147-48, 176, 207-8
    environmental mystique and, 27-30
    fund reduction for, 35-36
    misplaced attacks on, 26-27
    psychological services in
        guidelines for, 199-201
        models of, 206-7
        to serve lower-class children, 197-98
        types of problems encountered in, 201-6
Health Education and Welfare, Department of, 199, 205, 206, 301
Healy, W., 486
Hebb, D. O., 126
Heber, 145
Herford, Oliver, 517
Heredity, cognitive development and, 133-35
Heroin addiction, 104
    treatment of, 105
Hernstein, R. I. Q., 345
Herrenstein, 26, 27
Herrick, J., 310
Hersch, C., 464
Hirsch, J. G., 488
Hess, R. D., 159
Hidden Dimension, The (Hall), 344
Higgins, M. J., 145
High school students, 298-99
    drug use among, 99
    as mental health workers, 62-63
Higher education, 371-80
    institutions of
        creating new institutions, 374-77
        extending present institutions, 373-74
        legitimizing other forms of learning in, 377-78

Higher education *(cont'd)*
    in 1980, 378-80
    for post-school population, 372-73
Hirsch, J., 133, 134
Hitler, Adolf, 4, 9
Hobbs, Nick, 39, 508
Holt, J., 292
Home environment
    of black children, 313, 314
    cognitive development and, 128
Homestart programs, 34, 147
Home-visit model for infant development programs, 146-47
Home visitors, role of, 150-51
Homme, L., 247
Homosexuality, 366
    as crime, 422, 423
    in sex education, 457-58
Honig, Alice S., 142-67
Horn, 320
Horton, Margaret, 425-36
House, B. J., 74
Housman, Alfred E., 48
Howe, William, 254
H.R. 1 (Welfare Reform Act), 178
H.R. 11322, 239
Hubel, D. H., 126
Human science
    defined, 337
    radical structuralism as, 346
Human teachers, automated vs., 149
Humphreys, L. G., 122, 127
Hunt, E. E., 266
Hunt, J. McV., 119-41, 213
Hunting economies, status of women in, 426
Huntington, Dorothy S., 168-78
Husek, T. R., 129
Hyden, Helgar, 126
Hyperactive children, 229

Ideas
    generation of, 189-90
    implementation of, 190-91
Identity confusion, ego identity vs., 393-99
Identity crisis of adolescents, *see* Identity Group Psychotherapy
Identity formation, 393-95
Identity Group Psychotherapy, 391-414
    contemporary techniques of, 399-400
    ego identity and, 392-93
    ego identity vs. identity confusion, 393-99
    illustrative cases of, 400-13

Identity Group Psychotherapy *(cont'd)*
  role of therapy in, 413-15
Identity search, aims of, 399-400
Idiots, IQ of, 120
Ignorance, rising, reasons for, 371-72
Illegal abortions, number of (prior to 1967), 433
Illegitimacy
  laws on, 22-23
  legalized abortions and, 433
  premarital sex and, 420-22
  prematurity and, 270
  teenage, 446-47, 456
Illegitimacy: Myths, Causes and Cures (Cutright), 420
Illinois, credit plans in 374
Illiteracy, U.S., 297
  functional, 296
Images, cognition through, 181, 186
Imbeciles, IQ of, 120
Imitation
  by infants, 123
  learning by, 181
Imparied adaptive behavior, *see* Maladaptive behavior
Income level
  drug use and, 99
  education and, 305
  nutrition and, 279-80
Individual competence
  promotion of, 224-39
    in children, 227
    as goal of Head Start programs, 27
    schools and, 227-28
    strategy and plan for action in, 235-39
    through symbols, 232-35
    teachers in, 228-31
  of youth, 225-26
Individualized programs in Family-Style Program, 218-19
Inequality: A Reassessment of the Effect of Family and Schooling in America (Jenck), 304
Infant development projects, 142-62
  assessment of, 156-62
  historical problems in, 142-44
  planning problems in, 144-48
  program operation in, 152-56
Infant mortality rate
  1964, 267-68
  non-white, 268, 281
Infants
  anemia among socially disadvantaged, 280, 281
  goal orientation of, 125
  imitation by, 123

Infants *(cont'd)*
  See also Infant development projects
Inference, as basic process of cognition, 182
Inhumanity, examples of, 3-4, 8, 9, 16, 18
Inner city schools, percentage of black children in, 301
Innovative curricula, 299-301
Institute for Advanced Study in Rational Psychotherapy, 243, 246, 248
Institutionalized children, 25, 64, 65
Institutions
  of higher education
    creating new institutions, 374-77
    extending present institutions, 373-74
    legitimizing other forms of learning in, 377-78
  state
    conditions in, 11-13
    decentralization of, 36
    need to close, 63-66
    punitive attitudes in, 23
    staff of, 53-55
Integration, 293-94, 301-2, 305
Intellectual experience sought by drug users, 103
Intellectual genocide, testing of black children as, 320-22
Intelligence
  changing concepts of, 121-24, 191-92
  IQ as only one variation of, 333-37; *see also* IQ
  maladaptive behavior and, 74-78
  Piaget's view of, 192-93
  prevailing notions of, 119-21
Intelligence and Experience (Hunt), 121
Internal-external control, defined, 384
International University for Independent Study, 375
Interest Group for Clinical Child Psychology, 463
Internship, 472-74
Interpersonal experience sought by drug users, 102
Interpersonal phenomenon, intelligence as, 335
IQ (intelligence quotient)
  alternatives to
    contextualizing of behavior as, 339-42
    radial structuralism as, 337-39
  criticized, 337, 346-47
  to determine response capabilities, 68-69
  genetic inferiority concept derived from, 343-46
  longitudinal validity coefficients of, 127-28

IQ (intelligence quotient) *(cont'd)*
  as only one variation of intelligence, 333-37
  predictions derived from, 193-95, 313, 321-22
  prevailing notions about, 119-21
  revised strategies for measurement of, 128-30
  social development and, 124
Interviewing approach for assessment of child's behavior, 82-83
Invitational routines in Famly-Style Program, 219-20
Iron deficiency, 280, 283
Irrational thinking, effects of RET on, 244-45
Irvine College (University of California), 375
Iscoe, Ira, 507-14
ITPA (test), 157

Jablonsky, A., 293
Jacobson, Lenore, 316
James, G., 267, 281
Jenck, Christopher, 304, 305
Jensen, A. R., 27, 325, 327, 345
Jensen Report, 26
Job career patterns of youth, socioeconomic factors in, 383
Job opportunities for women, 429-31
Johnson, Lyndon B., 28, 29
Johnson, M. S., 83
Joint Commission on the Mental Health of Children, 22, 382, 383, 494, 507
  advocacy concept endorsed by, 42-43, 45
  recommendations of, 35-44
Jones, Richard E., 254, 280
Journal of Applied Behavior Analysis (journal), 88
Journal of Behavior Therapy and Experimental Psychiatry (journal), 88
Jung, Carl, 365
Juvenile courts, punitive attitudes of, 23
Juvenile delinquency, *see* Delinquency
Juvenile Psychopathic Institue, 486

Kagan, Jerome, 144, 179-96
Knafer, F. H., 94-95
Kapfer, S., 147
Karnes, M. B., 147
Karno, M., 329
Kass, E. H., 277,278
Katz, L. G., 151, 158

Katz, P., 123
Keister, M. E., 143, 145, 153
Keller, Helen, 14, 232
Kempe, C. Henry, 445
Kennedy, John F., 39, 508
Kentucky, infant mortality rate in, 268
Kerner Report (President's National Advisory Commission on Civil Disorders 1968), 37, 59, 292
Key Integrative Social System (KISS), 227, 231, 232
Keys, A., 286
Kidder, J. D., 77
Kipling, Rudyard, 126
Kirschner Report, 26
KISS (Key Integrative Social System), 227, 231, 232
Klaus, R. A., 147
Klein, D. C., 235
Knaus, W., 248
Kohen, A. I., 382, 384
Kohlberg, L. 124
Kpelle (tribe), 183
Krasner, L., 39, 75, 491
Krathwohl, David R., 254
Krech, D., 126

Labor, Department of, 384, 432
Labor force, mothers in, 180, 431
  need for child care programs and, 171-72
Labor unions, re-evaluating role of, in relation to youth, 23
Labov, W., 344
Lafferty, J. C., 247
Lally, J. Ronald, 147, 150-52, 154, 155, 159, 160, 213-23
Lambert, N., 235
Language
  as basic symbol, 233-34
  difficulties of, for Mexican-American children, 326-27
  nonstandard negro, 344
  thought and understanding shaped by, 119
Language development, 133
  in Family-Style Program, 222
  infant, 157
  mediating persons in, 234-35
  memory and, 182-83
  problem comprehension and, 188
Lanham Act (Community Facility Act; 1941), 169
Lantz, C. E., 91, 92
Large-Muscle Room, 214, 215, 218
Larson, C., 228

Laws
  adoption, 25
  on illegitimate children, 22-23
Lay, M. J., 144, 157
Lazarus, A. A., 246
LD children, *see* Learning disabled
  children
Learning
  by conditioning, 156
  effects of childhood experiences on,
    179-80
  environment and, 110, 126
  by imitation, 181
  intelligence as ability to learn, 336
  by mentally retarded children, 75-76
  nutrition and, 278-79
  problems of, 258-65
  See also Education
Learning disabilities, specific, defined,
  258
Learning disabled children (LD children),
  258
  brain defects and, 343
  classroom situation and, 260-61
    implications, 261-65
  defined, 259
Leonard, G., 247
Le Page, A. L., 95
Levenstein, P., 147, 151
Levine, J., 123
Levitt, E. E., 493
Lewis, M., 150, 156
Lezine, I., 142
Liberated women, liberated children and,
  425-36
Lieberman, James, 446
Lieberman-Bernhardt, 376
Liebow, Elliot, 438
Lief, R., 491
Life and Times of Frederick Douglass
  (Ashton-Warner), 233
Lifton, Jay, 438
Lilienfeld, A. M., 269
Limbacher, Walter J., 254
Lincoln, Abraham, 39
Lindemann, E., 235
Lindstrom, D., 155
Linney, Thomas, 363-70
Living School, RET at, 242-51
  effectiveness of, 246-50
Livson, N., 157
Local (regional) Child Development
  Councils, 45-46, 48
London, University of (England), pro-
  grams offered by, 373
Longfellow, Henry Wadsworth, 438, 439

Long-term effects of day care centers,
  143-44
Look (magazine), 456
Louttit, C. M., 486
Lovaas, Ivar, 39
Lovaas, O. I., 77
Lower-class children
  IQ of, 194
  psychological services for, 197-98
  rearing, 180
Lower class families
  family planning and, 443-45
  illegitimacy in, 447
Luther, Martin, 393

McCall, 509
McCance, R. A., 272, 278
McCarthy, Eugene, 364
McDonald, N. F., 197
McGanity, W. J., 275
Macht, L. B. 386
McKay, G., 247
McLuhan, Marshall, 185
McMahon, B., 269
Mahler, Gustav, 364
Mainardi, Pat, 434
Maine
  Child Advocacy Bill in, 43
  external credit plans projected in, 374
Maladjusted children (maladaptive behav-
    ior)
  assessing, 68-69
  educating, 296
  etiology irrelevant to
    problems of, 71-74
  intelligence level and, 74-78
  need to avoid labeling of, 70-71
Malcom X, 232, 322
Malnutrition
  among socially disadvantaged children,
    278-84, 313
    effects on learning, 284-87
    reasons for, 283-84
  among socially disadvantaged mothers,
    272-75
Manifest Anxiety Scale, 328
Mao tse tung, 9
Marien, Michael, 371-80
Marriage, anachronistic views on, 419-20
Martinez, G. A., 280
Marston, A. R., 94-95
Maslow, Abraham H., 247, 394
Mass media
  aggressive behavior stimulated by, 22
  effective intervention on mental health
    problems through, 58-59

Massachusetts
  child advocacy in, 43
  external credit plans projected in, 374
Massachusetts State College System, 375
Massimo, J. L., 387
Masturbation, 421, 457
Match, problems of the, 121-23, 213
Materials used in Family-Style Program,
    214, 216-18, 222-23
Maternal care, 159-60
Maturation, experience and, 126-27
Mature reaching, 131-32
May, Rollo, 394
Mayer, Jean, 283-84
Mead, Margaret, 395
Medicare, 37
Meditation, symbols and, 233-34
Mees, 77
Mellanby, 272, 273
Memory
  anxiety and, 189
  cognition and, 182, 188-89
  language development and, 182-83
Menninger Foundation, 477, 495-96
Mensh, I. M., 225
Mental age (MA), 119-20
Mental disorders
  diagnosis and prevention of, 110-15
  effective intervention in, 58-60
  preventive mental health check-ups, 41
Mental Health Facilities Act (1963), 508
Mental health professionals
  most needed, 60-62
  in state institutions, 53-55
  See also Pediatricians; Psychiatric nur-
    ses; Psychiatric social workers;
    Psychiatrists; Psychologists
Mental health research, 36-38
Mental Health Survey (Los Angeles
    County), 231
Mental health workers
  clergy, high school students and police
    as, 62-63
  need to train, 53-54, 56
Mental retardation
  brain damage and, 70, 74-75
  defined, 119
  nature of, 67-68
  as result of socioeconomic conditions,
    60
Mentally Retarded Child, The (Robinson
    and Robinson), 71
Mentally retarded children
  attention capacity of, 74
  cognitive development of, 135-37
  educable, 72-74, 326

Mentally retarded children (cont'd)
  learning by, 75-76
  need to destroy concept of, 15-16
  neglected, 22
  treatment of, 9-15
  See also State institutions
Mercurio, Robert, 159
Merleau-Ponty, Maurice, 344
Metera Baby Centre (Greece), 132-35
Methadone programs, 105
Methods in Human Development (Bessell
    and Palomares), 254
Metropolitan Reading Test, 29
Mexican-American children, testing of,
    326-31
  foreign cultural values present in tests
    and, 327-28
  language difficulties and, 326-27
  need for new tests, 330-31
Mexican-American Civil Rights Move-
    ment, 326
Meyer, W. J., 144, 155, 157, 491
Meyerson, L., 75-76
Middle-class children
  home environment of, 314
  IQ scores of, 194
  rearing of, 180
  tests geared to, 310, 312
Middle-class families, illegitimacy in, 447
Middle-class fathers, 440
Milgram, N. A., 312-15, 320, 321
Military-industrial complex, 60
Miller, W. D., 237
Miller Analogies Test, 330, 331
Milne, D. C., 91
Mineral deficiency
  calcium, 283-84
  iron, 280, 283
Minneapolis General Hospital, 276
Minnesota Multiphasic Personality Inven-
    tory (MMPI), 328
Minimum functional levels, defined, 297
Minority groups, see Black children;
    Mexican-American children
Mississippi, infant mortality rate in, 268
Mischel, W., 82
Mishler, E. G., 491
MMPI (Minnesota Multiphasic Personal-
    ity Inventory), 328
Mobilization for Youth Program, 387
Mondale-Brademus bill (Comprehensive
    Child Care Act; 1971), 177-78
Mood, Alexander M., 375
Morgan Community School, 302
Morons, IQ of, 120
Mortality rate

Mortality rate *(cont'd)*
  infant
    1964, 276-68
    nonwhite, 281
  of mothers in childbirth (1930; 1960), 268
  legalized abortions and drop in, 434
Moses, Stanley, 244, 377
Mother-child relationshp
  cognitive development and, 125
  development of, executive processes and, 183-84
  effects of day care centers on, 142-43
Mothers
  in labor force, 180
    need for child care programs and, 171-72
  maternal care, 159-60
  meaning of family planning to, 449;
    See also Family planning
  as psychotherapists, 91-92
  socially disadvantaged, 268-75
    deficient diet of, 272-75
    obstetrical care of, 276-78
    perinatal risk run by, 271-72
    prematurity and obstetric complications among, 268-71, 273-74, 445, 446
Motivation
  cognition and, 122-24, 195-96
  compensatory education to stimulate, 27
  to drug use, 100-1
  effects of childhood experiences on, 179-80
  effects of malnutrition on, 286-87
  pre-school learning and, 184-85, 195-96
  of socially disadvantaged children, 294
Motivational autonomy, cognitive development and, 124-26
Movies (films), aggressive behavior stimulated by, 22
Moynihan, Daniel Patrick, 168
Multi-campus programs, 374
Multiple baseline design for data gathering, 83
Municipal Orphanage (Athens; Greece). 132-35
Mussolini, Benito, 9
"Mystique of Parenthood" (article), 439
Myths about drugs, 98-99

Naive Overburdened syndrome in Head Start programs, 201-2
Najarian, P., 142

NASW (National Association of Social Workers), 47, 48
National Advisory Committee on Handicapped Children, 258
National Association of Social Workers (NASW), 47, 48
National Baccalaureate Examinations, 376
National Center for Child Advocacy, 43
National Institute of Mental Health (NIMH), 54, 198, 331, 382, 446, 470
National Job Corps, 385, 386
National Research Council, 283
National University, 376
Native son (Wright), 233
Naturalistic observation of infants, 156-57
Naturalistic studies of role of work, in adolescence, 384-85
Nature of man
  inhuman side of, examples of, 3-4, 8, 9, 16, 18
  need to change, 17
    by personal confrontations, 5-6
Negroes, *see* Black children
Neighborhood Youth Corps, 37, 385-87
Neill, A. S., 247
Neurological development
  development of central nervous system, 126-27
  prematurity and disorders of, 269
New Careers Program, 385
New York External Degree, 378
New Frontier programs, 37
New York Hospital-Cornell Medical Center, Division of Pediatric Psychology of, 112, 113
New York State
  abortion laws of, 435-36, 460
  adoption laws of, 25
New York State Regents, 375
New York Times (newspaper), 30, 293, 305
Newland, T. Ernest, 318-20
Newman Report (Report on Higher Education 1971), 376, 378, 382, 384
Newsletter (Interest Group for Clinical Child Psychology), 463
Newsweek (magazine), 363
Newton, Huey P., 322
Newton, M. R., 235
Nicotinic acid deficiency, 284
NIMH (National Institute of Mental Health), 54, 198, 331, 332, 446, 470
Nimnicht, G. P., 147
Nitko, A. J., 129
Nixon, Richard M., 43, 177, 178

Non-drug users, alternatives discovered by, 104

Non-obtrusive measures in infant development projects, 160

Nonstandard negro English, characteristics of, 344

Non-Traditional Study, Commission on, 378

Nonwhite mortality rate
of infants, 268, 281
of mothers in childbirth (1930; 1960), 268

Nonwhite women, stature of, 271-72

Nonwhites, distribution of birthweight among whites and, 269-71

Norm-reference tests, 129

Norms
of reaction, 132-34
age of, 132,133
heredity and, 133-34
social, drug use as, 99

Norris, George W., 39

Norris, R. C., 237

North America, University of, 375

North Carolina, Child Advocacy Bill of, 43

North Carolina University Hospital, 271

Nursery for Children of the Poor, 169

Nurses, psychiatric, 55

Nutrition, see Malnutrition

"Nutritional Status of American Negroes, The" (Mayer), 283

Oberlin College, 456

Observation approach to assessment of behavior, 82

Obstetrical care received by socially disadvantaged mothers, 276-78

OEO (Office of Economic Opportunity), 199, 205, 206

Off-campus learning, need to legitimize, 373

Ojemann, Ralph, 254

Oklahoma external credit plans projected in, 374

Oliver, M., 76

Olshansky, S., 60

"On the Origin of Family, Private Property, and State" (Engels), 438

On Understanding Science (Conant), 128

Ontario Institute for Studies in Education, 377

Open University (England), 374-76

Operant behavior modification techniques, 75-78

Oral-genital contacts, as crimes, 422

Ordinal Scales, 129-30, 135

Osofsky, H., 145

Osofsky, J., 145

Outer-directed responses of educable mentally retarded chilren, 74

Painter, G., 146, 155

Pakter, J., 270, 278

Palmer, F. H., 146

Palmer, J. O., 486

Palomares, Uvaldo, 254

PAR (Pre-school Attainment Record), 220, 221

Paradise, N. E., 129

Paraskevopoulos, J., 123, 132, 135

Parental deprivation, working mothers blamed for, 431

Parental participation
in Head Start programs, 147-48, 176, 207-8
in Welfare Reform Act, 178

Parent-and-Child Center (Mt. Carmel, Ill.), 132, 135, 136

Parent-child Centers, 35, 41, 147, 148

Parent-group model in infant development programs, 147-48

Parenthood, education for, 33-34, 40

Parents
opinions of, on Head Start programs, 27
as psychotherapists, 84-85, 88-92
See also Children; Mothers

Parnes, H. S., 382, 384

Pasamanick, B., 269

Patterson, C., 155

Patterson, G. R., 77

Pavenstedt, E. A., 162

Peabody Picture Vocabulary Test (PPVT), 157, 220, 221, 321

Peace Corps, 58, 62

Pedersen, F. A., 125, 128

Pediatric psychology, 111-15

Pediatricians in diagnosis and prevention of mental disorders, 110-15

Peer relations, effects of day care centers on, 144

Peers, as psychotherapists, 86

Perception, as basic process of cognition, 126, 182

Perinatal risk among socially disadvantaged, 271-72

Perloff, B. F., 77, 95

Personal identity, ego identity transcending, 395

Personality, intelligence and, 336

Personality adjustment, as useless concept, 41; see also Maladjusted children

Personality changes, effects of malnutrition on, 286-87
Personality development, environment and, 110
Personalized classrooms, 261
Persuasion, as educational tool, 196
Perversions
anachronistic view of, 422-24
in sex education, 457
Peterson, D. R., 82
Peterson, R. F., 77, 83
Pickett, Robert S., 437-42
Phillips, J. S., 95
Philosophical experience sought by drug users, 103
Physical defects treated in Head Start programs, 26
Physical development, nutrition and, 278-81
Physical experience sought by drug users, 102
Piaget, Jean, 130, 131, 185, 187
Pittsburgh, University of, 376
Plakos, J., 326
Planned Parenthood World Population, 443, 449
Plasticity in cognitive development, 131-33
heredity and, 133-35
Platt, B. S., 278
Podell, Lawrence, 444
Polarization, dangers of, 31
Police, as mental health workers, 62-63
Political action needed to establish child care programs, 173
Political experience sought by drug users, 103
Politics of Housework, The (Mainardi), 434
Poor, the, as victims of racism, 60; see also Black children; Lower-class children; Mexican-American children; Socially disadvantaged children
Popham, W. J., 129
Population
percentage of U.S., using drugs, 99
school
percentage with learning problems, 258-59
post-school population, 372
See also Students
Pornography, 424, 458
Porteus Mazes, 72
Post-school population, 372
Poverty, families headed by women living in, 432

PPVT (Peabody Picture Vocabulary Test), 157, 220, 221, 321
Pratt, Jeanine, 122
Pregnancies
risks in frequent, 445-46
See also Illegitimacy
Premarital sex
adolescent, 351
anachronistic views on, 420-422
Prematurity, 268-71, 273-74, 445, 446
Pre-School Attainment Record (PAR), 220, 221
Pre-school education, 179-96, 213-23
academic performance and, 313, 314
child rearing practices and, 180-81
cognition and, 181-82, 185-91
executive processes and, 182-84
Family-Style Program, 213-23
discussion on, 221-23
preliminary findings on, 220-21
program for, 214-20
innovations in, 39
learning new structures and skills, 193
motivation and, 184-85, 195-96
promotion of individual competence through, 224-39
in children, 227
as goal of Head Start programs, 27
schools and, 227-28
strategy and plan for action in, 235-39
through symbols, 232-35
teachers in, 228-31
See also Head Start programs
President's National Advisory Commission on Civil Disorders (Kerner Commission; 1968), 37, 59, 292
Preventive mental health check-ups, 41
Price-Williams, D. R., 328, 329
Princeton University, 430
Problem comprehension, cognition and, 188
Problem solving
as most valued competence, 333
by mentally retarded children, 74
processes necessary to, 188, 189
Professionals
mental health
most needed, 60-62
in state institutions, 53-55
in youth programs, 22
See also Child care specialists; Teachers
"Protean Man" (Lifton), 438
Protein deficiency, 281, 283-84
Provence, S., 162
Psychedelic drug users, 99, 104
treatment of, 105

Psychiatric nurses, disappearance of, 55
Psychiatric social workers, 61-62
Psychiatrists, distribution of, 55
Psychological effects of work, 388
Psychological identity, adolescent development and, 381
Psychologists
  deprofessionalization of, 343
  function of, 67, 68
    in Child Development Councils, 48
    as lobbyists, 177-78
  need for more Mexican-American, 330-31
  TCCP and identity development of, 498-501
  training of, 463-82
    application of development concept, 471-74
    background to, 465
    overview on, 479-80
    post-doctoral training, 476-79
    present state of academic programs, 469-70
    present state of practicuum training, 466-69
    Standards for pre-doctoral training, 474-76
Psychology, see Clinical child psychology; Traditional clinical child psychology
Psychology Today (magazine), 431
Psychotherapy
  behavior assessment in, 82-84
  best psychotherapists, 84-87
    children, 86-87, 92-95
    parents, 84-85, 88-92
  goals of, 81-82
  as purchase of friendship, 58
  RET as, 242-51
    effectiveness of, 246-50
  specific therapeutic interventions of, 87-88
  See also Identity Group Psychotherapy
Public behavior, acquisition of, 181
Public Health Service, 466
Pygmalion in the classroom (Rosenthal and Jacobson), 316, 319

Rachman, Arnold W., 391-416
Rachman, S., 89
Racism
  damage done by, 60
  as mental health problem, 59
Radical structuralism, 337-39, 346
"Rainbow Series" (Head Start series on psychology), 200n
Ramirez, Manuel, III, 326-31

Randolph, Norma, 254
Rapaport, J., 398
Rational-emotive psychotherapy (RET), 242-51
  effectiveness of, 246-50
"Rational-Emotive Therapy: Confirmation of Its Principles and Practice" (Ellis), 247
Rettich, P. 247
Reaction, norm of
  age of, 132, 133
  heredity and, 133-34
Readership of comic books, 351
Radiness, what is, 296
Re-Ed (project), 39
Reformatories, 23
Regional child development centers, 35
Regional (Local) Child Development Councils, 45-46, 48
Rehabilitation of drug users, 105
Reinforcement
  for maladjusted children, 68-69
  for mentally retarded children, 77
  self-reinforcement, 95
Reiss-David Child Study Center, 478
Rejected Children, 445
Relationship therapy, 58
Remedial education, 296-99
Report on Higher Education (Newman Report; 1971), 376, 378, 382, 384
Retardation, see Mental retardation; Mentally retarded children
Ribicoff, Abraham, D., 43
Riboflavin deficiency (vitamin B^2 deficiency), 283-84
Ricciuti, H., 157
Richard, R. C., 83
Richmond, Julius, 29, 145, 154
Rie, H. E., 491
Riesen, A. H., 126
Rieu, E. V., 516
Right to education, 343
Rights of mentally retarded, 11-13
Risley, 77
Roberts, P. V., 91,92
Roberts, Robert E., 65
Robins, L. M., 225-26
Robinson, H. B., 71
Robinson, Jackie, 233
Robinson, N. M., 71
Robinson, Sugar Ray, 233
Robles, B., 286
Rockwell, Norman, 520
Rod and Frame Test, 328, 329
Rogers, C. R., 247, 394
Roos, P., 76
Roosevelt, Franklin Delano, 39

Rosenthal, Robert, 309, 310, 314, 316, 319
Rosenthal Effect, 309, 314-16
Rosenzweig, M. R., 126
Ross, Alan O., 35-45, 48, 67-80, 469, 486
Rossi, Alice, 439
Rubens, Peter Paul, 191
Robenstein, Judith L., 125
Rules
   cognition through, 182, 187-88
   used in Family-Style Program, 214, 216
Rumpelstiltskin Fixation, 70, 71
Ryan, William, 62

Salaries of women, 429, 431
Salber, E. J., 280
Salk, Lee, 110-15
San Francisco Health Department, 448
San Francisco program of family planning, 447-49
Sanford, N., 224
Sarason, Seymour, 39
Sarason Scale, 248
Saturday Review (magazine), 437
Sayl, E. B., 276
Schaeffer, B., 77
Schaefer, E. S., 146
Schemata
   as basic unit of cognition, 181
   described, 185-86
Schendel, H. E., 280
Scherl, D. J., 386
Schickedanz, David, 132
Schofield, William, 58, 112
School entrance regulations, 237-38
School population
   percentage of, with learning problems, 258-59
   post-school population, 372
   See also Students
Schools
   community, 302-3
   delinquency prevention in, 230
   individual and social competence promoted in, 227-28
   and needs of community, 21
   re-evaluating role of, 23
   sex education in, 453-60
   See also Curricula; Education; Students; Teachers
Schrupp, M. H., 229
Schorr, Alvin, 443
Schulman, R., 498
Schultz, T. R., 123
Schwartz, E. K., 398
Schweid, E., 77
Schweitzer, Albert, 233

Science (magazine), 36
Scribner, Harvey B., 305
Second World War (1939-1945), perinatal risk during, 273-75
Segner, L., 155
Self-administered behavior analysis, 95
Self-concepts
   as cognitive construct, 123
   of black children, 58-59
Self-confrontation technique, 95
Self-control, techniques of, 94
Self Enhancing Education (Randolph and Howe), 254
Self-esteem, youth's need for, 21
Self-monitoring technique, 95
Self-punishment technique, 95
Self-reinforcement technique, 95
Self-treatment programs, 93-95
Self-understanding through education, 252-56
Sense-Perception Room, 214, 216, 217
Sensory experience sought by drug users, 102
Sex
   in communes, 366-67
   premartial, 351
Sex education
   comic books for, 351-61
   in schools, 453-60
Sex roles
   child's concept of, 124
   freedom from stereotyped, 429, 435
   motivation and, 195
Sexual behavior
   anachronistic notion of, 419-24
   laws relation to, 23
Shanker, Albert, 300, 305
Shapiro, S., 270, 277
Shaw, George Bernard, 393, 419, 424
Shipmen, V. C., 159
Shirley, Mary, 130
Shore, Milton F., 19-34, 381-89
Siberian camps, as example of inhumanity, 4
Sickness model of disturbed or deviant behavior, consequences of, 53-54, 56
Sigel, I., 145
Simon, 119
Sinai Hospital, 456
Skelly Wright Decision, 293
Skinner, B. F., 94
Skolnick, Arlene, 438
Skolnick, Jerome, 438
Slavery, as example of inhumanity, 4, 8
"Sleeper" effects in infant development projects, 161
Slobin, D. I., 157

Small-group consultations in Head Start programs, 206-7
Small-Muscle Room, 214, 217-18
Smith, 508
Smith, C. A., 274, 275
Smith, Lucille, 213-23
Social class, breast feeding and, 280; see also Lower-class children; Lower-class families; Middle-class children; Middle-class families; Middle-class fathers
Social competence, 224-25
    promotion of
        in children, 227
        as goal of Head Start programs, 27
        in schools, 27-28
            strategy and plan for action in, 235-39
        through symbols, 232-35
        by teachers, 228-30
        of youth, 225-26
Social development, IQ and, 124
Social environment, dehumanization of, 59-60
Social experience sought by drug users, 102
Social norm, drug use as, 99
Social unrest, major causes of, 59
Social work, child advocacy concept in field of, 46-48
Social workers
    Code of Ethics of, 47
    in family planning, 443-45, 447, 450-51
    lack of, 55
    psychiatric, 61-62
Socially disadvantaged children, 29, 266-91
    education of, 292-306
        in community schools, 302-3
        examples of wasted funds, 293-94
        false assumptions about, 294-96
        innovative curricula in, 299-301
        integration and, 301-2
        need to change approach to, 313
        remedial programs in, 296-99
    malnutrition of, 278-82, 313
        effects on learing, 284-87
        reasons for, 283-84
    mothers of, 268-75
        deficient diet of, 272-75
        obstetrical care of, 276-78
        perinatal risk among, 271-72
        prematurity and obstetric complications among, 268-71, 273-74, 445, 446
    See also Black children; Lower-class children; Mexican-American children

Socially disadvantaged youth, work programs for, 383
Society, U.S., menacing nature of, 7-9
Society of Pediatric Psychology, 112
Society for Research in Child Development, 125
Socioeconomic factors
    development and, 29
    in job career patterns of youth, 383
    in mental retardation, 60
    See also Education; Environment; Income level; Social class; Socially disadvantaged children
Solitary confinement of mentally retarded, 11
Solomon, Harry C., 64
Somerville, Addison W., 19-34
Song My (Vietnam), as example of inhumanity, 4
Sophisticated Slicker Syndrome in Head Start programs, 204-5
Sowa, J. M., 269
Spearman, 128
Specific learning disabilities, defined, 258
Speech development, conditions of, 181
Sperber, Zanwil, 19-34, 208
Spinster (Ashton-Warner), 233
Spiritual-mystical experience sought by drug users, 103
Spock, Benjamin, 238
Stalin, Josef, 4, 9
Staats, A.W., 77
Stanford, Helen P., 449
Stanford-Binet Intelligence Scale, 220, 221, 317, 321
Stanford Research Institute's Educational Policy Research Center, 372, 430
Starr, R. H., Jr., 150
State institutions
    conditions in, 11-13
    decentralization of, 36
        need to chose, 63-66
        punitive attitudes in, 23
        staff of, 53-55
Stature of white and nowhite women, 271-72
Stern, C., 147
Stern, Wilhelm, 119
Stevenson, M. B., 143
Stewart, W. H., 267
Stress, environment and ability to tolerate, 110
Strickland, S. P., 145
Students
    high school, 298-99

Students *(cont'd)*
    drug use among, 99
    as mental health workers, 62-63
    number of U.S. (1970), 377
Subsidized adoptions, 25
Sullivan, Anne, 15, 232, 234
Sumter Child Study Project, 235-38
Sumter South Carolina Child Study Project (Newton and Brown), 235
Symbols
    cognition through, 182, 186-87
    individual and social competence and, 232-35
Syracuse University, Children's Center of, 157-158

Taft, L. T., 72
Tally's Corner (Liebow), 438
Tannenbaum, J., 143, 157
Tashnovian, P., 228
Taxonomy of Educational Objectives: Affective Domain, The (Krathwohl), 254
Taylor, Harold, 376
TCCP, *see* Traditional Clinical Child Psychology
Teachers
    approach of, to socially disadvantaged children, 296, 300-1
    authority of, challenged, 253-54
    development of self-understanding and, 255
    in Family-Style Program, 214, 216-18, 222
    goals of education and, 252
    human vs. automated, 149
    in infant development projects, 151-52
    at Living School, 248
    in promotion of individual and social competence, 228-31
    testing and, 309-11
Teaching Program in Human Behavior and Mental Health, A (Ojemann), 254
Teenagers
    family planning program for, 447-49
    illegitimacy among, 446-47, 456
    See also Adolescence; Youth
Television (TV)
    aggressive behavior stimulated by, 22
    intervention on mental health problems through, 58-59
Tennessee, infant mortality rate in, 268
Terman, 120
Test-intelligence, defined, 333-35; *see also* IQ

Test Service Bulletin, 317
Tests
    for black children
        attacked, 309-11, 324-25
        defended, 315-20
        as intellectual genocide, 320-22
        viewed as secondary problem, 312-15
    for Mexican-American children, 326-31
        foreign cultural values present in tests and, 327-28
        language difficulties and, 326-27
        need for new tests, 330-31
Texas Research Institute of Mental Sciences, 65
Therapeutic studies on role of work in adolescence, 385-88
Therapy
    group play, 93
    relationship, 58
    self-treatment programs, 93-95
    work as, 385-88
    See also Identity Group Psychotherapy; Psychotherapy
Thiamine deficiency (vitamin B¹ deficiency), 283-84
Thinking, irrational, effects of RET on, 244-45
"This Child Labelled X." (TV program), 25
Thomas, A., 491
Thomas Edison College, 374, 375
Thomson, A. M., 270, 271
Thorndike, Robert L., 316
Thought, *see* Cognition
Thurstone, L. L., 128
Thurstone's Test of Primary Mental Abilities, 72
Tomkins, S. S., 503
Tough, Allen, 377
Toverud, G., 274
Traditional clinical child psychology (TCCP), 485-506
    contemporary *Weltschmerz* and possible pseudo-obsolescence of, 498-501
    obsolesence in, 487-98
        changes in concepts of children's disorders, 490-92
        children and, 488-90
        effectiveness of non-TCCP methods and, 494-97
        questionable effectiveness of TCCP and, 492-94
    social climate and viability of, 497-498
Training

Training (cont'd)
  of child care specialists, 31-33, 36, 41,
      50-52
  of infant testers, 158
  of mental health workers
    clergy personnel, 62
    in institutions, 53-54, 56
  of parents, as psychotherapists, 88-92
  of pediatricians in child rearing prac-
      tices, 110-12
  of psychologists, 463-82
    background of, 465
    development concept in, 471-74
    overview of, 479-80
    post-doctoral training, 476-79
    present state of academic programs,
        469-70
    present state of practicuum training,
        466-69
    standards of pre-doctoral training,
        474-76
  of teachers, 40
  vocational, 383
Training opportunities for women, 429,
    430
Turnure, J., 74
Tutorial model of intervention in infant
    development programs, 146
TV, see Television
Tyler, R., 310

Ullman, L. P., 75, 491
Understanding
  imitation and, 123
  of others, 253
  self-understanding, 252-56
  shaped by language, 119
Unemployment among adolescents, 382
United Federation of Teachers (UFT),
    305
United Nation (UN), 11
United Nations Charter on Children
    (1959), 24
United States population, percentage of,
    using drugs, 99
U. S. Riot Commission Report (Pres-
    ident's National Advisory Com-
    mission on Civil Disorders; Kerner
    Commission; 1968), 292
Universal Declaration of Human Rights
    (December 1948), 11
University Exploiter Syndrome in Head
    Start programs, 203-4
University-Without-Walls, 374-76
Upchurch, B., 155
Upstart (project), 157

Utku child rearing practices, 180-81
Uzgiris, Ina C., 122, 123, 125, 127, 130,
    131

Valley, John, 376
Valverde, F., 126
Vanderbilt Cooperative Study of Maternal
    and Infant Nutrition, 275
Venereal disease prevention, 454, 455,
    457, 458
Vernon, 320
Veterans' Administration hospitals, 466
Video University, 375
Vietnam War, 4, 198, 499
Violence, 22, 499
Virginity, 420-22
VISTA programs, 63
Vitamins, deficiency in, 280-84
Vocational training, 383
Vogel, F., 398
Von Eckartsberg, R., 339
Von Hilscheimer, G., 247

Wahler, R. G., 69
WAIS (Wechler Adult Intelligence Scale),
    338
Waltereck, 132
War on Poverty, 37
Warkany, J., 273
Warren, Earl, 39
Warsaw Ghetto, as example of inhumani-
    ty, 9
Washington Post (newspaper), 168
Washington Report (magazine), 36
Watson, J. S., 125, 149
Waxler, N. E., 491
Wechsler, D., 321
Wechsler Adult Intelligence Scale
    (WAIS), 338
Wechsler Intelligence Scale for Children
    (WISC), 72, 321, 326
Wegman, M. E., 268
Weikart, D. P., 147, 151
Weinstein, Laura, 237
Weizmann, F., 122
Welfare Reform Act (H.R. 1), 178
Werkman, Sidney, 38, 39
"What Kids Still Don't Know About
    Sex" (T. and A. Fleming), 456
White, Burton L., 124, 127, 131, 155
White, Mary Alice, 35
White, Robert, 125
White House Conference on Children
    (1930), 24

White House Conference on Children and
       Youth (1970), 171
   position paper of, 19-34
White women, stature of, 271-72
Whites, distribution of birthweight among
       nonwhites and, 269-71
Whitten, P., 144
Whorf, Benjamin, 119
Wickman, E. K., 228
Widdowson, E. M., 278
Wiesel, T. N., 126
Wikoff, R. L., 315-18, 320, 322
Wilkerson, D. A., 293
Williams, Gertrude J., 44-49, 419-24, 515-
       22
Williams, Robert L., 309-12, 315-18, 320-
       22, 324
WISC (Wechsler Intelligence Scale for
       Children), 72, 319, 321, 326
Wisconsin, external credit plans projected
       in, 374
Witkin, H. A., 328
Witmer, J. Melvin, 255
Wohlford, Paul, 197-209
Wolf, A., 398
Wolf, M. M., 76, 77
Wolf, S. W., 77
Wolfe, J. L., 244, 246, 247
Women
   as conservative force, 441
   liberated, liberated children and, 425-36
   stature of white and non-white, 271-72
   See also Mothers
Women's Movement, 429, 435, 458
Wood, M. O., 273
Work
   adolesence and, 381-89
       naturalistic studies of, 381-85
       as therapy, 385-88
   in communes, 367-68

Workers
   mental health
       clergy, high school students and po-
           lice as, 62-63
       need to train, 53-54, 56
   social
       Code of Ethics of, 47
       lack of, 55
       psychiatric, 61-62
Working hours of average housewife, 428
Work-study programs, 383, 385
World War II (1939-1945), perinatal risk
       during, 273-75
Wright, C. M., 143
Wright Richard, 233
Wycoff, Deborah, 376

Yale University, 430
Yarrow, L. J., 125, 128
Young, Whitney, 37
Youth
   alienation of, 19-20, 363-64
   delinquency and
       individual and social competence and,
           224-26
       prevention of, 230, 287
   need for participation by, 20-21
   role of labor unions in relation to, 23
   sex education for, 351-61
   socially disadvantaged, work programs
       for, 383
   See also Adolesence, Teenagers

Zeaman, D., 74
Zigler, Edward F., 24-34, 43, 68, 74, 77,
       123, 124, 199

THE LIBRARY
OF THE
WASHINGTON SCHOOL OF
PSYCHIATRY